Promoting
Your
Medical
Practice

Promoting Your Medical Practice

MARKETING COMMUNICATIONS FOR PHYSICIANS

Stephen W. Brown
Andrew P. Morley, Jr.
Sheryl J. Bronkesh
Steven D. Wood

Anne-Marie Nelson, Editorial Coordinator

Medical Economics Books
Oradell, New Jersey 07649

Library of Congress Cataloging-in-Publication Data

Promoting your medical practice.

  Includes bibliographies and index.
  1. Medicine—Practice. 2. Medical care—Marketing.
I. Brown, Stephen Walter, 1943– . [DNLM:
1. Marketing of Health services. 2. Practice Management,
Medical. W 80 P965]
R728.P77 1988   610′.68′8   88-23092
ISBN 0-87489-494-8

ISBN 0-87489-494-8

Medical Economics Company Inc.
Oradell, New Jersey 07649

Printed in the United States of America

To contemporary health care professionals and the patients they serve,
with the hope that this book helps them meet the challenges
of an industry in the throes of dramatic change

Contents

About the Authors

Stephen W. Brown, PhD, is professor of marketing and executive director of the First Interstate Center for Services Marketing at Arizona State University, Tempe; past president of the 50,000 member American Marketing Association; 1988 recipient of the prestigious Philip Kotler Award for Excellence in health services marketing; and a member of various boards and advisory groups. A recognized authority in services marketing, Dr. Brown is a popular speaker to physicians and other audiences, frequently quoted in the national business and health care publications, and the co-author of six other books and over 100 articles on various marketing topics.

Andrew P. Morley, Jr., MD, is managing principal of the Atlanta office of Health Services Marketing, Ltd. A recognized authority in medical marketing since 1980, Dr. Morley has conducted numerous workshops and seminars throughout the country. He has written many articles on the topic and has co-authored (with Dr. Brown) the best-selling book, *Marketing Strategies for Physicians.* As a practicing private physician, he remains active in state and national medical societies. Dr. Morley also has extensive media experience, having served as a medical editor and commentator for television and radio.

Sheryl Bronkesh, MBA, has specialized in the health care industry since 1973. She has extensive experience in public relations, communications, advertising, marketing and physician relations. Currently she is a principal with Health Services Marketing, Ltd., managing the firm's Scottsdale, Arizona office. Previously, she worked in administrative capacities for hospitals and a multi-hospital system. Ms. Bronkesh has been recognized for achievement in program planning, promotion and public relations with a number of national awards. She is a frequent speaker on the topic of physician marketing and serves on the board of directors of the American Society for Hospital Marketing and Public Relations.

Steven D. Wood, PhD, is professor and associate dean for graduate programs in the College of Business at Arizona State University, Tempe. He has been an active researcher, educator and consultant in the health services industry for nearly two decades. A frequently featured authority on health-care product/service packaging and joint venture relationships, Dr. Wood concentrates on developing and implementing strategic options for medical professionals. He serves on the board of directors of the Decision Sciences Institute and is a past president of the organization's western association.

Acknowledgments

Writing a book like this generally involves many people pulling together to achieve a common goal. While the authors assume the high profile in the eyes of the reader, others have contributed significantly in writing, researching, and keyboarding. This team approach is an accurate description of how this book developed.

Collectively, we recognize and appreciate the influence of our colleagues at Arizona State University, Health Services Marketing, Ltd., and the Decatur Clinic.

Most importantly, we recognize the substantial contribution of Anne-Marie Nelson of Health Services Marketing, Ltd. (HSM). In serving as the book's full-time editor, she strengthened and polished the work, while also researching and writing many of the initial drafts of the chapters. Throughout the process, she has been an inspiration to the authors through her diligence and the quality of her work.

Special mention goes to Don Jones, MBA, and Claire Botsch, MBA, of HSM, and to Debra Morley, RN, who researched and wrote drafts of several chapters. The conscientious assistance of Carol Moore, Mary Rugg, and Jeri Sluder of HSM was also important in moving this book to a finished product. Consultant Pat Kleisley provided much helpful data and material for a number of the chapters. Carrie Martz of Martz and Associates reviewed and provided valuable input to the radio and television chapter. Special appreciation is extended to Alice Macnow, John Chapman, Joyce Freid, Phyllis Gold, Thomas Bentz, and the fine staff of Medical Economics Books.

A book of this kind would not be effective without real-life examples. We acknowledge the contributions of the many physicians who offered insights and promotional materials. The Neurology Center in Maryland and the Indiana Center for Hand Surgery & Rehabilitation were especially helpful.

Finally, we offer our deep and enduring thanks to our families for their love and encouragement.

Preface

Recent American Medical Association and *Medical Economics* studies have found that for the first time since they began tracking financial data, physician income is decreasing. Patient visits per doctor have dropped. More and more physicians are dissatisfied with their practice and with the medical profession.

The above situations reflect a profession in the midst of dramatic change. Increasing numbers of physicians, hospitals and even business entities are competing, often aggressively, in the health care marketplace for limited patients and diminishing dollars. Government regulations (present and proposed) strangle and threaten. Health plans in the form of HMO's, IPA's and PPO's are altering delivery systems and dictating physician behavior. And finally, consumers, as employer-payers and/or patients, are further reshaping the health care industry by learning to make better-informed decisions about treatment alternatives.

Within this volatile environment, physicians are actively seeking ways to protect and expand their practices and practice services. In seeking this growth, increasing numbers of doctors are turning to marketing and promotion.

When we first started helping physicians market their practices in the early 1980's, we were confronted with many misconceptions and sometimes even hostility. Yet, the increasing competition of this decade has made physicians more interested in and favorably inclined toward marketing. Marketing books, seminars and articles, and work with practice marketing consultants have made physicians more knowledgeable about marketing. Many now recognize marketing as a professional discipline in its own right, offering the logic for ethically enhancing one's practice.

Our work with doctors over the years has convinced us that they are looking increasingly for hands-on guidance in promoting their practice. A desire to respond to this need served as the catalyst for us to write *Promoting Your Medical Practice.* Our approach to promotion is to anchor the subject within an overall practice marketing effort. We view promotion not as a single action, but all the communications activities that help generate and retain consumers. These communications range from the interpersonal, one-to-one contact between doctor and patient to practice brochures, publicity and even advertising.

This book is written for the practicing physician. While grounded in the logic of the marketing discipline, the content is highly pragmatic and replete with examples and exhibits of practices successfully engaged in promotion. Included are illustrations of actual media coverage doctors have received, brochures and newsletters, print advertisements, and suggestions on how to involve your staff in marketing the practice.

This volume is a companion to our 1986 best seller, *Marketing Strategies for Physicians*. The earlier publication was the first book ever written on the topic and continues to serve as an excellent introduction to medical marketing. *Promoting Your Medical Practice* is a more targeted discussion, offering far more specific strategies and examples of ethical ways to successfully promote one's practice. Together the two books provide a set of comprehensive resources for the enlightened physician.

Besides physicians, others in the health-care industry will also find this book of value and use. "Marketing to and through the medical staff" has become a major priority for hospitals, health plans, pharmaceutical companies and other vendors. Thus, hospital executives, as well as their managers in the areas of marketing, physician relations, planning and public relations will benefit from its contents, as will clinical department heads and nurses responsible for marketing specific programs that involve physicians. Managers of health plans and other professionals (e.g., dentists, nurses) will also be able to use the practical insights provided by the volume. Finally, vendors will find the book attractive in understanding today's medical practices and in helping physicians succeed.

The approach taken in this book synthesizes our professional backgrounds in marketing, medicine and communications, and our work conducting seminars, developing other educational materials for physicians and consulting in the area of health care marketing. This book is a melding of our working and learning together over the years. This collective growth has enabled us to bring medicine, marketing and promotion together in a pragmatic way to help you meet today's competitive challenges.

Setting the Stage for Action

Chapter 1

The Challenge of Change

In its transition from a cottage profession to a $400 billion industry, health care has experienced profound changes. In our first book, *Marketing Strategies for Physicians: A Guide to Practice Growth,* we tried to capture many of these changes and relate them to the challenges facing practicing physicians. Yet, in the ensuing years, the list of change factors once considered mere possibilities have become realities that are having a profound impact on the practice of medicine.

THE REALITIES

"I simply will not allow the practice I started 25 years ago to enter into contracts with any business which is trying to take away my patients!"

This statement captured the frustration of a 55-year-old internist. He had listened as his three partners discussed the new health maintenance organization in town, and was becoming increasingly angry that they were even considering "signing up."

"But we really have no choice," countered one of his partners. "More than 10 percent of the patients in our practice work for the big manufacturer in town and it's providing incentives to entice employees into using a prepaid system."

"Well, I guess the next thing on the agenda will be becoming participating physicians with the federal government!"

There was a long silence. "We have no choice," came the reply. This admission signaled a dramatic change in direction for these Massachusetts internists and their once secure and profitable independent practice.

"What's next?" mumbled the older physician as he left the meeting. "What's next?"

Six months later, he accepted a position with a large insurance company.

This scenario is being replayed in one form or another by an increasing number of practices across the country. The changing health care environment is forcing many physicians to rethink the way they practice medicine. As Donald O. Hayen, MD, of Oceanside, Calif., wrote in the Sept. 7, 1987 *Medical Economics,* "I'm not a slick operator selling medical hope. I'm a gray-haired physician who's accepted the reality that medicine will never be the way it used to be."

He adds, "Many of us think all we have to do is be good doctors, and patients will beat a path to our door. But almost every other physician is trying to be a good doctor too. Our services need to be something special."

Not only must the services be special, physicians must let the public know these services are available. That's what marketing communication is, and that's what this book is all about. In our previous book, *Marketing Strategies for Physicians: A Guide to Practice Growth,* we explained *how* marketing applies to medical practice. In this book, we'll help you apply the marketing communication principles we touched on in *Strategies* to your practice.

A PREVIEW OF WHAT'S TO COME

In the chapters that follow, we'll discuss the importance of communication in all forms—the one-to-one communication you engage in with a patient and his or her family, the telephone communication by your receptionist when a patient calls for an appointment for the very first time, the message that comes through in your practice brochure or payment policy handout. Every time you or anyone in your practice has contact with a patient or potential patient, something is being said about your practice. We'll help you say good things, because a basic premise of marketing that's especially true in medical practices is that current customers are your best source of new customers. So pleasing your patients should be a primary goal of any marketing strategies you engage in.

Many physicians hear the term *promotion* and their immediate response is, "I want a brochure." We'll help you take a step back, look at your practice, your personal and professional goals and the marketing objectives you've set for your practice. Then you'll assess all of the promotional strategies available to you for meeting your objectives, strategies such as:

- Personal communication
- Practice image and logo
- Positioning
- Referral source promotion
- Media contact and publicity
- Practice brochure
- Newsletter
- Advertising (newspaper, magazine, radio and television)
- Health education materials
- Yellow Pages
- Ad specialties
- Direct mail
- Community involvement and special events

Once you're acquainted with these strategies, you'll learn how to determine which are appropriate for you. You'll learn how to develop a promotion piece—a newsletter, a brochure, an ad—according to specific objectives.

You'll find within this book examples of what other physicians have done. We hope you'll take away ideas, incentive, and innovative approaches from what you read and see.

MARKETING BENEFITS YOUR PRACTICE, YOUR PATIENTS

Over the years, as we talk to physicians who attend our seminars and read our books and articles, we've found that the best thing about practice promotion is that patients as well as doctors benefit from the enhanced communication that results. Patients become more knowledgeable about health and fitness and the importance of professional medical advice, and more likely to follow your instructions. And that means you gain productivity and a feeling of accomplishment. You have less concern about dissatisfied or noncompliant patients, and more time to spend managing your patients. You'll worry less over what new changes will occur next week, next month, next year.

THE CHALLENGE OF CHANGE

The changes that have occurred in medicine have descended like an avalanche over the past decade, threatening to bury the private practice of medicine as we know it. Many physicians, reacting to actual and perceived threats to their livelihood, have taken drastic measures—leaving private practice for the safety of administrative medicine or going to work for large firms. Others have turned to marketing in one form or another. Some have approached it cautiously, testing the concept with communication efforts that whisper and, therefore, are not heard at all. Others have shouted about their practice from the mountaintop to everyone within range. As a result, some of their colleagues and their intended audiences have turned away from the blare of their messages.

Our contention is that before a marketing communication effort can be implemented, the medical practitioner must understand the changes that are taking place, the effect these changes will have on health care and private practice, and how a marketing plan and communication strategy can make change a positive force.

THE CHANGES

Traditionally, medicine in this country has been delivered by independent practitioners receiving fee-for-service from their patients and third-party payers. However, several important trends are changing the face of practice patterns forever. These trends are occurring both within medicine and from the external environment.

INTERNAL CHANGES

The internal factors center on technology, physician manpower, medical education and indebtedness, the current liability crisis, new practice modalities, and changes in real income.

Technology. The health care industry has experienced technological advances seen in very few other professions. Its evolution is not unlike the computer industry that has advanced from the simple silicon chip, to artificial intelligence and, now, the semiconductor.

Look at the field of urology. Several years ago urologists had plenty to do. There were many patients with urological problems such as kidney stones. Traditional urological training gave these specialists all the skills necessary for their practice. Then technology in the form of the lithotripter created a totally new emphasis on a machine very few physicians could afford, yet which many patients were demanding. The challenge for physicians was to learn the use of this new technology—which is how they have traditionally responded to such advances—and to explore innovative ways in which they might expand its role in their specialty field.

It's also up to physicians who will use this new technology to inform their patients and the public about it in a manner that is understandable, professional and mindful of collegial reaction. Promotional approaches are appropriate, but must be thoughtfully implemented. Traditional responses to technology now require both professional and business skills.

Similar considerations exist in the field of cardiology with advances in imaging and echocardiography. The need for skills in one procedure, such as catheterization, might lessen with procedurally-oriented cardiologists having to seek alternative services and sources of patients.

With technological change, urologists, cardiologists and other specialists will need to communicate their new services to their target markets.

Physician Manpower. There appears to be increasing disagreement over whether or not there is a physician manpower problem in today's health care system. The 1981 report from the Graduate Medical Education National Advisory Committee (GMENAC) created the focal point for a debate which has been waged publicly and privately.

To illustrate, from 1970 to 1983, the number of physicians increased by 54 percent. During these same years, the U.S. census rose by only 15 percent. If current projections hold, there could be 220 physicians per 100,000 population by 1990, compared with 156 doctors per 100,000 population in 1970. The projections for the next 5 to 10 years do not indicate a decline in the overall physician surplus. A 49 percent increase is predicted between 1981 and the year 2000. This translates to almost 667,000 physicians in the U.S. as we enter the 21st century.

Others have questioned the predicted surplus. There have been several articles in the *New England Journal of Medicine* contradicting the

GMENAC report. They suggest that trends such as increased demand created by new technology may actually result in greater need for physician services. Further, many physicians will be retiring, a fact not considered in the report.

Uwe Reinhardt, PhD, a professor of political economy at Princeton and one of the country's leading health care economists repeatedly warns that even the new reports do not accurately reflect the future. Noting that it's hard to pin an exact number to future demand, Dr. Reinhardt goes on to explain that the uncertainty of the future demand creates equal uncertainty regarding supply.

The problem is much deeper than the numbers indicate. Other factors, including an aging population, specialty and geographic distribution, and assumption of physician roles by paraprofessionals, are important factors as we interpret the impact of the GMENAC report.

For instance, there appears to be a significant surplus of certain specialties on the horizon. At the same time, the need for primary care physicians continues to be emphasized by the American Medical Association and other leading organizations. Additionally, physicians see more and more of their responsibilities—such as life insurance physicals, routine exams and other medical tasks—being taken over by RNs, nurse practitioners, physicians' assistants and other allied health professionals.

Nevertheless, the actual or predicted surpluses have some significance to you, the practicing physician. Certainly one immediate result is that most physicians are seeing fewer patients because of these increasing manpower figures. In many areas, there are simply more physicians available to treat the population, and therefore, fewer patients for each physician.

Medical Education and Indebtedness. After more than two decades of steady growth, medical education only recently appears to be experiencing a slowdown. The number of medical school graduates rose from 7,743 in 1967 to an estimated 15,872 in 1987. This represents nearly a 50 percent increase in just 20 years. However, according to the American Academy of Medical Colleges, the number of applicants has begun to decline, down 1,570 from 1985–86 to 1986–87. Meanwhile, the average student indebtedness has grown steadily, from $5,500 in 1971 to close to $34,000 for current graduating students.

This has to have an impact on younger physicians. With the cost of setting up a new practice and medical school indebtedness, physicians with loans in the $100,000 range are commonplace. Many, therefore, are seeking ways to eliminate or reduce their debt through alternative practice modalities such as employment rather than private practice, involvement with groups rather than solo practice, and other options that ultimately affect medicine as a whole. Those who opt for private practice become quite aggressive in seeking to attract patients.

The Liability Crisis. Much has been written about the current liability crisis, its impact on health care and on the way physicians practice medicine. It is not our purpose to review this issue here. However, the all too common 50 to 100 percent insurance premium increases place additional pressure on the new physician as he/she enters practice. The increased inclination by patients to sue has had an attendant psychological, time and economic impact on every physician in every specialty. As we shall see, communication—or the lack of it—has been implicated in patients' perception of medical quality and ultimately, their decision to seek a malpractice judgment.

Changes in Practice Modalities. Although more than 50 percent of all physicians continue the independent practice of medicine, the curve is beginning to shift. More and more younger physicians, faced with what appears to be an insurmountable debt, are opting to go into salaried positions. A 1984 survey by the American Medical Association found that 27 percent of physicians with less than six years of practice were in salaried positions, and the trend is growing.

There has also been a dramatic trend toward group practice arrangements. Between 1970 and 1980 the number of group practices increased 36 percent and from 1980 to 1984 the number increased another 44 percent.

Changes in Real Income. On the surface, it appears that physician incomes have increased. However, when compared to the cost of living, the figures are very misleading. *Medical Economics* in 1988 reported that the 1987 net practice earnings of office-based physicians scored a gain of $3,650, or 3.2 percent, while the cost of living went up 4.4 percent. (See also Figure 1-1.)

For the decade of 1975 to 1985, the real median income for physicians declined by 5 percent. All primary care specialties experienced a decline, while only a few specialties saw an increase, such as surgeons (8.3 percent), radiologists (5.9 percent), and anesthesiologists (17.5 percent).

FIGURE 1-1   Percent of Increase in Physician Income Compared with the Inflation Rate, 1978–1987

Year	% increase	
	Practice net	Cost of living
1978	4.0%	9.0%
1979	12.8	13.3
1980	9.1	12.4
1981	3.0	8.9
1982	8.2	3.9
1983	1.4	3.8
1984	7.8	4.0
1985	0.5	3.8
1986	10.0	1.1
1987	3.2	4.4

EXTERNAL CHANGES

There are also many external forces which will affect the way medicine is practiced in the future. The complex matrix of proliferating managed care systems, government intervention, an aging population that will need increased federal commitment, and changes in hospital/physician relationships all require decisions that directly affect medical practice growth. Like "Alice in Wonderland", physicians are not only being challenged to get through the maze of decisions, but also to follow the rules at a time when key players continually change them.

Physicians who have confronted these forces with a long-range marketing plan, and a communication strategy that acknowledges present and future changes, have seen growth in their practices. They have attracted new groups of patients to services they enjoy providing, and they have found that quality care is possible even in times of turmoil.

Managed Health Care Systems. Once thought of as a trend that would be done in by the economic strain of providing capitated care, health maintenance organizations (HMOs) have become a major entity in the health care system. If projections hold up, by 1990 over 44 million Americans will be enrolled in an HMO.

The trend continues toward consolidation of HMOs with the top companies having the greatest market penetration. Currently, the top 15 plans have well over one-third of all enrollees.

Likewise, preferred provider organizations (PPOs) have grown. Some 600 PPOs enroll over 19 million Americans. If these statistical trends are not startling enough, there are other players, in the managed care arena, such as utilization review organizations, third party administrators, and others who contract with managed care systems such as freestanding diagnostic centers, hospitals, and large group practices.

Despite income losses and a significant disenrollment by their membership, HMOs still maintain a steady growth rate. A federal government movement to provide HMO coverage for the Medicare-eligible segment of the population is another new factor.

What does all this mean to the practicing physician? Perhaps everything if you practice in areas such as Minnesota or Illinois where the share of the market dominated by managed care programs is between 30 and 40 percent. In these states, physicians must evaluate the percentage of their present and potential patients who might be covered under managed plans and determine what the potential loss of these patients might mean to their practice income. Many physicians, having made these calculations, have opted to devote at least a portion of their practice to managed care. In California, close to 80 percent of physicians are members of at least one plan.

On the other hand, if the managed care penetration in your area is less than 5 percent, as it currently is in such states as Georgia, New Jersey, Iowa, and North Carolina, your decision will be based on what you anticipate future penetration rates may be. There are no clear-cut answers, only questions. What impact, if any, do managed care plans have on your practice now? What impact will they have in the future, and are you willing to risk loss of patients in a competitive environment? Have you calculated the percent of your current patients affected by these plans, and the economic impact of their potential loss?

Government Intervention. Diagnosis related groups (DRGs), federal government pressure for physicians to accept Medicare assignment, and the new emphasis being placed on a system to determine the relative value of services provided by physicians, along with talk of a quality rating system for Medicare providers, all shape directly and indirectly the reimbursement future of the private practice of medicine. These pressures make it increasingly important to seek ways of becoming less dependent on government-mandated reimbursement—or to live with, and be profitable, under the inevitable lower payment schedule.

Our Changing Demographics. Demographic trends have a dramatic impact on how physicians view their present and future practice patterns. The one we can expect to most influence physician practice patterns is the shift in age groups of America's population.

The most rapidly growing segment of our population will be those 65 + , projected to increase from 28.5 million in 1985 to 34.9 million in 2000. By the year 2020, the growth rate of the elderly is expected to surpass that of physicians. Primary care physicians such as family physicians and internists, as well as specialists such as surgeons, ophthalmologists, urologists, cardiologists, anesthesiologists and radiologists can expect significantly increased demands for their services from this age group. A greater demand for physicians specializing in geriatrics is already being met by the American Boards of Internal Medicine and Family Practice, which began offering certification exams in geriatrics for the first time in 1988.

The anticipated decline in the birth rate will have a strong impact on other specialties. We can expect a decline in the need for both obstetrical and pediatric services in the 1990s. Women, however, will continue to be the major health care consumers in the 1980s and 1990s; their needs should herald a significant number of practices that emphasize women's health. Finally, primary care physicians (with the exception of obstetricians) and psychiatrists will be in demand. Proactive physicians and their practice managers must keep up with these and other demographic trends and tailor their practices accordingly.

Hospital-Physician Relationships. During the 1980s, many physicians began to view hospitals as competitors. This viewpoint was primarily fueled by a hospital tactic called "unbundling." Hospitals began to realize that many of their traditional in-hospital services could generate more patients and greater profits if they were "unbundled" or moved out of the hospital and made free-standing. Primary care centers, diagnostic centers, and facilities with targeted markets such as women's health centers became commonplace.

Thus the perceived competition between practicing physicians and hospitals has intensified. Furthermore, the efforts of many hospitals to bond their patients more closely to them was interpreted by some physicians as efforts to shift the patients' loyalty from physicians to hospitals.

However, recently there have been movements by hospitals to reconsider their relationships with their medical staffs. Many hospitals have created or are considering physician relations programs. These programs include everything from management/marketing assistance to sharing computer systems. Hospitals are once again investigating business relationships in joint ventures such as office buildings and outpatient diagnostic centers. In spite of the perceived competition, physicians and hospitals are seeking ways to grow together rather than separately.

PRACTICE PROMOTION: A NEW CHALLENGE

With all these changes come significant opportunities for innovative, proactive physicians. The American Medical Association Center for Health Policy Research has documented a trend to practice promotion. In its 1987 publication, *Socioeconomic Characteristics of Medical Practice,* physicians were reported as saying they expect to utilize the following responses to competition:

- Increased participation in alternative delivery systems
- Increase in housecalls made
- Increased evening and weekend office hours
- Advertising

The unfortunate aspect of their responses is not that physicians cite advertising as a competitive strategy, but that they often regard it as a stand-alone. Rather, we suggest that communication and promotion (of which advertising is an optional component) are part of a comprehensive marketing plan that is inevitable and invaluable to physicians in every specialty.

Fortunately, over the past several years we have seen general acknowledgment that, if properly utilized, the marketing discipline is ethical in health care. Physicians are seeing that the effective incorporation of patient-oriented programs within a practice enhances compliance and thus improves patient care. Physicians are evaluating their practices, they are utilizing ethical and innovative management techniques, and they are making their services more accessible to their patients.

Now, however, comes the NEW CHALLENGE: How can I tell patients about these changes I am making, and about my product, pricing, and availability, and how can I accomplish this while still preserving my own ethical standards and those of my profession?

The answer: through the use of ethical, creative, carefully thought out communication strategies. That is the purpose of this book. It provides a detailed look at the various marketing and promotional strategies available and describes how to carry them out in accordance with your personal and professional standards, the needs of your patients and the public, and your practice objectives.

Our objective is to help you better respond to change by utilizing effective strategies and, in turn, enhancing your practice and personal growth.

First, let's agree on what marketing is. Our premise is simple:

- *Marketing* is nothing more than focusing on the needs and wants of those who use or could use your services—patients, other physicians and referring agencies . . .
- . . . then delivering the program and services and developing the pricing to meet those needs and wants
- And, finally, *communicating* these programs and services to existing and potentially interested users of your practice. (This communication component of marketing is also referred to as promotion.)

Next, look at Figure 1-2, which illustrates a series of perspectives that will help you understand where medical marketing stands today and where it is headed. These perspectives provide a foundation for much of the book, and will be familiar to anyone who has read *Marketing Strategies for Physicians: A Guide to Practice Growth*. In this chapter we also hope to show you how to put that brochure or newsletter you've been considering into a marketing context *before* you write and print it.

The following observations form a perspective that's both sobering and

FIGURE 1-2 A Five-Point Marketing Perspective

---

1. **A Narrow View.** Marketing is viewed and implemented too narrowly. (This is the "marketing is advertising" or "marketing is a brochure" perspective.)

2. **Undertrained and Inexperienced Personnel.** Most medical-services marketers have little training or experience in marketing. (This is gradually improving, however.)

3. **Negative Image.** In the minds of many physicians, negativism and skepticism still surround the practice of marketing.

4. **Oversimplification and Overselling.** Marketing has been oversimplified and oversold in many health and medical situations. It is **not** a panacea.

5. **Everybody's Business.** Most importantly, within a practice setting, marketing is everyone's business, not just the responsibility of the doctor and/or the office manager.

---

enlightening: Sobering because we're beginning to recognize that marketing isn't a cure-all or quick-fix for all the major dilemmas facing health and medical-services organizations. But enlightening because these perspectives serve as a springboard for initiating realistic and achievable strategies for your practice.

The tendency of many marketing novices is to become preoccupied with only one or two components of marketing. It's natural that marketing's most visible components, advertising and promotion, are often mistaken for marketing as a whole. Marketing is not just a less offensive term for advertising; rather, advertising is one component of marketing. Promotion or communication is another. Marketing also involves planning, research, strategy, evaluation and analysis (Figure 1-3). As Dick McDonald, president of McDonald Davis & Associates, Inc., pointed out in a *Medical Economics* article, "When I go to a doctor, he takes my history, does tests, makes a diagnosis and finally prescribes treatment. He never goes straight to treatment. Doctors who just want to advertise—without developing an overall marketing strategy—are in effect going straight to treatment. They often waste money by treating the wrong problem."

GET EDUCATED

If the subject of marketing is new to you, we strongly encourage you to increase your knowledge by taking a marketing course or seminar and reading as much about practice marketing as you can. More and more hospitals are offering marketing or practice enhancement seminars for their medical staffs; if yours hasn't, why not suggest it? Many medical specialty societies, such as the American Academy of Family Practice and the American Academy of Dermatology, also offer practice marketing programs to

FIGURE 1-3. Components of the Marketing Umbrella

- **Research and Analysis.** Gathering and digesting pertinent information from outside your practice, and assessing its impact, e.g., patient survey, demographics, economic trends.
- **Strategic Planning.** Articulating goals and the actions necessary to help realize them in marketing strategy planning; includes identifying priority areas of practice opportunity, e.g., geriatrics, sports medicine, adult acne.
- **Product/Service Development, Modification and Elimination.** Infusing a market with new services and modifications, and possibly deleting certain existing services.
- **Pricing.** Imposing market-based input on fee setting and presenting your prices to users of your services.
- **Distribution and Accessibility.** Viewing the services of your practice from the user's perspective (patients and referral sources) and developing methods to improve access e.g., office hours, location(s), parking.
- **Communications: Personal Selling, Advertising and Public Relations.** Informing existing and potential patients of your services through a variety of methods, e.g., face to face discussions, newsletters, community involvement.
- **Evaluation and Control.** Monitoring your progress and modifying strategies when necessary.

members. These are very beneficial because they are specific to the needs of the individual specialties.

In addition, a variety of print and professional resources are available from the American Medical Association, pharmaceutical firms and health care marketing consultants. These include such publications as *Marketing Showcase for Physicians* published by Health Services Marketing, Ltd.; *Physician Marketing,* a newsletter published by American Health Consultants; and the *Journal of Health Care Marketing.* In addition, less specialized publications such as *Medical Economics, Physician Management, The Internist, Group Practice Journal* and *AAFP Reporter* often feature articles on marketing and practice management topics.

For those who want a broad-based view of how marketing affects business, we recommend enrolling in mini-courses. They are available at almost any college, since marketing is one of the most popular majors today.

Also, you can join in the activities of the American Marketing Association, and its Academy for Health Services Marketing. Finally, there are many practical periodicals, such as *Marketing News* (American Marketing Association, 250 South Water Drive, Chicago, IL 60606) and *Advertising Age* (Crain Communications, Inc., 740 North Rush Street, Chicago, IL 60611), as well as numerous books on the subject.

INVOLVE OTHERS

In addition to educating yourself, you can and should look to your staff and others to bolster your marketing and communication efforts. Begin with your staff. The physician who tries to develop and implement a marketing and promotional campaign without the help, support and perspectives of his staff is asking for trouble—and an unnecessary workload.

But your promotional effort may need to go beyond your practice for assistance. Seek outside advice and help from friends and associates, professional writers and artists, public relations consultants. Get a fresh perspective, creative thinking, new ideas and approaches from those who can be objective. Marketing is a big job. Take all the help you can get.

While it may be referred to by some other names—practice enhancement, public relations, promotion—marketing has been utilized to some extent by doctors and the health care industry for decades. But now competition and other external forces have suddenly made marketing crucial for everyone in the health profession. Thus, the issue today is not whether health and medical providers engage in marketing, but how they can do it well.

BE INNOVATIVE, NOT REACTIVE

Ever wonder who coined the phrase "We care for you" in reference to providing health or medical care? The slogan is now so overused it has been adopted by car dealers, grocery stores and the whole gamut in between—as well as physicians, hospitals, therapists, dentists and home health agencies.

There's a lesson to be learned. Don't react to what your competitors are doing by imitating them. Your practice is unique; you are unique. You have services and qualities that no one else has. Be as original as your practice. Study what the competition does, but don't do what they do. Try to convince consumers, through your communication efforts, that there are very distinctive reasons for selecting you over the physician down the street or across town.

Research, covered in Chapter 3, will help you determine the distinctiveness in your practice, or your "Unique Selling Position." We like to compare what marketing professionals do in developing a marketing plan and related strategies to what a physician does when he or she encounters a new patient with an ailment or medical complaint. The first step is *research*—taking the personal and family medical history, asking questions about the duration and intensity of symptoms, possibly ordering tests if more information is needed.

Once the test results are in and the information is evaluated, you'll take *action,* arriving at a diagnosis and treatment plan. Then you must *communicate* with the patient, explaining your diagnosis and the treatment you're recommending. If you've prescribed medication, you may tell the patient to take the medication for a week and then return to your office for a visit so that you may *evaluate* the results. If little or no improvement is seen, you may adjust the medication or try a new approach.

Marketing works in the same fashion. The first step in developing a marketing plan for a practice is *research:* a thorough analysis of the practice, the service area demographics, the competition and other pertinent factors. A patient survey will likely be administered to determine current attitudes and satisfaction levels.

After the research is completed and analyzed, it's time for *action.* Objectives and strategies are determined based on the data, then implemented. If the objective for an ob-gyn practice is to increase the number of women patients from a certain zip code, the strategies may include generating additional appointments for annual pap tests and breast exams. You can use a media-directed educational effort about the need for annual pap tests and breast exams, a direct mail effort to women age 25+ in the targeted zip code, evening or Saturday seminars, and/or ads in the feature and food sections of the daily paper. The strategies involve *communication:* the public and patients must be informed about these efforts.

Following a reasonable period of time and ongoing tracking of the origin of new patients, the results are *evaluated.* Did the strategies generate new patients? Which efforts were most effective? Retain them. Which did not work? Modify or don't repeat them.

Whether marketing or medical care, the basic approach is the same: Research, Action, Communication, Evaluation.

GET CLOSE TO THE CUSTOMER

One message continually emphasized throughout this book and in our seminars and articles, is that marketing is everyone's business, not just the concern of the physician, the office manager, or someone with the word marketing in his or her job title.

To instill new ways of thinking and behaving in your employees, you must begin at the top—with yourself. A report by McKinsey & Co., one of the world's most prestigious and pragmatic consulting firms, led to the best-selling book, *In Search of Excellence.* The report reviews the characteristics and unique features of some of America's most successful corporations, such as Hewlett-Packard and McDonald's. A hallmark of most of these firms is a "closeness to the customer" that permeates the organization and all its employees. It's common for many of the top executives in these companies to spend a number of days each month in contact with current and potential customers. These experiences help them monitor the ever-changing marketplace while they're implicitly or explicitly selling the customers on the firm's products.

Each of these companies has a marketing department with personnel specializing in research, promotion/advertising, personal selling, distribution, and other activities. Yet, by their actions and words, the top executives are constantly demonstrating that marketing is everyone's business, not just the focus of the marketing department. These companies are "customer driven."

And so it should be in the increasingly competitive medical environment of the 1980s. With you as a role model, all of your staff must recognize that the very existence of the practice—and therefore their jobs—depends on their customers.

AND FINALLY . . .

In marketing, as in most endeavors, balance and harmony are essential. Don't go off in one direction to the exclusion of all others. Just as you would recommend to your patients a mix of physical, emotional and intellectual stimulation, so your marketing and communications program requires the variety and diversity that results from weighing all options and incorporating all of the elements that comprise a sound strategy. It's best not to put all your promotional dollars into one marketing tool, for promotional efforts complement each other. Marketing is a many-faceted activity; it cannot be oversimplified.

It's what you do as well as how you do it that matters. Determine through research and analysis what you want to communicate, and then don't let yourself be distracted. Be sure everything you do relates directly to your objective.

Measure your results. Don't be married to a medium or a strategy. If a particular promotional technique is not working, modify or discontinue it. Be sure the dollars you invest are paying returns. If not, find a better way to spend your money. Know where you're going; make intelligent decisions backed up with adequate resources.

The communication component of marketing is the most visible aspect. It takes time, planning and effort, but the satisfaction of seeing your practice grow in an orderly fashion, with the kinds of patients you want seeking the kinds of services you offer, makes the effort well worth it.

Chapter 2

An Overview of Practice Promotion and Communication

"Promotion is for cars and laundry soap," Dr. Getwell said scornfully one day as he drove by a billboard advertising a local urgent care center. His comment was for the benefit of his partner, young Dr. Fitt, who had recently brought up the subject of developing a practice newsletter for their patients.

"By the way," Dr. Getwell continued, "have you sent Dr. Crane a thank you letter for referring Mrs. Peterson to us? That's the third patient he's sent us this month."

"Yes, and I also asked Mary to schedule lunch meetings with the directors of the senior centers and retirement centers near our office," Dr. Fitt said. "By the way, don't forget we have a Rotary meeting tomorrow."

"I have it on my calendar. Have you seen Ed Brown yet? At the last meeting, he was having a problem with his knee and said he was going to see you."

"I believe he's coming in next week," Dr. Fitt said. "You know, I've been thinking, if we had a practice newsletter, we could send it to our referral sources as well as our patients. I've had several of them say they weren't aware of our new treatment for joint problems. It would help them to know what we can do for their patients."

"You have a point," Dr. Getwell said somewhat grudgingly. "But I still think promotion doesn't belong in medicine, and you'll never see it in our practice!"

QUALITY CARE AND PRACTICE PROMOTION

Practice promotion . . . a small step up from the patent medicine peddlers who hawked their wares from the backs of brightly painted wagons? Or a legitimate and necessary means of attracting and retaining patients to well-run, high quality medical practices in an increasingly competitive era of health care?

In April 1983, *The Internist,* a publication for internal medicine specialists, editorialized that "hard-sell marketing (is) practiced by fringe rather than mainstream professionals and is overt, immodest, crass and clearly designed to steal patients from colleagues." In addition, the editor said, this form of marketing is "epitomized by advertising, especially when it fudges the truth a little, or glorifies credentials, or offers cut-rate prices."

Fortunately, we've come a long way in a relatively short time. We believe that the vast majority of physicians who engage in practice marketing and promotion are ethical practitioners who wish to provide needed medical care, but who see the need to let the public know who they are and what they have to offer. They don't "fudge the truth," glorify their credentials or promote cut-rate prices. Those who do will not last long in most communities. In the Fall/Winter 1986 issue of the *Journal of Professional Services Marketing,* McDaniel, Smith and Smith wrote, "It is apparent that it would be economically disastrous, in the long run, for a physician offering poor quality medical service to advertise heavily. . . . If the advertised health care provider performs poorly, then the consumer will tend not to patronize that service provider again, especially when he or she is constantly reminded of that particular physician through advertising."

The health care provider who seeks to attract patients to a practice offering inferior services, "assembly-line" medical techniques, care without concern, and a staff that exhibits little regard for the comfort or convenience of patients is not our intended audience. Moreover, we suspect that physicians who attempt to promote substandard care will find their practice losing patients and referrals, as dissatisfied patients rapidly spread the word about the less-than-quality care.

PROMOTION FINDS FAVOR WITH CONSUMERS

For high quality practices and providers, promotion is an increasingly favored method for generating and retaining patients. Study after study has shown that the public not only wants health care information, they rely on advertising and publicity to provide much of it. Ten years ago a study of consumer attitudes toward professional advertising found they reacted favorably toward it, and did not feel it lowered the image of the professional. Eighty percent felt it could be tasteful and would provide useful information; most wanted to see more professional advertising. In another study six years later, it was found that consumers with high income levels had a more favorable perception of physician advertising than consumers with low income levels.

In fact, every physician who wishes to see his or her practice grow engages in some form of promotion, whether it's sending thank-you letters to referring colleagues or speaking to the local Breakfast Club. It's not a new concept; it has simply been formalized and tied to specific goals and strategies.

EVERYTHING OLD IS NEW AGAIN

Back in the days when opening a medical practice meant hanging a sign out in front of your office, the term used wasn't marketing or promotion. It was just plain common courtesy. Like calling or visiting a patient after surgery or a severe illness, opening your office on Saturday or during the evening to accommodate your patients, or decorating your office so that it was pleasant and comfortable for patients.

That's what marketing is—attention to customer wants and needs. You know it as patient satisfaction. Your "customer" may be your patients, potential patients, and referring physicians, among others. And many of the things doctors have always considered a routine part of running a practice well are, in reality, the communication element of marketing.

For instance—do you belong to social clubs or civic organizations partly because it will help you develop contacts for patients or referrals?

Do you instruct your staff regularly about how best to handle patients in person and on the telephone?

Does your Yellow Pages listing include additional information, such as your hours, services, and a map showing your easily accessible location?

Do you meet for lunch or breakfast with doctors who refer to you— or who could refer to you?

If so, you're practicing promotion.

If you want to continue to thrive and grow in your practice, you probably plan and carry out your promotional efforts in a consistent, thoughtfully executed manner. You've probably developed a marketing plan for your practice, with short- and long-range goals that help you see and plan what lies ahead for you.

You know that promotion consists of a multitude of methods for communicating with those who use, or could use, your medical services. You know that patients and the public want to know not only about their current state of health, but also how they can maintain good health for themselves and their family. Referring physicians want to know about the program of care or treatment you provide their patient—and they want to be assured you'll return the patient to them.

The goal of a marketing communication campaign is to maintain and increase your patient base by providing information about medicine and your practice to individuals and groups who have the potential to use or refer others to your services, and to convince them that your practice will meet their medical care needs.

While a short-term increase in patients and income is desirable, other long-range objectives are achieved with practice promotion. Some strategies (like Yellow Pages advertising) reach those in immediate need of your services. Others will serve as a source of information, helping consumers make more knowledgeable decisions. Still other approaches will serve as image builders, creating a presence for your practice in the consumers' minds. Then when the need for medical care arises, your practice is the one they'll recall.

SAY IT AGAIN, SAM

The adage, "If it isn't broken don't fix it," applies to advertising and promotion as well. If a particular message or approach works, use it until it doesn't. To be effective, promotion must be repetitive. The more often people are exposed to your message, whether it's via a newsletter, an ad, or staff attitude, the better the chance that it will be remembered and acted upon. Your aim is to inform and convince, and repetition is how you accomplish that goal. Consumers are bombarded with messages. The ones they recall are those they hear again and again.

THE ROLE OF THE STAFF

Physicians who have a successful practice generally involve their staff heavily in all aspects of the day-to-day operation. They know they can't function alone; they rely on the competent and experienced people they've hired to accomplish many of the non-medical and health education tasks of the practice. That's also true of those who have a marketing plan. The staff works closely with the physician(s) in implementing the targeted strategies in the plan. This involvement accomplishes two objectives: it frees physicians for direct patient care, and it helps the staff become more committed to the practice because they have a greater understanding of the goals and direction it's taking. (It's important, however, to be careful not to overload your staff with ancillary responsibilities. You risk losing good employees if you ask them to do more than they have time for.)

The steady decline that has been reported in office visits to all types of specialists is not expected to reverse itself until the year 2010, when the postwar baby-boomers reach age 65 (see Figure 2-1). You've seen how some of your colleagues have used marketing and advertising to achieve a thriving, patient-oriented practice. They know that consumers demand information, reading newspapers and magazines, listening to radio and TV programs, voraciously seeking the latest medical reports and current health tips. They use the media, through paid advertising and public relations efforts as well as special events, classes and other educational forums to reach beyond current patients to individuals in the community.

PROMOTION: A VITAL PART OF DOING BUSINESS

Promotion encompasses all the communication techniques available. And that covers a wide range, for there are techniques you may never have thought of. Before getting into the major techniques, let's look first at the times and circumstances when you will draw on promotional strategies in your practice:

NEW SERVICES AND PROGRAMS

When Dr. Landis, an internal medicine specialist, was certified by the FAA to provide physical exams for pilots, he wanted to let his patients know about this new service. But he also wanted his referring colleagues and private pilots to know. He sent a letter notifying patients and physicians

FIGURE 2-1   Patient Visit Rate versus Practice Earnings

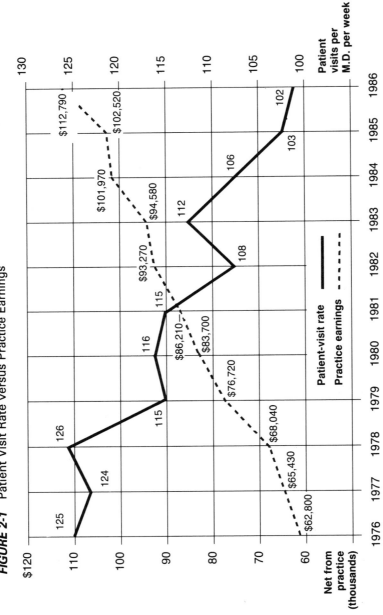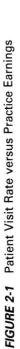

Patient visits are the total of times the physician personally saw patients in the office, hospital, and other locations during a typical week last spring. For unincorporated physicians, net is individual practice income minus tax-deductible professional expenses, before taxes; for incorporated physicians, it's total compensation from practice (salary, bonuses if any, and retirement set-asides) before taxes. Data in this and the charts and tables that follow apply to individual office-based M.D.s. Pathologists have been excluded from all patient-visit tabulations. Where no year is specified, figures are for 1987. Source: the MEDICAL ECONOMICS Continuing Survey.

that he was now certified to do FAA physicals. Then he mailed a similar letter with additional information about his background, experience and training to flying schools and local airports, following up with phone calls and personal visits to some of the larger schools. He also regularly runs a small ad in the weekly newspaper that's distributed at the private airport in the area. Dr. Landis knew that his FAA certification would be of no value if he didn't let those who would need the annual physical know he was available to provide it.

Whether you add a service, expand your hours or location, or add a new staff member with specialized skills, it's important to inform those who stand to benefit. This may include your patients, referring physicians, the public, or selected groups in your community.

ASSURING AUDIENCES YOU'RE RESPONSIVE TO THEIR NEEDS

Many of today's consumers want instant gratification. When they have a problem or a need, they want to solve it or fill it. The health care provider who can anticipate the needs of patients or specific target groups is a step ahead. But it's not enough to meet the need; you must communicate to all these audiences that you are serving their needs by offering a variety of services with a courteous and caring staff, by convenient location and hours, and by filing insurance for them, accepting Medicare or offering payment plans.

When you keep your target audiences informed, when they see that you are responding to their needs, they will turn to your practice when a health care need arises. When there is a record of trust, people will seek health care advice or referral from the physician whom they feel they know.

COMMUNICATION OFFERS A FEEDBACK MECHANISM

Communication techniques such as practice newsletters, print or radio advertising, direct mail, community events and practice-sponsored classes give you the opportunity to learn from a broad audience what their health care needs and wishes are. Through feedback from referring physicians, patients and others, you learn whether your services are adequate and appropriate, whether enough information is available about them, whether they are offered conveniently, whether your staff is perceived as caring and friendly.

While it is true that you can learn what patients think of your services by asking them directly, you will not gain such broad information, nor will you learn whether there are unmet needs among audiences and groups who are not represented by your patients. Your promotional strategies— depending on the types(s), frequency, message content, and audience can give you some of the feedback you don't get from your patients. A well-designed promotional effort provides information while encouraging a re-sponse from the recipient. Your audience wants to feel that their opinion is valued and useful—and it is, for you can use it to modify or add new services to meet the needs of current and potential patients.

A surgeon we know sends a simple two-page typewritten survey to every one of his surgery patients. The survey asks how they feel about the office environment, the ease of scheduling an appointment, the staff, the surgery, the physician, the treatment they received; every aspect of their care is covered. The survey was developed by his surgical RN, who takes great pride and ownership in it, and responses are mailed to her. She compiles the answers and uses the results both for Medicare quality assurance documentation as well as to bolster staff pride and determine if any problems are developing. Patients who return the forms indicate they are delighted to be asked their opinion, and their written comments are read aloud during weekly staff meetings as incentive to keep up the good work.

TECHNIQUES WE'VE KNOWN AND YOU'LL LOVE

Promotion encompasses a variety of communication methods with all of your actual and potential audiences. An important part of developing a marketing communication plan is to clearly define the *position* your practice has with your audiences. Positioning and perception is discussed in detail in Chapter 4. You should be aware, however, that the *perception* people have of your practice is as important as the reality. Your communication strategies, and the message in them, will help define your position and create a perception to match.

A wide variety of promotional strategies is available to the physician who is implementing a marketing plan. In the succeeding chapters, we will identify the most commonly used methods as well as some of the newer ones, and we will describe the variations available in marketing a medical practice. For now, let's take a quick look at what is available to you.

INTERNAL MARKETING

Internal marketing refers to all of the activities aimed at meeting the needs of, and communicating with, your staff, your patients and your referring physicians. These three groups are your most important audiences. Ignore any of them with your marketing efforts and your practice may suffer. Your staff, as we will show you, is crucial to your practice promotion efforts and to developing a close, positive affiliation between you, your practice and your patients. Fortunately, there are a number of ways to communicate with your patients, referral sources and your staff. Equally as important, effective use of these promotional techniques provides you with valuable insight into how you, your services and staff are regarded by those who use them.

Interpersonal communications. The one-to-one communication between physician and staff, physician and patient, and staff and patient is the most important promotional technique utilized in a medical practice. All of the other promotional techniques we will discuss in this book, no matter how creative or costly, supplement personal communication. Although brief in duration, the quality, courtesy and content of face-to-face communication carry great weight with the new or existing patient.

Patient survey. This is one of the most frequently used and helpful techniques for communicating with your patients. Not only does a survey provide you with feedback about what patients think of you, your staff, your office and services, it's also an excellent device for assuring patients that you care about what they think of your practice.

Patient education material. Either purchased or developed by you, health education materials are valuable both in keeping patients informed and to help assure compliance with verbal instructions for medication, therapy, exercise or treatment. It also can be used in your advertising and direct mail to encourage requests from the public.

Business package. This includes your letterhead, business cards, invoices and other imprinted stationery that make up your professional image. This may be the first introduction a patient or referral source has to your practice, so you'll want to give careful consideration to its cohesive and professional appearance.

Other forms of communication. All other communication you have with your patients or referring physicians is also part of your internal marketing promotional material. This includes telephone conversations, thank-you cards, letters and notes, small gifts and other methods you may have for keeping in touch with patients, such as recall or appointment reminder cards, birthday cards. No matter how insignificant these items may seem, they help form a perception of your practice in the recipient's mind.

EXTERNAL MARKETING

External marketing encompasses all of the activities aimed at influencing potential patients, opinion leaders and influential groups or organizations in the community. There are countless ways you can reach audiences who may be the intended markets for your care and services, or who can influence those who are. We'll highlight some of the more well-known and commonly used techniques here; they'll be discussed in depth later.

Media publicity. Health information through the media is a primary promotional technique. Media coverage is one of the most credible links between you and your public. The implied endorsement from the media when it does a favorable, factual story on a business is a powerful persuader and motivator. News and feature stories (such as in Figure 2-2) and interviews on television, radio, and in newspapers and magazines have much to recommend them when they are initiated and followed through ethically. Media coverage offers these benefits:

FIGURE 2-2 Media Publicity
Newspaper features like this help to educate the public, while enhancing the image and credibility of the physician who is interviewed. Source: Jo Griffiths, *Harrisburg Patriot News*, September 7, 1987.

Cataracts: *Eye affliction is common among older people*

By Jo Griffiths
Patriot-News

Joe Gonglowski will always remember the vivid colors of a box of cotton swabs he saw shortly after the cataract in his right eye was removed and replaced with an artificial lens.

"That box had the prettiest blue and purple in it I have ever seen in my life," Gonglowski said. "It was so vivid, so beautiful."

Buford "Mac" Ambrose doesn't recall any one particularly striking sight after removal of his cataracts and artificial lens implantation. He said he just remembers "looking around at everything to see what I could see."

For 79-year-old Florence Grimm, who underwent the same procedure, it was seeing clearly again the stars on a moonlit night.

Mildred Dietrich, just two weeks after her eye operation, delights in the view from the kitchen window of her hilltop home.

None had fears the surgery wouldn't work.

"I never gave it a thought," Ambrose said. "All I had in mind was I was going to see again."

All four in recent weeks have had intraocular lens implants following cataract removal. They are patients of Dr. Bennett Chotiner, ophthalmologist and director of The Memorial Eye Institute, a free-standing, outpatient eye surgery and eye-care center on Linglestown Road.

CATARACTS are a common eye condition in older adults. Most people over 60 have some cataract formation. By 75, virtually everyone has the condition to some degree.

Understanding how the eye works is helpful when talking about the vision problems cataracts cause. Ophthalmologists compare the eye to a camera, and the analogy is a good one.

Just like the camera, the eye's various components — when working properly — transform light rays entering the eye into images that are sent on to the brain for interpretation. That, in a nutshell, is how we "see" whatever it is we are looking at.

Cataracts occur as an opacity or "clouding" of the lens, the tiny, crystalline, oval capsule about an eighth of an inch thick and convex (curved outward) on both sides that sits behind the pupil — that black "dot" in the middle of the eye that opens and shuts to help regulate the amount of light entering the eye — and the iris, the colored part of the eye.

THE LENS is one of two parts of the eye — the cornea, the transparent covering of the pupil and the iris, is the other — responsible for focusing light rays so they converge on light-sensitive cells in the retina.

The retina is the lining of the back of the eye responsible for changing the rays into images and then sending them to the brain via the optic nerve.

Muscle fibers attached to the lens contract or relax, causing the lens to flatten for seeing distant objects or fatten (thicken) for seeing objects up close.

However, as the body ages, the lens loses its elasticity, those abilities to flatten and fatten, and its clarity, that crystalline quality.

Chotiner explained it this way: The lens' tissue — similar to the skin — lays down fibers beginning almost from the day we're born. That's all fine and quite normal, except for one thing. The capsule's only so big, and there's only so much room for so many fibers. So, eventually, the lens becomes dense — hard — and opaque from fiber accumulation and chemical changes occurring in the tissue.

And that, Chotiner said, is what is called a cataract.

MOST CATARACTS are a natural result of growing older, but there are other conditions that can cause them.

For example, diabetics are at greater risk of developing cataracts because of the disease's effects on the body, including the eye.

Certain eye diseases, eye injuries or toxic substances can make cataracts more likely in susceptible persons.

Some children are born with cataracts or develop them later on because of congenital deformities. This is rare, however.

Cataracts tend to develop as tiny spots near the center of the lens or in its cortex, or outer portion, Chotiner said. The condition generally affects both eyes, although the cataract usually grows faster in one eye than the other.

IN THE DISEASE'S early stages, there are few symptoms to alert the person to the trouble ahead.

But, Chotiner said, there are some classic signs as the disease progresses.

"Second sight" is one. Nearsightedness increases as the cataracts develop, Chotiner explained, and frequently people who previously needed eyeglasses to read or do close work, find they can see up

See CATARACTS — Page C3

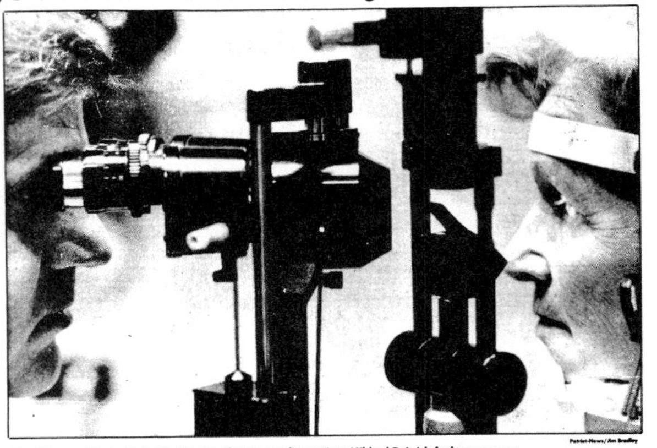

Patriot-News/Jim Bradley

Harrisburg ophthalmologist Dr. Bennett Chotiner readies patient Mildred Deitrich for laser surgery

close without their glasses.

A gradual blurring or fuzzing of vision is another symptom. Ophthalmologists say cataract patients often describe it as trying to peer through a filmy veil.

Other signs include objects appearing dimmer and less bright when viewed through the affected eye (cataracts are yellow-brown in color and so tint everything the patient looks at with a yellow hue, according to Chotiner) or distortion of printed images, something Chotiner said patients often attribute to dirty or smudged glasses.

Also, cataracts scatter light, so glare from bright lights or night vision difficulties, such as accurately seeing headlights from oncoming cars, are two more common indications of cataracts' presence, he said.

Mac Ambrose said he started developing cataracts eight years ago, but knew he was headed for real trouble when he began seeing double and everything "looked like I was looking through a pair of sunglasses."

Oncoming traffic would blend in with the road, and one day Ambrose said he mistook the white divider line for an actual barrier.

Gonglowski said his retirement from the Postal Service seven years ago was due in part to his fading vision. By 1983, he was relying completely on his left eye and could see only light or dark images through his right eye.

"I stopped driving," Gonglowski said. "I would drive down a street, and it would look like it was completely blocked from a distance. But when I got up closer, I could see it was just cars parked on both sides of the street."

Deitrich had to stop driving, too, but while many cataract patients have problems initially with nearsightedness, she had trouble with distance vision.

"I couldn't see the street signs," Deitrich said. "I would go past the sign and then turn around and go back."

The final straw for Grimm was when her sight became so bad she no longer could easily work her beloved crossword puzzles.

"The eye was always cloudy, and it kept getting worse and worse," she said.

By the time she went in for a check-up last spring, Grimm was more than ready to listen to her eye doctor's recommendation she have the cataract removed and an artificial lens placed in her eye.

THERE ARE no pills or eye drops for controlling cataracts, Chotiner said. There is the option of replacing the bad natural lens with a plastic artificial one, however, he said.

Called intraocular lens implantation, the surgical procedure, when combined with appropriate prescription glasses, has made it possible for millions of cataract patients to see clearly again.

Eye surgeons used to remove the entire lens within its capsule, so-called intracapsular cataract surgery (ICCE), Chotiner said. But this removes the natural barrier the lens capsule creates between the front and back parts of the eye.

Also, with intraocular lens implantation, if the entire natural lens capsule is removed, the implant must be placed in front of the iris rather than in the natural lens position behind the iris.

Most surgeons now prefer a technique called extracapsular cataract extraction (ECCE) because this procedure leaves the natural lens capsule in place to separate the front of the eye from the back and to support the lens implant in the natural position behind the iris, Chotiner said.

AN EVEN newer technique — and the one he likes best — is phacoemulsification, Chotiner said. It involves a smaller incision than ECCE and use of a special probe with an ultrasound tip that allows the surgeon to fragment the hard lens and suck out the particles. The implant then is inserted, the eye bandaged for 24 hours, and a plastic shield is worn for several weeks while sleeping to protect it from bumps or rolling on to the eye.

Patients are mildly sedated prior to surgery, and the eye anesthesized or put to sleep with a local anesthetic. Because any surgery can pose risks, an intravenous line is started, and blood pressure, heart rate and respiration monitored throughout the procedure.

The surgery itself takes 30 to 45 minutes, Chotiner said.

However, patients can count on spending a good two to three hours at the center the day of their surgery because of pre-and post-operative care, he said.

THE ARTIFICIAL lens eye surgeons use is made out of polymethylmethacrylate, a subtle yet firm plastic. It is circular in shape, with tiny wire-like appendages that anchor it in place inside the lens capsule.

Other materials being looked at include silicon lenses, which can be made into different refractory powers and are bendable for insertion through even smaller incisions, and hydrogel lenses, which absorb fluid when placed in the eye and then expand to their full size. Both are investigational, Chotiner said, and not currently widely used.

While artificial lenses can give cataract patients back good vision, bidding one's old eyeglasses goodbye forever is unlikely.

Unlike the eye's natural lens, the artificial implant is a single-focus lens, which means it can't adjust its shape for sharp distance and near vision.

"We can get them [cataract patients] to be either 20/20 distance or 20/20 near, but not both," Chotiner said.

That's why implant patients almost always need prescription lenses to enhance one or the other vision skill.

Also, an artificial lens doesn't necessarily mean the end of the cataract patient's eye problems. Sometimes the capsule membrane becomes cloudy. When that happens, surgeons can use a laser or another surgical technique to destroy the bad tissue.

Chotiner said 95 to 99 percent of cataract surgeries are successful. Patients say they experience little or no pain or discomfort, and most report vastly improved vision within days of the operation. There may be some inflammation and astigmatism while the sutures are in place, but this dissipates when the eye is fully healed, about six to eight weeks following surgery.

THERE ARE risks with any surgical procedure, Chotiner said, and patients should understand that while serious complications from cataract surgery are rare and while most can be successfully treated, some can leave the patient with permanent visual impairment.

However, the potential for visual improvement makes cataract and lens implant surgery well worth the minimal risk for most people, he said.

Ambrose had his right eye done on June 17 and his left eye Aug. 20. When he wakes up each morning, he delights in seeing only one button on the light fixture in his bedroom and the vivid colors of the foliage outside his window.

Gonglowski, who admitted he worried about the outcome of his Aug. 13 surgery, is so pleased he's thinking about getting the cataract in his right eye worked on.

"I think this will change my lifestyle," he said.

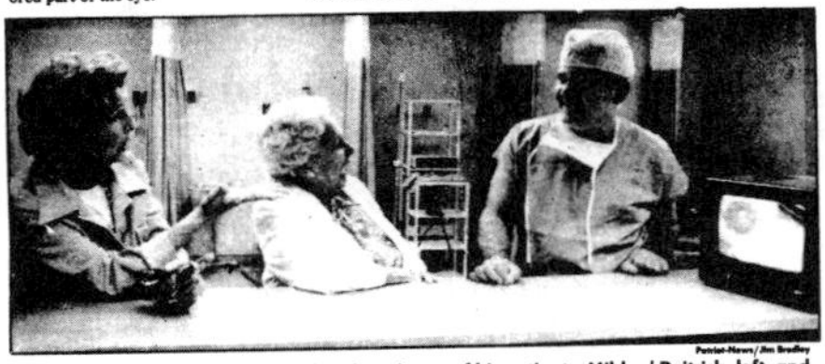

Patriot-News/Jim Bradley

Dr. Bennett Chotiner enjoys a laugh with two of his patients, Mildred Deitrich, left, and Florence Grimm, center. Chotiner replaced the cataracts both women had with artificial lens.

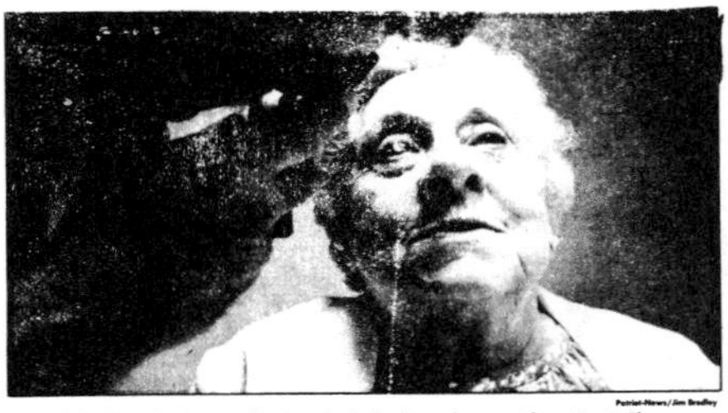

Patriot-News/Jim Bradley

Ophthalmologist Dr. Bennett Chotiner checks for signs of cataract formation in Florence Grimm's right eye. Chotiner removed a cataract from Grimm's left eye Aug. 20 and replaced it with an artificial lens.

- It's credible. People believe what they read or hear in the news.
- There is no direct cost. However, don't forget your time, or your staff's time, or that of a public relations consultant you may hire.
- The public wants health and medical information, and the media wants believable, reliable sources.
- Media coverage gives you added authority.
- It enhances your other promotional techniques.

Public speaking. This technique gives the public an opportunity to meet you and assess you, your knowledge and your background in a more personal way. If you are an effective public speaker (or willing to become one), here's a chance to become well-known to targeted groups on self-selected topics. You can double your impact by generating publicity before, during or after a speaking engagement.

Advertising. Advertising is a paid promotional technique that allows you to select the media and control your message and timing. A carefully planned advertising campaign with a reasonable budget can help you establish yourself among new audiences with new or existing services. Backed up by other public relations strategies and a strong internal marketing program, effective advertising will more than pay its way in new patients (see Figure 2-3).

Direct mail. A form of advertising, direct mail is a personalized way of reaching a select group to provide them with information about you and your practice. Direct mail is controllable; you create the message, the medium (post-card, letter, brochure, newsletter, etc.), and the mailing list, and you determine how, where and when the piece will be mailed. Because it is more personal, direct mail is often regarded as more acceptable for medical professionals than more overt advertising methods.

DUAL-FUNCTION COMMUNICATION STRATEGIES

Some of the marketing communication efforts you develop meet both internal and external marketing needs. They will reach your current patients as well as new audiences who may become patients in your practice if they are impressed with what they learn from you. Here's a brief rundown of these dual-function efforts:

Practice newsletter. Newsletters allow you to keep your patients, potential patients and referral sources informed about what's going on in your practice, provide new information on health care and remind them of the need for regular contact with you. But if you're going to the effort and expense of developing a newsletter, why limit it to your internal audience? With a practice newsletter, you can also reach a very broad external audience, including the public, the media, community leaders, health care professionals and physician referral sources with news about your practice services and health care updates.

Practice brochure. A practice brochure allows you to create a com-

FIGURE 2-3   Educational Ad with Coupon
An educational ad like this not only gives new information to the public; the coupon offers a response measurement device for the physician. This ad generates from 10 to 30 responses a week for the doctor and is well-accepted by his colleagues.

WHAT HAPPENS WHEN A KNEE REPLACEMENT FAILS

Mr. Oscar Saari is a 71 year old gentleman who lives in the Finnish community in Lake Worth. He had had a total knee replacement which lasted for 5 years but failed when the bone cement cracked around it. (Nothing in this world is 100%.) His walking became so painful that something had to be done or face a wheelchair existence. The bone around the implant had become so eroded away that putting in a new one would have been near impossible. Not all was lost because the knee could be saved by another surgical operation called a fusion.

WHAT IS A KNEE FUSION

When the ends of two bones are held against each other, they will join together like two pieces of steel welded one to the other. In this case the two surfaces of the knee, femur and tibia, were fused together. It was technically difficult, however, because there was a large gap left in the knee joint where the old prosthesis had been installed. The problem was solved by modern medical advances. In this case bone grafts were obtained from the Miami Medical School Bone Bank. They were used to fill in the gap as well as take up the space which would have ordinarily collapsed making his leg almost two inches shorter. Four months after his surgery he was walking pain free with the use of only a cane for moral support.

WHAT HAPPENS AFTER A KNEE IS FUSED

To some patients a fused knee means terrible things, the end of the line. On the contrary, a successfully fused knee can be quite a blessing. Look at how well "Chester" did as sheriff's deputy in the TV series Gunsmoke. He strutted around with the best of the characters, riding horses and capturing those mean outlaws. However, there are a few drawbacks. If a fusion is done on his right leg, the patient must learn to drive his car with his left leg crossing over the pedals, or have a special extension attached to the right pedals. (No big deal.) Riding in airplanes does require some advanced planning to reserve a bulkhead seat so that the fused leg can be stretched out comfortably. Once the fusion becomes solid, the pain is gone completely forever. Some patients can even run on their leg just as Chester did. A fused knee is not all that bad.

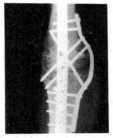 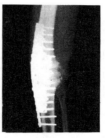

The photograph on the left is taken with the patient front to back while the one on the right is side view. Achieving a fusion in the knee is a technically difficult operation. There are a number of ways of doing this. A recent article published in the "Journal of Bone and Joint Surgery" showed that the most successful method is to fix the two bones together by special heavy-duty bone plates. This is the technique used by Dr. Tronzo in Mr. Saari's case. As seen in the photogrtaph, the metal knee joint implant has been removed. The hole left in the bone has been filled in by bone grafts in such a way that the length of the leg has been reestablished. The femur and tibia are held together by two heavy steel plates and especially heavy steel screws. Once this is accomplished, the grafts become congealed into one solid mass of bone making the femur continuous with the tibia as one long piece of bone. This then allows the patient to bear full weight on the leg without pain.

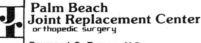

Palm Beach
Joint Replacement Center
orthopedic surgery

Raymond G. Tronzo, M.D.

Raymond G. Tronzo, M.D.
1114 N. Olive Avenue, West Palm Beach, Fla. 33401
Telephone: (407) 655-7858
Please send me your BROCHURE ON ☐ Knees ☐ Hips ☐ Series
Name _____
Address _____
City _____ State _____ Zip _____

---

prehensive, factual picture of your practice. You should never make a personal contact of a professional nature—whether in the office or in a group—without offering copies of your practice brochure to the individual or group members. A practice brochure also can be part of a direct mail package, and it can be mailed or handed to all new patients. A brochure offers information about your practice, staff, policies and services and, through the graphic look and message, it also helps create the perception or image you want your patients and potential patients to have.

Advertising specialties. Advertising specialties such as imprinted pens, magnets, stickers, notepads and other "giveaways" provide patients and the public a physical remembrance of your practice. Don't downplay the effectiveness or significance of a carefully selected specialty item as part of a total promotional campaign.

Special events. Open houses, health fairs, classes and seminars are worthwhile ways to get you in the public eye and to familiarize a relatively large group of people with you and your services. Special events are valuable because they position you as community-involved. They give patients and the public an opportunity to meet and assess you (and your staff, who represent you); and they allow you to meet a relatively large number of people, hopefully leaving them with a favorable impression.

Signage. This is another seemingly insignificant item that, taken in combination with all the other visible means of practice promotion, creates a unified and positive image. Your office's exterior sign and all of the internal signs and messages that direct, inform or instruct your patients give a strong message to everyone who sees them. Do you know what kind of message you're sending?

KNOW THE RULES OF THE ROAD

There is one major error that can occur in marketing a medical practice. That is to implement a promotional strategy without first familiarizing yourself with the guidelines of the American Medical Association, the American Osteopathic Association, and those of your state medical association and local medical society.

In its 1979 ruling against the American Medical Association and two Connecticut medical societies, the Federal Trade Commission wrote that advertising restrictions by the AMA "have served to deprive consumers of the free flow of information about availability of health care services, to deter the offering of innovative forms of health care, and to stifle the rise of almost every type of health care delivery that could potentially pose a threat to the income of fee-for-service physicians in private practice. The cost to the public in terms of less expensive or even perhaps more improved forms of medical services are great."

Following the FTC decision, which was upheld by the U.S. Supreme Court in 1982, the AMA and local medical organizations have attempted to spell out what is considered to be "appropriate" or ethical advertising by physicians. The guidelines specify certain restrictions regarding use of testimonials, discussion of past treatment successes, high-pressure advertising and, of course, misleading, false or deceptive statements. See Appendix E for the AMA guidelines on advertising.

It's recommended that you become familiar with these guidelines as well as the FTC advertising regulations in Appendix E before starting an advertising or promotional program. It's also wise, we believe, to review your proposed promotional efforts with your medical organization and with your attorney in order to avoid after-the-fact censure or peer criticism.

AND FINALLY . . .

The communication component of marketing takes time, planning and effort, but the satisfaction of seeing your practice grow in an orderly fashion with the kinds of patients you want—patients who seek the services you offer—makes the effort well worth it. You'll see that your professional medical skills and approach to the practice of medicine are enhanced when you establish a direction of growth for your practice, then implement the promotional strategies for your chosen path. Moreover, we believe you'll see that practice promotion actually gives you *more* time for your patient—as well as patients who are more satisfied with your practice and more educated about their roles in maintaining good health.

BIBLIOGRAPHY

Guide to Advertising Media. *Boardroom Reports* 1981; August 10: 10.

Physicians Marketing Showcase, Vol. I, No. II Scottsdale, AZ, Health Services Marketing, Ltd.

Why Doctors Need a Healthy Dose of Public Relations. *Private Practice* 1983; July.

Bellizzi & Hite: Consumer Attitudes Toward Accountants, Lawyers and Physicians with Respect to Advertising Professional Services. *Journal of Advertising Research* 1986; June 7.

Gray: The Selling of Medicine 1986. *Medical Economics* 1986; January 20.

McDaniel, Smith L, Smith K: The Status of Physician Advertising. *Journal of Professional Services Marketing* 1986; Fall–Winter.

A Discouraging Forecast for Office Visits. *Medical Economics* 1987; October 5.

II

Building Your Practice Identity

Chapter 3

Assessing Your Practice

You've heard enough about the competitive medical environment in which you and other physicians attempt to fulfill your professional oathes. Given this setting, it's apparent that those who do the most communicating with their existing and potential patients are more likely to retain current patients and generate new ones.

However, before initiating a marketing communications program, you must do some research. Research comes *before* developing your patient newsletter, before offering an educational seminar or considering a more substantial Yellow Pages ad. Starting your marketing communications program without research is guaranteed to result in the waste of many dollars, and could hurt your practice in other ways.

The research we recommend (and the focus of this chapter) includes an evaluation of yourself and your practice, and an assessment of the marketplace, your competition and other factors.

While research may sound like an imposing and formidable task for a physician with little marketing experience, once you understand the process and the steps involved, establishing this capability within your practice is not that difficult.

Actually, research is nothing more than the orderly and objective process of understanding your practice and its users . . . the people upon whom the success of your practice ultimately depends. Too often the process is seen as a costly one involving a large or extensive surveys and studies. But marketing research does not necessarily have to be complicated or expensive.

THE MARKETING RESEARCH PROCESS

While many volumes have been written about how to establish a research program, the process involves the same basic steps regardless of the sophistication of your endeavor. What may differ is the means by which you carry out the research process.

Personal/Professional/Practice Evaluation. The first step is to understand yourself and your practice. What are your personal goals and needs vis-à-vis yourself, family time, vacation time, time off? What strengths and weaknesses do you and other physicians in the practice have? What skills—both technical- and people-oriented—do you possess? What services do you provide and what services do you plan—or would you like—to provide? What goals do you and other physicians in the practice have for yourself and the practice?

What about the practice itself? What is the office ambience, physical appearance, technical and equipment capabilities? What is the image of the practice? What makes it unique, sets it apart from other practices? Does your staff reflect your image, or are they capable of supporting your desired image? Are you receiving maximum support from your staff? What are their strengths and weaknesses? What is your existing patient profile, and what do your patients think of you, your staff, your services and your office environment?

Marketplace Demographics and Target Market. It's critical to know exactly who you are trying to reach. You must define and describe the narrow community of actual and potential patients and referrers who have the most likelihood of using or recommending your services. This includes individuals, groups, employers, health plans, physicians and other professionals. From a geographical standpoint, solo practitioners generally draw patients from within a three- to five-mile radius of their offices. For larger group practices, multi-office practices, and certain other types of solo practices, this guideline does not necessarily apply.

What is the ethnic make-up, the proportion of working to non-working women, the number of retirees, of children? Is your community primarily white collar, blue collar, or a mix? And which of these groups does your practice attract or would you like it to attract? How you shape your communication message is ultimately determined by the value systems, needs and lifestyles of those you need to communicate to.

Competition. You should also know who your competitors are. What are their strengths and weaknesses? What is their image in the community? What kinds of patients do they attract? How does your practice stack up against the competition from the vantage point of the consumer? How much do you think they invest in practice promotion and how effective are they?

Budget. How much should you allocate for marketing your practice, and where can those dollars be most profitably spent? You are making a considerable investment in hopes of a larger payback in increased business and profitability. To realize a maximum return on your investment, you must plan your expenditures and monitor the results very carefully. (Promotion budgeting is discussed in depth in Chapter 20.)

Media. These are vehicles that will carry your message. What is available in your community in terms of newspapers and magazines, radio and television stations? Who are their audiences and what are their rates? What about coupon distribution services and newcomer welcoming programs?

Where can you find a mailing list of newcomers and other target groups in your area?

PERSONAL AND PRACTICE EVALUATION

No two physicians conduct themselves or their practice exactly the same, nor does every physician enjoy working with the same type of patient. So it's important that you carefully assess yourself and your practice so you can target your communications to the patients you seek.

Begin by looking at your practice as a patient would. Your communications efforts should project an image consistent with your practice. If it does not, you create dissonance. The patient feels misled, and the doctor-patient relationship begins on a note of discord.

As you evaluate yourself and your practice, remember too that there are no right or wrong answers. You are merely trying to gain a clear view of your practice so that you may establish a logical focus for your communication strategies. When you determine the image or character of your practice, you can make that into a positive selling point in your promotional endeavors. You'll find forms in the appendix for completing the physician, practice and community assessments. Before you turn to these forms, however, let's take a look at your practice from the vantage point of the patient.

Office Ambience. One of the first impressions a patient gains is of the office environment or ambience. What kind of non-verbal message does your decor communicate? Does the decor exude an image of wealth and class? Or is it more relaxed, family-oriented? What type of reading material is provided? Does it address the interests and values of your typical patients? Or is it a mishmash of outdated subscriptions contributed by you and your staff? Are the signs you have posted negative or positive?

Take a tour of your office. As the patient goes through a complete visit, what does he see and hear? Begin with what the patient sees from the time he arrives. This means you should consider outdoor signage and directories that indicate your office location in a complex. Once inside and beyond the reception area, can the patient see cluttered work areas? Other patients being treated? Storage areas? Can he or she hear the staff talking among themselves? Can exam room conversations be heard? From the patient's vantage point, does equipment appear modern and non-threatening?

Practice Staff and Personality. Now let's turn to the "people" aspects of your practice, the elements that give your practice character, personality and, hopefully, warmth. Look at yourself and your staff as well as anyone else who has contact with your patients . . . including your answering service. How developed are your interpersonal skills? Do you deal with people effectively? Are you outgoing and communication-oriented? Do you have empathy with your patients' needs? Do you exude confidence and efficiency? How much time do you spend getting to know your patients and discussing their health care needs?

In considering the people side of your practice, include appearance, dress and speech. Patients immediately form opinions based on these factors. Do you fit the image of the traditional physician, or are you extremely casual in dress and speech? Does your staff dress professionally? Do they look like they all work in the same practice?

Is there a visible rapport among office staffers? Such factors are clearly perceived by outsiders and set the tone for the visit. Are they warm, personable, courteous and thoughtful toward patients?

Services and Features. Consider specific services and features for your practice that can be used as tangible and effective promotional points in your marketing communications. What about extended hours, multiple locations, specialties, amenities? Ancillary services such as diabetes or hernia screenings, nutrition or CPR classes, or parent-child sex education classes all offer promotional opportunities.

Quality of Service. Would your care be considered very high-quality from the patient's point of view? Do you stress quality and service rather than price? Do you enhance the patient's perception of value with educational materials and an attentive staff? Are your services as broad and varied as those offered by competing practices? What do you do better than or different from other physicians? What makes you a good physician besides your clinical skills?

Accessibility. Are you accessible to the public? Is your practice located on a busy street with lots of traffic, or in or near a major medical building? Are your hours convenient to working patients seeking early morning or evening appointments? Is parking a problem? Do you offer handicapped access? Do you maintain a high public profile? Are you well-known and respected in your community?

Patient composition. The image of your practice is also characterized by the patients you currently treat. Is there a predominance of men or women in your patient base? What about seniors, teenagers? Is the income level of your patients high, medium or low? Do most of your patients live within a three-mile radius of your practice, or do they come from a larger geographical area? Are there certain employers who are well-represented among your patients? Do you have a high percentage of patients from health plans?

Are the patients you are getting the patients you want? If not, try to profile or describe the patient you want.

Is the makeup of the residential area near your office changing? Are families getting older, or are more young families moving in? Why do people come to you? Do you know why your best patients continue to see you? Could their positive reasons be featured in your marketing communication as benefits? Do these reasons help you view your practice image more objectively? Have you ever asked former patients why they stopped seeing you?

The answers to all these questions are valuable as a starting point in your self-evaluation. The more you know about your practice, the more effectively you can communicate to your staff and others on whom you will depend to help institute your marketing program. They need to know as much as they possibly can about your practice, your goals, your patients and your target audience. You may also find the self-assessment forms in Figure 3-1 and the Appendix helpful.

It is also important to realize that the assessment process is ongoing. It's easy to become too close to what you are doing and thus lose your objectivity. Review the questions with other physicians in your practice and your staff on a periodic basis so you will not lose touch with your practice—or your patients.

FIGURE 3-1 Self-Assessment Form

Self-Assessment

How would you rate yourself? Base your responses on patient comments and complaints (if any); your observations and perceptions, and comments you've heard from your staff. You can also give this evaluation to your staff and ask them to rate you anonymously. Their judgments can be valuable.
(Make a copy of this page before taking the test, since you'll use the same assessment for your staff members.)
Give yourself from 1 (low) to 5 (high) for each attribute depending on how strongly it is exhibited.

_____ Friendliness

_____ Concern for patient's welfare

_____ Awareness of your patients' values/needs

_____ Tact

_____ Promptness

_____ Courtesy

_____ Cooperation

_____ Knowledge

_____ Positive attitude

_____ Humor

_____ Dependability

_____ Enthusiasm

_____ Professional appearance

_____ Attention to detail

A score of 3 or lower for any attribute indicates an area that needs improvement.

PATIENT SURVEYS

An excellent way to ascertain valuable information about your practice is to ask your patients. No one knows the image you project better than the people who utilize your services. Most would be happy to cooperate if asked in a non-threatening manner. The patient survey is an excellent vehicle for this purpose (see Appendix D).

Administering a patient questionnaire is a responsibility you can delegate to your staff so they can begin getting involved in your marketing endeavors. The survey will not replace your interaction with the public as a means of soliciting information, but will complement it. It will give you a broader base of input, though it may not have the depth. Insure confidentiality by having the completed questionnaires deposited in a closed box, or by having patients seal them in an envelope before returning them to you.

Preface your questionnaire with a statement of purpose that expresses appreciation for their input and explains that the answers will help you to continue providing the best possible service.

Your questionnaire should cover areas such as your patients' satisfaction with your office environment; staff attitude, courtesy, assistance; waiting time; quality of medical care; your attitude, courtesy, treatment and professionalism; as well as patient demographics (sex, age, income, employer/occupation, geographic location). You may wish to give or send your questionnaire to patients after an office visit or outpatient procedure, or administer it annually as a "practice check-up." Another option is to develop a brief post-visit questionnaire specifically for distribution after a visit. (See Figure 3-2.) The briefer post-visit format, however, will not provide the comprehensive information gained from a lengthier questionnaire.

By analyzing returned questionnaires, you can gain information about your current patients as well as groups not represented in your practice whom you should target with your communication efforts.

From the information, or from your patient records, you can determine where your current patients come from. Using a map and colored pins, indicate your patients by location, drawing concentric rings extending in one-, two- and three-mile radii from your practice. Look for bare areas and areas of mass coverage. This procedure can also be easily accomplished with your practice computer if you have one, by zip code sorting. Whichever method you use, it is necessary to chart about 10–15 percent of your patients to identify your primary service area(s).

YOUR PRACTICE IMAGE

Now that you've taken a magnifying glass to your practice, put it aside temporarily and turn to the mirror. What does all this information say about the image of your practice? People are forming impressions of you and your practice and acting on those impressions every day. For a mar-

FIGURE 3-2 Post-Visit Patient Questionnaire

POST-VISIT PATIENT QUESTIONNAIRE

1. How long did you wait in the reception area? _____
2. Did you consider the waiting time:
   _____ Brief _____ Reasonable _____ Excessive
3. Were you greeted promptly and courteously by the receptionist?
   _____ Yes _____ No
4. Was the doctor knowledgeable? ___ friendly? ___ helpful? ___
5. Did the doctor spend enough time with you? ___ Yes ___ No
6. How would you rate our staff in terms of courtesy and service?
   _____ Excellent _____ Good _____ Fair _____ Poor
7. Would you recommend this practice to others? ___ Yes ___ No
8. We welcome your comments or suggestions:
   _____
   _____

keting communication program to be effective, you must determine what your image is, then polish it or change it so that you can achieve your desired goal.

It's best to develop an image that reflects who you really are. You want to attract people who will be comfortable with you, who feel that you are comfortable with your external image, and who will stay with you and refer others. Not every physician, not every patient, would feel comfortable with the approach used by the big city plastic surgeon who achieved a mood of muted elegance with suede-cloth chairs in exam rooms in which medical equipment is hidden behind brass-handled cabinets.

This is an example of image created primarily through office decor. That's one important image determinant. Office decor sends out a non-verbal message about how the physician acts and runs his or her practice. But other elements also go into creating your practice image. Whether you wear a traditional white coat or dress more informally will also contribute to your image. Image is the composite of everything from your speaking mannerisms to your practice policies.

The point is that every medical practice has its own unique image and identity, something that puts it in a class of its own, something that can be projected through a marketing communications program to enhance the success of that practice.

MARKETPLACE ASSESSMENT

When physicians decide to promote their practice, many immediately wonder what to say in their communications rather than whom to say it to. It may seem backward to put creative development last, but your message doesn't mean a thing if you don't get it in front of the right audience—the people who are most likely to need your services, in the media where they are most likely to see it. All this at a cost you can afford.

You need to find out the demographics of the marketplace so you will know what ages, incomes, ethnicities, types of employment and household groups are increasing or decreasing. A pediatrician or a specialist in children's diabetes needs to know school district enrollment projections. You need to know in what zip codes families with children live. You want to know where other doctors are located if your practice depends on physician referrals, because you want to be located near them. Looking into the demographics of your area will help ensure that your marketing effort is indeed on target. It's not enough to assume your area is populated with young families and children just because you pass through a few school zones on the way to work. You may want to know how many children, and their age ranges. You want to know if their mothers are out in the work force and, if so, where they work.

This kind of information will guide you in allocating your marketing communication budget for the biggest return.

Sources of Information. The information you need to make these decisions is available from a number of sources. Start with your local Chamber of Commerce. Most provide research on city population and income levels by district. The local office of your state's Department of Economic Security also has population statistics and labor market analyses that can tell you the percentages of white-collar and blue-collar workers by area.

You can gain information from the latest census, from the city planning department, local school districts and utility company projections. The larger banks and newspapers along with universities conduct research as well. In many cases, the research departments of these institutions will be able to give you information about the present as well as what to expect in coming years. The Small Business Administration compiles bibliographies listing a variety of available sources. And don't forget the hospital where you have staff privileges; its planning or marketing department should have demographic information they can share with you.

You'll want to look at the information on educational levels, income levels, age groups, ethnic groups, number of children living at home, number of retirees, number of newcomers and part-time residents, occupational status, and major employers. You want as much insight into your marketplace as you can get. Compare the population demographics in your service area with your own patient records. In this way, you can determine if you're missing a large segment or group you ought to be capturing. If so, the next step is to determine why.

After that, when a radio advertising representative tells you her station delivers a 35-plus age group, you'll know if a high percentage of your potential patients will be reached, or if your target market is predominantly younger or older. Media reps can and will provide you with reams of research pinpointing who they reach, but you must view this information against facts you have researched for it to have meaning.

Target Marketing. Targeting. Market segmentation. Positioning. We'll cover them all by the time you've finished reading this book, but essentially they all have to do with identifying and then zeroing in on specific portions or groupings of the population. The idea is to decide what particular markets you would like to reach based on your research and your practice analysis, goals and specialty interests. Find out what is important to those who comprise the selected markets, then tailor your practice and promotional endeavors to meet their needs, values and desires.

This strategy is especially important for physicians. Unless you're part of a very large group practice or multi-specialty clinic, your patients come from a rather narrowly defined geographic area, or are attracted by the nature of your practice or by what friends or family tell them. Primary care practices usually draw from their immediate area, often populated by a specific socio-economic group. Specialists generally appeal to particular markets such as the elderly, or those with a particular disease or problem. Unless you're located in a small community, it is normally not cost-effective to try to appeal to everyone in your city. By determining those market segments predominant in your service area, or by determining what segments you would like to attract, you can "target" your message and promotion dollars to reach the audience most likely to respond.

Target marketing is an effective way to offset the chasm between your marketing budget and the major companies whose messages you compete with for consumers' attention. When you're outnumbered, you have to outsmart the competition. By developing a very precise knowledge of your practice and your patients, by identifying the unique aspects of your practice, you will have a basic undersanding of where you are and, hopefully, where you would like to be in the future. To target to the specific groups most likely to use your services, you must discover their interests and needs, adjust your practice to reflect those needs, and then communciate in terms they will understand and relate to (see Figure 3-3).

ASSESSING THE COMPETITION

Increased competition has driven growing numbers of physicians into at least rudimentary marketing programs. Successful practices are no longer assured without some attempt to communicate practice strengths.

As more and more physicians acquire marketing savvy, those with high-quality medical practices geared to patient satisfaction and who do the best job of communicating the benefits their practices offer will be most successful.

But how can you expect to compete successfully unless you know what you're up against?

FIGURE 3-3 Target Marketing Illustration

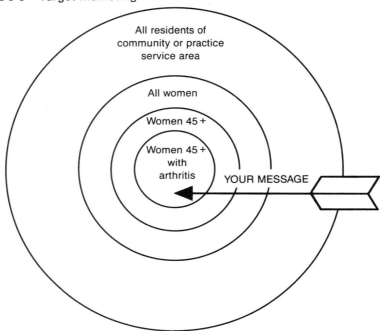

Any assessment of the competition must necessarily be conducted from the vantage point of the consumer. It doesn't matter how you see your practice relative to your competitors. It doesn't matter that you are better qualified than the average person on the street to judge the capabilities of other medical practices. The only thing that matters is the perception of those who make the decision to see you or the physician down the street.

Even if your practice is the most successful in your marketplace, it's imperative that you keep a close watch on the competition. Satchell Paige, the legendary baseball pitcher, used to attribute his longevity to the fact that he never looked over his shoulder because something might be gaining on him. That approach may have worked for Satch, but you need to know who may be gaining on you. Circumstances change. Competitors challenge. Complacency can be fatal.

You can judge your competition by a variety of methods. The easiest is to monitor their marketing programs. What are they telling the consumer? How are they communicating? You may pick up some valuable tips.

Other competitor assessment methods include telephone calls to inquire about rates and services, actual appointments by staff members (who, incidentally, will also benefit from seeing the inner workings of another practice), and simply talking to other physicians in your area. Often your competitive colleagues' practices will come up for discussion. Don't neglect to talk to your patients. Find out what's important to them. Ask how you can better meet their needs. Truly listen to what they say; don't inwardly disparage their comments and opinions. Remember, what they're telling you reflects their own needs and desires vis-à-vis your practice.

Your ultimate objective is to develop unique features that will strengthen your practice. To improve or maintain your position, it is essential to make the consumer's perceptions work to your advantage. A competitive analysis based on the consumer's perception is an important step on the road to marketing sophistication and increased success.

Most importantly, you need to communicate as well or better than your competition. If you don't tell people why they should choose your practice in terms they can relate to, why should they choose you?

PATIENT CONVENIENCE

An important feature to the health care consumer is convenience. Compare your hours with those of the competition. If it's easier for a patient to see another doctor or group practice because he or she offers more flexible hours, you can rest assured that is exactly what some will do.

What about location, parking, or waiting time once a patient arrives for an appointment? Location may not be a factor you can do much about, but if it is seriously impeding the success of your practice, a change may be essential. With waiting time, steps can be taken to improve the situation.

What about emergency service? Are you as accessible as the physician or facility down the street? Do you make your accessibility known through your practice promotion? Do you make it easy for patients to reach you in case of an emergency or off-hours medical problem?

Do you offer convenient payment plans? Accept major credit cards? Assist patients with insurance paperwork? These are all non-medical factors patients consider important.

Most of all, be sure your promotional efforts state the advantages of your practice clearly, concisely and in terms the consumer can understand and appreciate. Remember, it isn't how you see yourself that matters. It's how the public sees you.

MEDIA SELECTION

Selecting the best media for your marketing communication program is not an easy task. There is a wide variety of media available, from the more subtle tools such as newsletters, practice brochures and patient-education pamphlets to print and broadcast media for paid advertising or publicity. The practice analysis you do will help determine the most appropriate media for your target audience(s) and your practice.

If you choose to advertise, each media representative you talk to will claim to have more efficiency and effectiveness than the competition. And in a sense, each is telling the truth. In one way or another, each medium can legitimately claim to be number one. One radio station, for example, may be dominant during the 6 to 10 A.M. time slot, while another may attract more female listeners over the age of 50. That's why practice analysis is important.

Radio and television audiences are measured by privately owned research companies based on samples of households or individuals in a market. Recognized statistical methods are used to make these measurements as accurate as possible. Exactly what these surveys will tell you depends on the company conducting the research, but they are all complete enough to give you insight into each station's audience characteristics and size.

With printed publications, you can obtain independently audited circulation statements from sales reps. Circulation audits examine subscription records or evidence of how nonpaid circulation is controlled. Audits do not determine readership, only circulation, so many publications will also have research on readership. Be sure to request such information.

Once you've assured yourself that you know what the media in your market can deliver, you're in a better position to make selections. You will obtain the best results if you limit the number of media you use, since you don't want to spread yourself too thin. On the other hand, don't put all your eggs in one basket. Chapters 14–19 provide complete information on the actual selection of media. Rate structures and suggestions for evaluating the major media are also discussed.

You need not always use paid advertising to get media exposure. As discussed in Chapters 9 and 10, the public's high interest in health care offers you many opportunities to be interviewed on radio or TV, hold an educational seminar or have an article about a patient or your practice appear in the newspaper. Furthermore, you can reach your own patients (and potential patients) through communications over which you have greater control, such as newsletters, patient brochures and, of course, the most effective communication of all—face-to-face communication.

BUDGETING

Once you have researched and evaluated your practice, your patients, your market, your competition, and the available media, you are ready to establish your marketing communications budget. This stage often makes the novice marketer nervous. But dollars allocated to promotion should not be viewed as an expense or as additional overhead. Marketing is an investment in the future, and a sound one. With marketing communications, the adage, "You have to spend money to make money," is especially true.

View your promotion expenditures the way you would the purchase of new equipment that allows you to treat more patients; you'll see that marketing is a means rather than an end. In part, it is a means of communicating important information to patients and referrers.

And it's important to realize that you have to stay committed to your allocated budget to the end. As the Eastman Kodak Company explains in its advertising guide, "Successful advertising isn't a hundred-yard dash. It's a marathon. You've got to go the distance to win." That's true not only of advertising, but of your total marketing plan. You must plan for the long run, and then stick with your plan. Keep this in mind when you're determining your budget. Plan for a whole year based on quarterly allocations. You'll need to remain somewhat flexible to take advantage of unpredictable circumstances, but a one-year plan gives you direction and stability.

Most periods of increased promotional expenditures are predictable. You can allocate extra money for events such as a cholesterol education seminar, diabetes awareness month, the semi-annual publication of your patient newsletter or other increased demand periods. Budgeting does not mean dividing your annual budget by 12 months.

Budgeting should also be linked to projecting where you want to be, realistically, in a year's time. It is best to base your projection in part on past performance. This gives you a degree of stability while allowing you to capitalize on market potential. Budgeting is discussed in more depth in Chapter 21.

AND FINALLY . . .

Many physicians who engage in marketing are initially anxious and impatient. They want to quickly develop a patient brochure, initiate an educational seminar or even begin advertising. Unfortunately, these beginners can end up wasting a lot of money and in some cases even hurt their practices in other ways.

Although this book presents a shopping cart full of exciting and effective ideas for marketing communication and promotion, we urge you to first do your homework. Understand yourself and your practice, assess the marketplace, learn about your competition and then formulate and implement your promotion strategies based on what you learn. You'll be rewarded by a better return on your marketing expenditures and a practice that steadily attracts and retains new patients—the kind of patients you want, and whose needs you are best equipped to meet.

Chapter 4

Positioning: Making Perception Reality

Suppose you were asked to describe the following in ten words or less: IBM, 7-Up, Crest, Helmsley Hotels. Could you do it?

In our practice marketing seminars when we've asked that question, most physicians have no trouble describing IBM as a computer manufacturer where excellent service is the hallmark, or remembering that 7-Up is "the Uncola." Crest is known as "the cavity fighter" and you stay at a Helmsley Hotel when you want to feel like royalty.

Now describe your practice in ten words or less. Could you or your patients characterize your practice in this same concise, specific manner? Probably not.

Each of the companies or products we've just described has done an excellent job of *positioning*. Each has created an image that is very clear, concise and simple. Positioning is creating an image in the mind of the consumer that defines, and differentiates from the competition, the perception of your product or service. In medicine, effective positioning can set your practice apart from others by giving it a valuable place in the health care marketplace. This is sometimes referred to as creating a *niche* in the market.

Positioning is a very basic and fundamental concept. In this chapter we will show you how a physician's practice or a specific medical service can be successfully positioned to define and enhance your marketing and communication efforts.

The selection of a position is a crucial strategic decision for any organization. Since customer perceptions of products and services influence the choices they make, shaping or controlling what perceptions they will have of your service becomes central to your success. Yet this concept is not simple to implement effectively, because it requires you to know yourself, your practice, your staff and your audience (patients and would-be patients).

DIFFICULTY IN DEVELOPING A POSITION

We are exposed to an incredible number of organizations each day, all trying to communicate their message. Newspapers, television, magazines, radio, direct mail, television, outdoor advertising, building signage, special event sponsorships, and other forms of promotion are all competing to be seen and heard. Closer to home, health care advertising is growing at a dizzying rate. Each advertiser is striving to differentiate its message from that of everyone else and be noticed by consumers.

Unfortunately, not all messages are heard. Thus, as we attempt to lift our communication above the clutter, we must be very selective not only in our message, but also in choosing whom to target.

Positioning seems to work best when it is focused on narrow target markets or audiences. In this way, you can more easily tailor the message to the people you want to reach and increase the likelihood of being heard. What we are talking about is *market segmentation,* or the division of a market into smaller sections with like characteristics. For example, the people residing in a particular city can be segmented by the zip code in which they live. Or the population can be segmented by gender, with women forming the market segment targeted by an ob-gyn. This doctor might further segment women by age, targeting women over 35 years of age for a new mammography program and women under 40 for a program geared to first-time mothers. By looking at the size of each segment in the population, the physician can determine the potential demand for each of the services he/she offers or is considering offering (see Figure 4-1).

Now let's look at how positioning and segmentation can be used in developing a marketing plan for your medical practice.

POSITIONING AND SEGMENTATION

Developing the best position for your practice requires that you answer several questions. You'll need to know who you are going to serve and what services you'll feature. Developing a positioning strategy may mean selecting a specific segment of the market to serve, or featuring an aspect of your specialty that's needed by only one segment of the population. For example, an allergist may decide to concentrate on children's asthma and position the practice to appeal to parents of children with this conditon. A dermatologist may wish to feature aspects of his or her practice that deal with cosmetic procedures such as dermabrasion. This physician may adopt the practice name: Metropolitan Institute for Cosmetic Dermatology.

Examples of positioning and segmentation are frequently seen outside of health care. Package goods marketers have been doing it for years. More recently banks have adopted positioning strategies. In one South-western metropolitan area a large bank has positioned itself as the bank that caters to small- to mid-sized businesses. Another bank has adopted the position as the most convenient bank by putting branches throughout

FIGURE 4-1 Segmentation of the Adult Female Population
Rather than deal with females in general, segmentation enables physicians to divide
up this population into subsets, each of which can then be targeted for special programs
and services.

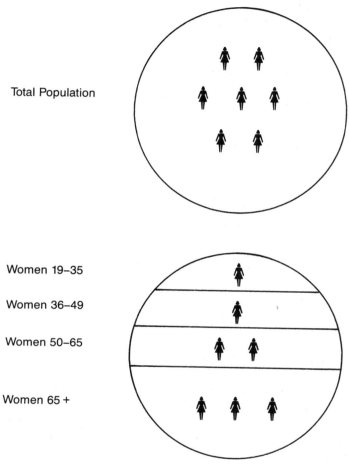

Total Population

Women 19–35

Women 36–49

Women 50–65

Women 65 +

the state and even in grocery stores. Other banks are positioned as financial
institutions for big business or for household customers.

Each of the banks offers similar services. Yet each has selected a segment of the market in which to concentrate. Thus, through its advertising,
hours of operation, location(s) and services offered, a bank can become
known as *the* bank for a particular group of people or businesses.

Automobile manufacturers have demonstrated superior positioning
awareness. Chevrolet has adopted the slogan "the heartbeat of America"
in order to maintain its all-American image.

Import luxury cars such as BMW and Mercedes have been positioned as status symbols for many segments of the population. When Honda decided to target the upscale buyer with its Acura line, it decided not to allow existing dealers to sell the Acura, but instead established separate Acura dealerships to differentiate the new product from Honda's traditional position as a moderately-priced car.

DEVELOPING THE POSITIONING STRATEGY

Your goal in developing a positioning strategy should be to develop a *positional advantage,* that is, to be recognized as the provider with the ability to serve your chosen customers (patients) better than all others do.

While a position takes a considerable amount of time and effort to establish, once established it provides a reason for people to be receptive to you and your messages. For instance, if your group practice wants to compete in an area where HMOs are dominant, you might position your group as providing attentive, personal care by doctors who know their patients by name.

As discussed in Chapter 3, before you can develop a position that's appropriate for your practice and your patients, you must have a good understanding of yourself, your practice and others offering the same services. What do you like doing best? What are your unique capabilities? And where do you want to be in three years? In ten years? Be honest; skirting the facts won't accomplish your objective.

The practice and marketplace evaluation you described in Chapter 3 will help you determine what unfilled niche can define your practice.

With this information, you can begin to develop an appropriate position for your services. A midwestern dermatologist, for example, has a practice in which three-quarters of her patients are teenage acne cases, a medical problem and age group she enjoys treating. In a move to enhance her practice's focus, the physician investigated several new office sites. Her current location is a downtown high-rise medical building. One site which seemed promising was in a very accessible office, located in a suburb populated by young families. The other was several miles away in a hospital medical office building. The doctor selected the suburban site which was more convenient to the local high school. She also evaluated her office hours and found that she could tailor them to meet the needs of young people by focusing on after school, early evenings and Saturdays. When she decided to promote the acne services, her research found a weekly newspaper and a section of the daily paper most often ready by young people. School nurses, youth organization leaders and high school counselors became important potential referral sources, and the doctor and her nurses frequently communicated with these people by letter.

In contrast, a small group of family physicians decided to specialize in geriatrics. They made entirely different decisions in office location, hours and promotional strategies. They located in a small medical office complex near the downtown shopping area. Their office was on the first floor with easy access and visibility from the street. They opened early in the morning and closed earlier than they had been. They offered free blood pressure checks between 9 and 10 A.M. daily. They also held weekly mid-morning education classes on different topics. The staff filled out claim forms for patients, a service that always generated thanks and appreciation. While these doctors have not yet begun to advertise, they do write a regular column in a monthly senior newspaper and present programs frequently at the senior center near their office.

A pediatric subspecialty group with a successful practice based in a major midwestern children's hospital was seeing an erosion of their referral base. The physicians suspected that a suburban general hospital which recently made a substantial investment in upgrading its pediatric unit was attracting some of their potential rural patients. The doctors made a bold move by sponsoring a scientific symposium on childhood diseases with well-known experts as speakers. Pediatricians and family practice physicians in a 200-mile radius were attracted to the event, and awareness of the sponsoring pediatric group soared along with referrals.

Each of these practices very consciously targeted a specific segment of the market and then consistently implemented marketing efforts to reinforce its desired positions. Figure 4-2 depicts the steps you must follow to implement a positioning strategy for your practice.

USING THE MARKETING MIX

The marketing mix represents the elements of marketing strategy that are used to provide the right service or product in the right place at the right time and for the right price. There are five major elements of this mix: Product, Price, Place, Promotion and Preservation (or Patient Retention). Let's look at each of these elements and see how it can be featured individually or with another as the major element in a positioning strategy.

FIGURE 4-2. Developing Positioning Strategies

1. Internal Analysis

2. Practice Analysis

3. Competitive Analysis

4. Segment Current Patients

5. Demographic Analysis of Potential Patients

6. Select Desired Position(s)

7. Use Marketing Mix to Carry Out Selected Position

PRODUCT OR SERVICE

There are innumerable examples of product features used as the key to a positioning strategy. 3M's "Post-It" notes were promoted on the basis of the many uses and benefits of this sticky paper that requires no paper clip. In medicine, a specific procedure or treatment can be the featured positioning strategy. Examples of this include liposuction, laser surgery, hernia surgery and mammography. (See Figure 4-3.) There are practices across the country which are promoted as centers for laser surgery or hemorrhoid repair. A south Florida neurology group has successfully positioned itself as a center for the treatment of headaches. Through the use

FIGURE 4-3   Positioning Through Advertising
The medical practice that developed this ad chose to feature the treatment of a specific disease as a positioning strategy.

THIS COULD BE THE LAST SPOT...

(Scratch Here)

YOU EVER SCRATCH.

You'll get about as much relief from scratching your skin as you would from scratching the spot in this ad. But there is a spot you can go to, for real relief, where medical professionals specialize in treating only psoriasis.

If you're one of the tens of thousands of San Diegans suffering from psoriasis, you know that the discomfort and scratching is only half the problem. Having to hide the embarrassing, inflamed areas and flaky skin can be equally troublesome.

The Psoriasis Skin Care Medical Clinics use the most advanced medical treatments, including ultraviolet lightboxes and medicated whirlpool baths, in a home-like setting to help clear your skin. We emphasize relaxation and personal attention. Our hours are flexible, so you can come when it's convenient for you. For more information call today.

The Psoriasis Skin Care Medical Clinics
231-0399 ext. 33   **434-7177** ext. 23
239 Laurel St., #101, San Diego   2801 Jefferson St., Carlsbad

of a variety of marketing efforts, this group has become known in a two-county area as the specialists for this common problem. These physicians have used a two-pronged approach, marketing directly to potential patients as well as to other physicians. The doctors regularly communicate with family practitioners through educational letters presenting new research information in a friendly, conversational tone.

Another way to feature a specific service involves packaging several services into one specific offering. Health professionals have become very knowledgeable about the benefits of bundling existing services together to create a unified program. Sports medicine is a good example. In one southwestern city, a family practice physician who was an advocate of running long before it became popular has transformed his practice into one that is predominantly sports-related. In addition to complete physicals for would-be athletes, his offerings include dietary counseling, muscle strength and tolerance evaluation, cardiograms, treadmill tests, and other appropriate evaluation and treatment modalities. When his practice outgrew existing space, he built a three-story building with room for other physician offices. The first floor includes a small gym with exercise equipment and apparatus for measurement of total body fat. A large multipurpose room is rented to exercise groups for aerobic exercise classes. Other physicians in the building include an orthopedic surgeon specializing in arthroscopic surgery, a sports podiatrist, psychiatrist and dentist. Several of the physicians have joined together to sponsor an annual run, further establishing themselves as physicians for runners.

As you can see, positioning is not simply a matter of choosing a service or an approach and target audience, then communicating your chosen position. Rather, it concerns both *perception* and *reality*. If you choose to position your urology practice as serving people with incontinence and impotence problems, you must have the expertise and knowledge to provide the service. You and your staff must be knowledgeable not only about the physical affliction, but the emotional attitudes such patients bring with them. You must back up your positioning with educational material, technical expertise and the resources patients expect to find from someone claiming to meet their special needs.

PRICE

Until recently, price has been more commonly used as a differentiating or positioning feature outside of health care. Price, however, refers not only to the actual cost of a product or service, but also includes the ease of payment and the perception of value for the fee charged. Can your patients take care of their bill with a credit card? Do you provide educational material to back up verbal explanations and information?

Perceptions of value are formed also from non-financial matters such as how long a patient waits in the reception room. There is a psychological cost of waiting which often is just as important as the fee.

In the health care arena, hospitals have had more experience using pricing as a variable to set themselves apart from other facilities. Hospitals have introduced a myriad of discount programs for maternity care, senior citizens and outpatient programs. There are also facilities that have tried to position themselves as the Cadillac of care, with private suites, gourmet menus, in-room VCRs, and more. Now doctors are getting into the act. There are plastic surgeons who furnish their reception area with Louis XIV furniture, provide *Town and Country* and *Connoisseur* magazines as reading material, and train their staffs to be attentive to every whim of the upscale clientele they seek to attract.

In some areas where competition is fierce, doctors are using discount coupons mailed to thousands of homes. Results vary but an often-heard complaint from this sort of promotion is that the type of patient attracted by coupons is less than ideal. We have come across numerous examples of advertisements by physicians for $10 or $25 discounts for specific procedures. Such discounts can work well for services such as school physicals or camp exams; however, we must caution you that some patients may equate discounted prices for medical services with lower-quality care. Properly utilized, price positioning can attract new patients to a practice in other ways, such as the price-point advertising in Figure 4-4.

Attracting upper income patients can be a difficult balancing act. On one hand you may be offering luxurious office decor and plush services such as limousine transport to and from outpatient procedures. Yet, you do not want patients to resent charges and assume they are paying high bills for frills. One internist consciously decided to build a practice which catered to the wealthy. The office location was carefully selected. The ground floor suite had closed circuit cameras trained on the parking lot so patients could be recognized before they came into the office. Thus, the receptionist was able to welcome each visitor by name. The office was decorated like a finely appointed living room, complete with fireplace. The receptionist sat at a table with no counter or glass partition separating her from her patients. Refreshments included a variety of gourmet teas and coffees as well as biscuits. For this physician, concentrating on the physical attractiveness of the office was deemed necessary to appeal to a certain type of clientele.

PLACE

In the marketing literature the *place* element is also known as distribution. In health care, an even better term may be accessibility or the ease with which the consumer can obtain your services.

We live in a convenience-oriented society. Just look at the growth in fast food establishments, teller machine banking and 24-hour supermarkets. Yet convenience involves more than just location. In medicine, it also includes the hours and days services are offered, ease in getting an appointment, waiting time and even the availability of convenient parking.

FIGURE 4-4   Price Point Positioning
Price advertising can be effective in medical care, depending on the product or service.
Low-cost mammography is a service sought by many woman.

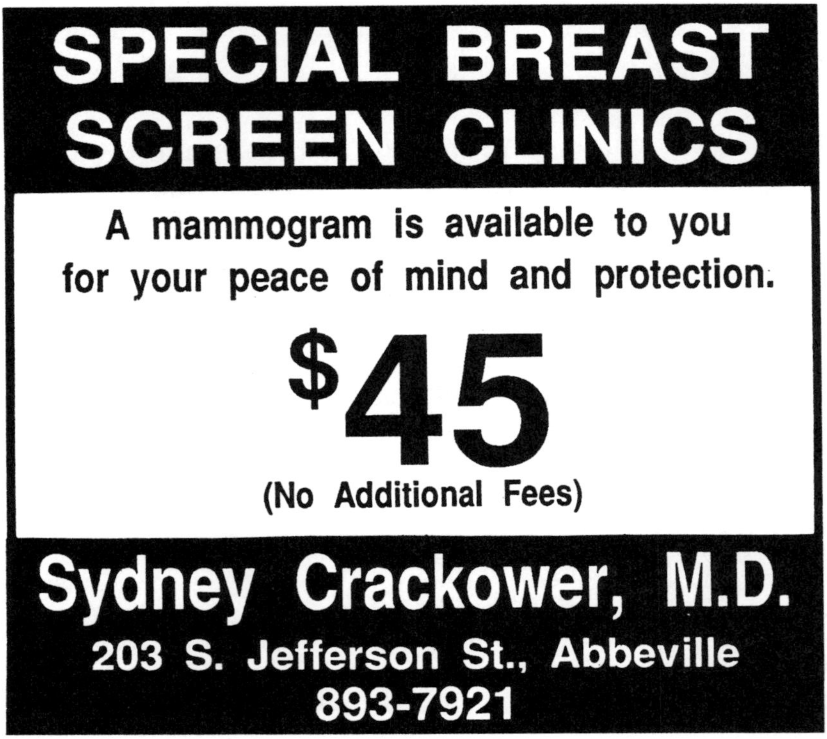

SPECIAL BREAST SCREEN CLINICS

A mammogram is available to you for your peace of mind and protection.

$45

(No Additional Fees)

Sydney Crackower, M.D.
203 S. Jefferson St., Abbeville
893-7921

Freestanding urgent care centers are an excellent example of health care services positioned for convenience. Open in the evenings and on weekends, these centers have been seen by some people as convenient alternatives to taking time off work to see their personal physicians, and as less expensive than hospital emergency rooms. In response to this type of competition, we are seeing more and more physicians (especially group practices) offering evening and weekend office hours. These providers can build their positioning strategy around the fact they are available when patients need care.

One northwestern multispecialty group began offering evening hours until 8 P.M. five nights a week, and added Saturday morning and Sunday afternoon hours. They informed patients and potential patients with flyers in the office and at area businesses, and by a direct mail promotion to residents in surrounding zip codes. They were surprised with the resulting practice growth. Not only did they better serve existing patients, they found they were attracting scores of new patients.

Another way to make your services more accessible is to take them on the road. Mobile diagnostic services such as CT scanners and MRIs now travel to different locations. There are laboratory services in vans and mobile mammography units. Similarly, in every major city, there is usually at least one physician practice specializing in house calls. Satellite offices, too, have become more and more common as physicians locate their practices to be more convenient to the market segments they wish to serve.

PROMOTION

Communicating information about a product or service, its price and its accessibility falls under the heading of promotion. While it is often thought that promotion equals advertising, there is much more to it than that. Advertising is only one element of promotion. Promotion also includes media publicity, special events, public speaking, direct mail, newsletters, educational seminars and specialty items.

Promotion is often used to help establish or reinforce a selected position. A neurology group in Maryland has positioned itself as "Innovators in Outpatient Care," and has established specialty clinics for headache, back and neck problems, Alzheimer's, Parkinson's, multiple sclerosis, epilepsy, stroke and neuromuscular disorders. Their promotional efforts have targeted the public and referring physicians with newsletters for each audience, public seminars on their specialty topics, special programs for patients and families, targeted brochures, Yellow Pages ads and advertisements in area medical society publications and directories. Because they have been extremely careful and professional in the wording and approach used in their communication materials and advertising, the 20 neurologists and radiologists have an ever-expanding referral base and have successfully attained their chosen marketplace position as "outpatient innovators in neurology" (see Figure 4-5).

A non-medical example of a positioning strategy that focuses on promotion is that of Converse, manufacturer of sport shoes. To promote their basketball athletic shoes, Converse relies on National Basketball Association stars. These well-known players appear in ads, make public appearances and wear Converse shoes during games. In honor of the retirement in 1987 of Julius Erving from basketball, Converse introduced the Dr. J, a "celebrity" version of their basketball sneaker. To promote the shoe, in each of the 23 NBA cities, Dr. J visited a Salvation Army center where he talked with inner-city children and gave out free shoes. The goodwill program drew considerable media attention and reinforced Converse's perceived expertise as a basketball shoe manufacturer.

Physicians are increasingly discovering the advantages of using a variety of communication methods in their promotional package. They publish newsletters, contribute to health magazines, produce medical broadcasts on television and radio and hold classes and seminars on medical topics. Together with other physicians or medical groups they sponsor walks, runs, triathlons and team sports and hold clinics for Little League coaches.

FIGURE 4-5 Sample Yellow Pages Ad
This Yellow Pages ad reinforces the Neurology Center's positioning strategy as "innovators in outpatient care" by listing all the group's specialty clinics and locations.

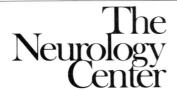

The Neurology Center

Comprehensive neurological care for adults and children in the comfort of a convenient, private office setting.

Innovators in Outpatient Care

Our specialty clinics include:

- **Back & Neck Center**
- **Epilepsy Center**
- **Headache Center**
- **Alzheimer Center**
- **Multiple Sclerosis Center**
- **Parkinson Center**
- **Neuromuscular Center**
- **Stroke Center**

FOR INFORMATION CALL
986-0777

CHEVY CHASE, MD	ROCKVILLE, MD	WHEATON, MD	WASHINGTON, DC	FALLS CHURCH, VA
Barlow Building	Physicians Building	Wheaton Plaza South Annex	University Medical Bldg.	Dominion Federal Bank
5454 Wisconsin Ave.	9715 Medical Center Dr.	11160 Veirs Mill Rd.	2141 K Street, N.W.	Building
652-3040	**424-5630**	**949-6655**	**223-1450**	7799 Leesburg Pike
				827-4090

The number of physicians advertising their practices has increased steadily. Many doctors are developing specialties within their specialty to serve particular market segments and then communicating these services to the appropriate people. There is increased use of the Yellow Pages to provide information about medical practices. With each new telephone directory, Yellow Pages advertising under physician headings is increasing dramatically. The content of the ads has changed as well, with more and more practices listing their hours, insurance plan coverage, and other special features.

An orthopedist we know, who had a long-standing interest and skill in athletic medicine, wanted to be perceived as the source of sports medical information for the community. He had a logo developed using a stylized runner, changed his practice name to "The Institute of Athletic Orthopedics," and created a bimonthly newsletter covering a wide variety of medical topics relating to sports and athletics. It was sent to patients who had been to the office within the past three years, as well as to school coaches and physical education instructors, fitness centers and gyms, exercise instructors, Little League and other children's and adolescent sports coaches, community athletic programs, tennis and golf clubs and residents in select zip codes. Each issue of the newsletter included a reminder that the doctor would be happy to address community groups on sports medicine issues; a variety of medical topics was listed to choose from. He contacted the sports editors and announcers in the local media and offered to provide information or comment whenever they needed medical expertise. By making himself accessible to civic and social organizations, and through related communications efforts, he gained valuable exposure as a medical resource.

Recognizing the importance of how they are perceived, the American Academy of Family Physicians embarked on a national advertising campaign to position its members as doctors who care for the whole person. "Physicans who specialize in you" was the slogan selected by the family practice physicians to communicate their message. The marketing program included a videotape on patient relations designed for use by physicians and their support staffs, educational programs on advertising, publicity in a variety of national media and an Academy-sponsored advertising campaign.

A Texas allergist cemented his position as an expert in the field of allergy when he volunteered to do a nightly report on the pollen count on a TV news program. This single but ongoing promotional effort helped develop his practice into one of the most successful in the metropolitan area.

PRESERVATION

This final element is the newest addition to the marketing mix, but in health care it may be the most important. Preservation is retaining the users of your services, be they patients, referring physicians or other groups. No matter how good your service is, how reasonable your fees, and how accessible your care, unless your practice is committed to patient satisfaction, patients will not stay. Quite simply, a consumer who is not satisfied with a product can elect not to purchase the same brand again; he or she has options. Similarly, dissatisfied patients will seek out another provider. They may also bad-mouth the practice to other existing and potential patients and, if extremely dissatisfied, initiate legal action. It is critical that strong attention be paid to this element in the marketing mix.

Practicing patient satisfaction techniques includes practicing good medicine, but it also goes further. It involves explaining treatment and findings so that patients fully understand, and spending what is perceived as "quality time" in the exam room. It means employing pleasant, empathetic, qualified staff and finding out whether or not patients themselves are satisfied.

One Arizona ophthalmology group we have worked with is especially adept at patient satisfaction. These doctors use it as the key to their positioning strategy. A well-designed and comfortable reception room is complete with telephones for patient use and a refreshment area with self-serve frozen yogurt, coffee, tea and soft drinks. A dozen red roses are delivered to the office every Monday, and on Friday patients are encouraged to take a rose home. Outpatient surgery patients and their spouses or relatives are picked up in the practice van the morning of surgery. During surgery the individual who accompanied the patient can watch the procedure on closed circuit television. Following recovery, the patient, family members or friends are reunited in a private dining room for juice and croissants before the van returns them home. That afternoon a nurse will call to check up on the patient just before the florist delivers a small green plant to his home. A formal written survey arrives about a week later. As you might imagine, patient satisfaction is extremely high. In fact, the practice has former patients who work as volunteers in non-clinical areas!

These successful surgeons have learned that designing systems that treat patients as special people, and incorporating monitoring measures, can be a rewarding strategy that yields numerous patient referrals, excellent reports to referring physicians and many repeat patients.

REPOSITIONING

Whether it was intentionally developed or not, most practices already have a position—at least in the eyes of their existing patients. *Repositioning* or changing the direction of an established position may be necessary when a market changes, when there are new competitive forces or when the behavior of a population changes. For example, hospital obstetric units of the 1950s were far different than they are today. In the late 1970s a few daring facilities updated these areas to become "family birthing centers." Now almost all hospitals have birthing suites with labor-delivery-recovery rooms all in one and a variety of birthing methods. These new approaches came about because of a change in consumer attitudes.

Some products have had to be repositioned because of new technology and competitive offerings. Baking soda was once used as tooth polish as well as in home-baked goods. With the popularity of cake mixes and toothpastes, baking soda sales were plummeting. Through promotion, however, the product was repositioned in consumers' minds as a necessary staple for fighting refrigerator odor.

Repositioning may also come into play when a physician decides to change the focus of a practice. An orthopedic surgeon who wants to concentrate on joint problems due to arthritis would be wise to select a name like "The Institute for Arthritis Joint Disorders," with a logo and stationery reflecting the change. His target audience would be the elderly population, so his marketing efforts (speaking engagements, screening programs, media coverage) would reach out to this group.

Similarly, we have consulted with several ob/gyns who have made the transition to practicing only gynecology, phasing out their obstetrical practice. Often this stems from the malpractice insurance issue coupled with a desire for a less time-intensive practice. Through positioning of the doctors as specialists in areas such as osteoporosis, PMS, hormonal imbalances or senior sexuality the change can be quite successful. Since older women are one of the fastest growing segments of the population, a doctor specializing in the needs of these patients can establish a recognizable position.

AND FINALLY . . .

Positioning is a concept that is applicable throughout the life cycle of a medical practice. While it is ideal for the new practitioner to have a clear position in mind when the practice is in the formative stage, doctors with well-established practices can implement a successful positioning or repositioning strategy as well. The key to success is the reinforcement of the desired position with all activities and elements of the practice. The perception that is created through positioning must be based on reality— reality developed and reinforced with the physical office environment, staff and physician attitude, expertise in the services offered, and the promotional materials and communication strategies that will convey the chosen position. Results are not noticeable overnight. But a consistently applied strategy will cumulatively build the image and reputation you desire.

BIBLIOGRAPHY

Aaker DA, Shansby JG: Positioning Your Product. *Business Horizons* 1982; May– June: 55–60.

Bronkesh SJ, Pritchard PJT, Wood SD: *Yellow Pages Advertising by Physicians: A Preliminary Analysis,* the Western Regional Meeting of Decision Sciences Institute, April 1988.

Kriegel RA: Positioning Demystified. *Business Marketing* 1986; May: 106–112.

Neal WD: Strategic Product Positioning: A Step-by-Step Guide. *Business* 1980; May–June: 34–41.

Ries A, Trout J: *Positioning: the Battle for Your Mind.* New York, Warner Books, 1981.

Ries A, Trout J: *Marketing Warfare.* New York, McGraw-Hill, 1986.

Timberman FL, Jr., If You Don't Position Your Bank, the Competition Will. *Bank Marketing* 1985; February: 10–12.

Chapter 5

Creating a Tangible Identity

Once you have decided on an image or positioning for your practice, you should translate that image into a tangible, visible identity. Your practice identity is created through your practice name, the graphic look of your name in print and on signage, and your logo.

How important is this seemingly superficial aspect of marketing? Simply put, your visible identity can influence consumer selection of your practice. Consider that, in many parts of the country, Yellow Pages are used by health care consumers not just to look up a name and telephone number, but to actually make the initial selection of a primary care doctor or specialist. The appearance, the *look* of your name and logo in a Yellow Pages ad or other locations will be one of the factors that influences these individuals. Well done, it will have a favorable impact, creating a positive impression of your practice.

Through your identity, you tell potential patients something about how you view yourself and your practice—and how you would like them to see you.

If you're wondering what influence your visual image may have, put yourself in the place of the Jones', a new family in your hometown. They know no one whom they can ask to refer them to a doctor. With three young children, Mrs. Jones knows how important a family physician is. She drives by a medical office building in her neighborhood, and one of the doctor's signs impresses her favorably. It reads, "I.M. Smith, MD, Personal and Family Care." The sign has large, visible lettering; it's brightly lit at night. She looks the doctor up in the Yellow Pages and finds the same distinctive type as the signage in an ad that offers a wealth of information. The logo in the ad is a flowering tree. She likes that; it seems to suggest health, growth and stability. The slogan beneath the doctor's name, address and logo is, "We help your family grow in health." So far, Mrs. Jones likes what she sees, and decides to call the doctor's office for an introductory appointment.

All of the elements Mrs. Jones evaluated—the sign, the name, the logo, the slogan, the appearance of the sign and ad—comprise the practice identity. Your practice identity is an integral part of your patients' perception of the quality of service and care you offer. Your graphic identity, professionally, creatively designed and consistently implemented in all your promotional material and signage, also helps your target markets—potential patients like the Jones family—to develop an *affinity* for you and your practice, even before they've met you.

This chapter will give you specific ideas and information on how to translate your name and image into a tangible identity. The two key areas we will discuss in detail are your practice name and your logo. These are vital components to the success of your promotional efforts. Together, your name and logo establish the theme—an ambience, if you will—for all your visual communications; they convey a cohesive message about you to your chosen audiences.

WHAT'S IN A NAME?

It may be true that a rose by any other name would smell as sweet. But if the rose was called stinkweed, it's doubtful anyone would have the inclination to get close enough to sniff.

You should give as much consideration to what you call your practice as you do to selection of your office location and furnishings. Of course, your name alone may be the choice you make: "Lee Jones, MD, PC." But for some practices, particularly group practices, and some specialties, a more descriptive or precise name may be helpful. The name you choose can be as descriptive and have as much impact as a line of poetry from Shakespeare. Or it can be as inappropriate and ineffective as calling a rose "stinkweed."

Your practice name should in some way communicate to the public, your patients and your referral sources what your services and/or scope of care are. Is there any doubt about the scope of services of a name like "The Children's Asthma Center" or "Georgia Center for Headache?" Your practice name may indicate your specialty or the positioning strategy you've chosen; it may include the names of physicians in your practice, or a combination thereof. It's important that your name stand apart from other practice names while communicating to potential patients something about what they can expect from you.

In today's competitive environment, more patients are finding you and your colleagues on their own, without a referral. They should be able to identify your specialty by more than a listing under your specialty heading in the Yellow Pages. Even if your name simply associates you with a hospital or medical center (Radiology Associates of Baptist Medical Center), you still derive benefit from that facility's perceived image. This association can influence a patient to use your services.

There are several options in the name you choose. You may use your name alone, "Pat K. Caduceus, MD, Internal Medicine". Or you can use both your name and a descriptive name, e.g., Pat K. Caduceus, MD, Anytown Dermatology and Skin Care Clinic.

Why should you consider a descriptive name?

- It immediately cues the consumer to the practice specialty. (See Figure 5-1.)
- It permits addition of more physicians without having to undergo a major name or letterhead or signage change.
- It creates instant identity for all physicians and personnel affiliated with the practice.

POINTS TO CONSIDER WHEN CHOOSING A PRACTICE NAME

1. What products or services do you offer now or might you offer in the future?
2. Have you positioned your practice toward a specific target market? (See Figure 5-2.)
3. Is there a possibility you may add partners or physician employees in the future?
4. What names are other physicians (in the same and competing specialties) using in your community?
5. If you are a solo practitioner, how much name recognition do you have among your referral sources and in the community? What do you stand to gain or lose by making your own name more prominent—or less so?
6. How distinctive and pronounceable is your name? A descriptive name may be better accepted as a practice name than one that's difficult to say or remember.
7. Do you have two or more distinctly different target markets? A descriptive name may make it difficult to appeal to all markets. For instance, a pediatric rheumatologist who also treats adult joint disorders might call his practice "The Center for Pediatric Rheumatology and Joint Disorders" in order to emphasize both aspects of the practice. However, this name could create confusion in the target audiences.

FIGURE 5-1 Descriptive Advertising
The name of this practice is descriptive, immediately telling consumers about the nature of the medical services offered. (Graphic artist: Stephen Baum, Fairfield, CT)

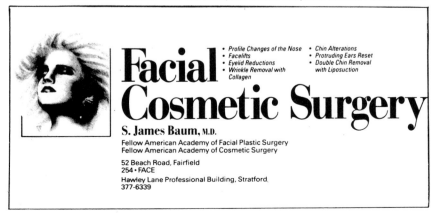

Facial Cosmetic Surgery

- Profile Changes of the Nose
- Facelifts
- Eyelid Reductions
- Wrinkle Removal with Collagen
- Chin Alterations
- Protruding Ears Reset
- Double Chin Removal with Liposuction

S. James Baum, M.D.
Fellow American Academy of Facial Plastic Surgery
Fellow American Academy of Cosmetic Surgery

52 Beach Road, Fairfield
254 • FACE
Hawley Lane Professional Building, Stratford,
377-6339

FIGURE 5-2   Womencare Breast Diagnostic Center
The target market—women over age 35—is immediately evident in this ad. The line art of the three women emphasizes the age group targeted. The educational copy is lengthy but informative. The topic warrants the extensive coverage and is likely to be well-read, since it is laid out in a graphically pleasing way.

The Facts About Breast Cancer Are Hard To Live With, But Harder To Live Without.

Breast cancer is every woman's fight. But avoiding it has helped make breast cancer a leading killer of women. It doesn't have to be. You can stop breast cancer.

At WOMANCARE, The Breast Diagnostic Center, we want you to know the facts about breast cancer, because knowledge is power and early detection saves lives.

Fact **1** Most women routinely have an annual PAP smear, yet cervical cancer (which a PAP smear detects) accounts for only 13% of cancer in women, while breast cancer accounts for 27% of cancer in women. A mammogram (breast X-ray) for every woman aged 35 can greatly reduce this alarming statistic through early detection.

Fact **2** Because of radiation, some women have feared a mammogram almost as much as the potential for a tumor. This is no longer a valid fear. Today's X-ray technology has greatly reduced the radiation dosage used and now the American Cancer Society recommends the use of mammograms.

Fact **3** The best first line of defense against breast cancer is a monthly self-examination. Not every lump can be detected with a self-examination, but you should make it as much a part of your life as brushing your teeth. Learn to do it correctly and do it every month. Ask your doctor, or call us for a free chart on how to perform the self-examination.

Fact **4** 95% of all breast lumps are discovered by women. Sadly, some women ignore the presence of a lump, fearing what it might be. If you feel a lump, don't panic, and don't wait, contact your doctor immediately, because

Fact **5** Not all breast lumps are breast cancer. Very often they can be a natural part of bodily changes over time. Even if a lump is breast cancer, 90% can be cured, without disfigurement, if caught early enough. The only way to find out which is which is by a thorough examination. A mammogram can determine the size of a lump, and newer

techniques, including light scanning and ultrasound can detect if it is merely a lump or a tumor, without the need for surgery.

Fact **6** Breast cancer can strike any adult woman. The fact is, the American Cancer Society recommends that all women at age 35 have a baseline mammogram, from age 40 to 50 have one every other year, and all women over 50 have one each year. Women with a family history of breast cancer should also have an annual mammogram.

American Cancer Society
Mammography Guidelines

| 35-40 Years Baseline Mammogram | 40-49 Years Annual or Biennial Mammograms | 50 + Years Annual Mammograms |

Fact **7** WOMANCARE, The Breast Diagnostic Center, is dedicated to the early detection of breast tumors, using the three most modern techniques: mammography, ultrasound, and light scanning. Each is painless, and combined will give the most thorough diagnosis possible.

In the Center's warm, unintimidating atmosphere our physicians and staff provide the full series of diagnostic tests and educational material, all from a woman's point of view. And because we're dedicated to winning the fight against breast cancer, the Center is open convenient hours for working women.

Don't wait. If you're 35, have a baseline mammogram. If you're 50, you should have a mammogram each year. Ask your doctor. Then call WOMANCARE for an appointment. Together we can win the battle against breast cancer.

Suite 106
4053 La Vista Rd.
Atlanta, GA 30084
491-6686

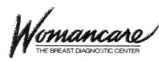

THE BREAST DIAGNOSTIC CENTER

If you use a descriptive name, be sure your patients understand the terms used. For example, "Arthritis Center" might be better than "Rheumatology Center" for the general public. "The Center for Digestive System Disorders" may be preferable to "Gastroenterology Treatment Center." At the same time, don't define too narrowly your practice services. A plastic surgery practice in the Southwest is called "The Nose Center." What if the physicians decide to do facelifts as well? Their name will mislead or turn consumers away.

You don't need to come up with a practice name by yourself. Try bringing together a mini-focus group to help you decide on one. Invite friends, patients, staff members, colleagues, your graphic artist or marketing consultant, and perhaps a member of your hospital public relations department to discuss possible names. You'll be amazed at the ideas that will come out of group dynamics. Guide the participants by explaining how you see your practice, what your research and patient surveys have revealed about its image, then let them tell you their views. Just listen; you'll hear some terrific ideas, not just for a name, but for other promotional efforts as well. (You can use this same group to evaluate your logo, practice brochure, etc.) Be sure to tape-record the session or have a staff member take notes so none of this creativity slips away. Just remember to thank, reward and otherwise recognize them for their time and ideas.

Once you've decided on the name of your practice, you must incorporate it into your identity "package" through the typeface and graphic treatment and logo. The graphic treatment should be used consistently on all printed materials and in your office signage. It's best to work with a professional designer or graphic artist to develop this as he or she can recommend a type style and look that will appeal to your target audience.

THE LOGO

Like your name, your logo helps people identify you and remember your practice. The logo does not create your image, but it can help perpetuate the image you create through your service and care.

Figure 5-3 contains examples of several practice logos and their applications.

WHY SHOULD YOU DEVELOP AND USE A LOGO?

1. Your logo can help create a recognizable, visible image for your practice, and helps patients and referral sources remember your practice name.
2. Your patients are more apt to read literature (newsletters, brochures, etc.) or information you send them when they can immediately identify it by your logo.
3. A logo distinguishes your practice from others who provide similar services.

FIGURE 5-3 Sample Logos
These logos represent some approaches for creating the appropriate image with the target audience. All are creative yet professional.

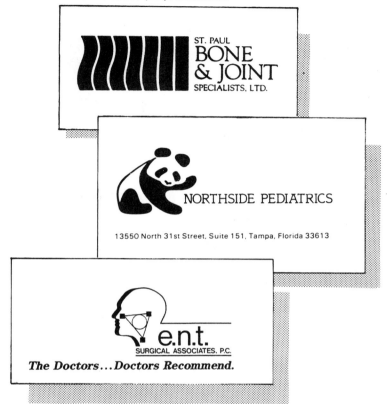

In addition to the reasons previously listed, a logo can reinforce the positioning strategy you've chosen for your practice, making it clear to the public what your "niche" in health care is.

Here are some tips for developing your logo:

1. Together with your practice name and the overall design of your name, your logo should project something about the perception you want the public to have of you and your practice.

2. Know your target audience(s) and what will appeal to them. Be original! Choose a design that's creative, yet professional. Avoid the obvious, the caduceus or cross, for example, as shown in Figure 5-4. These generic representations say nothing about the physician who uses them.

3. Avoid a design that duplicates the look of other specialists in your community. Look in your Yellow Pages directory for examples of what other professionals in your field are using. Then come up with something unique and creative for your practice.

FIGURE 5-4 Sample Caducei and Crosses
Avoid the generic cross and caduceus as a logo. They offer no personal or distinctive image for the physician.

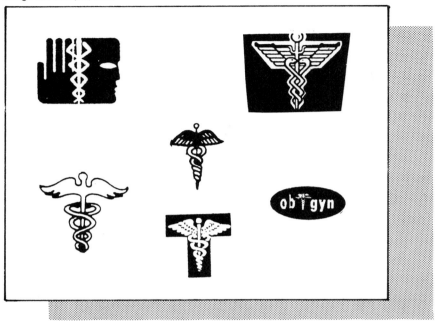

4. Hire a graphic artist or designer to create your logo. Your logo is an extension of your image and must be as professional as you are, so don't call in a would-be artist or try to do it yourself (unless you were a well-paid commercial artist before entering medical school!) Discuss with your designer the image you want to convey; provide examples of logos you like. They don't have to be related to medicine. This will give the artist a good idea of the "look" you are seeking and more insight into what would coincide with your own likes and dislikes.

5. Expect to pay anywhere from $750 to $2,000 for a final design if you live in an urban area. In smaller communities, you may find a good designer for less. Another option is to use logo design services offered through some physician marketing publications and consulting firms.

6. Your graphic artist should give you at least three logos from which to select. Take time in making a decision. Get your staff's and selected patients' reactions to the designs. But keep these criteria in mind:
   Professional quality
   Image desired
   Simplicity of design
   Message to be conveyed

7. A logo can be symbolic; it does not have to be an actual representation of a specialty or service. Ophthalmologists do not have to use an eye as a logo; a sports medicine center does not have to depict a runner. A symbol can do an excellent job of conveying an image. In addition, your logo can be your practice name creatively incorporated in a distinctive typeface. (Figure 5-5.)

FIGURE 5-5 Logo of the Joint Replacement Center
The doctor who developed the Joint Replacement Center hired an artist to create this logo, using the practice initials to create a distinctive design that also represents the medical specialty. This logo was an award winner for the artist.

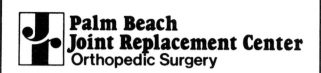

**Palm Beach
Joint Replacement Center**
Orthopedic Surgery

Raymond G. Tronzo, M.D.

8. Your logo should reproduce well in black and white as well as color. This is important because it will be used wherever your practice name is used in promotional material and signage, including advertisements in your local newspaper, Yellow Pages ad, and your practice newsletter. Have the artist show you how the logo will look in black and white and in the colors you choose for your stationery and brochure. He or she should be able to recommend appropriate colors.

9. Once you've selected a logo and the colors you will use when reproducing it, stick with it. Frequent changes in the design, color and placement on stationery cause confusion and lessen the effectiveness of your design. It also implies an uncertainty with your image which can convey that you aren't comfortable with the medical services you offer. Graphic consistency indicates consistency in care.

Your logo enhances your practice identity. It conveys to your patients and referral sources your image, products and quality of service. Keep these things in mind when developing a winning logo for your practice.

USING YOUR PRACTICE NAME AND LOGO

Your logo and practice name represent your practice identity in a tangible way. But the development of your identity does not end when the design work is through. Where and how you use your logo and practice name is equally as important in communicating a consistent quality image. Just as Lee Iacocca advertises that he will not put Chrysler's name on anything but a quality product, you cannot allow your practice name or logo to appear on anything less than high-quality stationery, newsletter, brochure, or business card. That means taking the time to assure that your stationery is quality stock, your typewriter or word processor produces a crisp, clean document, and your office signs communicate a professional image for your practice.

BUSINESS CARDS

Your business cards should provide a patient or referral source with general information about your practice. By now, you have chosen a name for your practice, a design theme and a logo. These are important elements to include on your business cards. In addition, since patients and referral sources will use your business card as a source of information about your practice, you must include such things as office location(s), phone number(s), the name and title of the card holder (Office Manager, RN, Lab Technician). Some physicians have found it helpful to place a map on the back of their business cards. By combining these two elements (information about your practice and directions), you can save patients valuable time and prevent unnecessary phone calls to the office for directions. In the medical profession, business cards are seldom kept by patients. By including your map, the patient has an added reason for keeping the card.

It's important to provide personalized business cards for all members of your office staff who come in contact with potential patients or referral sources. This is a cost-effective way of reaching people and heightening your practice visibility. It also creates a sense of belonging and commitment in your staff. It makes them feel they make a difference in the success of your practice (and they do!).

STATIONERY

Choosing stationery is more complicated than just picking a color for letterhead and envelopes that match. You must also be cognizant of the image you want to project to your patients, referral sources and colleagues.

The quality of paper stock and the color(s) you choose for your letterhead all communicate your practice image to the recipient. Again, they give a subtle message about the quality of medical services you provide. Most professional stationery is on 70- or 80-pound watermark bond in a neutral color (gray, beige, ivory) which is pleasing to the eye. Try to avoid the use of pure white for your stationery. This often produces a glare when reading under office lights.

Determining how and where to place your logo, practice name, address and physician name(s) on letterhead and envelopes is a decision that's generally made with the artist who designs your name and logo. As a rule, when an artist creates a logo, you should also request that he or she design your "business package." The business package includes your letterhead, envelope and business card, invoice, note paper or cards plus other stationery you may use. The business package layout shows exactly where and how your name and logo are to be placed.

One way to place your practice name and related information is at the top of your letterhead where it's easily read. Another is to break the address out of the logo and practice name and put it at the bottom of the letterhead. Either way presents a professional image; it's only a matter of preference and the design of your name and logo that will determine which you use. One suggestion is to list all physicians in the practice. Just as a business card for your office staff gives them a sense of ownership in your practice, all of the members of a practice (whether partners or employed physicians) are important in establishing your practice as a source of medical expertise.

Some practices are faced with a dilemma when they have more than one practice location. The stationery may look cluttered. One suggestion is to make one address on the stationery larger, with other locations in smaller, less dominant type. Another suggestion is to put the primary location at the top of the letterhead, with alternate locations at the bottom in smaller type.

SIGNAGE

It's easy to forget that both internal and external office signage help form an image of your practice. Yet your signs are important: they help people find you, reach people who are passing by your office, and—by their design and appearance—carry a message other than the wording.

External Signage. Your sign should be consistent with the tone and ambience of the surrounding architecture, landscape and nearby signs of other businesses. Your sign should be unique, but environmentally compatible. If your practice is in a mall or office complex, contact the property management to determine if a particular sign company has been contracted to do all tenants' signs. There may also be restrictions placed on signs by the management or by city zoning laws. Be sure to check local ordinances.

Considerations for exterior signs include the wording of your message, graphic elements, legibility and overall physical appearance. Graphic elements include layout of the message, color(s), lettering, logo and overall harmony. Your decision is simplified if you've had your practice name and logo professionally designed, because you'll simply carry through that typeface and graphic theme.

Legibility and visibility are imperative, and are affected by the style of lettering and color combinations. Some signs are difficult to read because of illumination problems such as glare from street lights, shadows caused by buildings and the signs of nearby businesses. Your goal is a sign that blends with the environment, has message impact and overcomes viewing problems both during the day and at night. To achieve this goal, keep these signage guidelines in mind:

- Avoid a cluttered, busy sign. Use no more than two typefaces. Gothic block letters work well if you are unable to reproduce your logo typeface.
- Use your own name as the dominant element only if it is well-known and established in your community.
- Use your practice logo on your sign. Logos are more easily remembered than names, and help create an impression in our visually-oriented society.
- A slogan or related wording is usually not recommended. Like billboards, signs should be kept to seven or fewer words.

■ If your address is not visibly displayed on your office building, consider putting it on your sign. It will save patients frustration and time.

Internal Signage. Have you ever taken the time to look at your office through your patients' eyes? Are your office signs clean, legible, pleasant and positive or do they just state rules? Is the lettering large enough for your elderly patients to read easily?

Which of these signs would you like to read when sitting in your attorney's or accountant's office?

■ DO NOT SMOKE	or ■ FOR THE HEALTH OF OTHERS, PLEASE REFRAIN FROM SMOKING
■ ALL BILLS MUST BE PAID IN FULL UPON COMPLETION OF YOUR OFFICE VISIT.	or ■ WE OFFER A VARIETY OF PAYMENT OPTIONS FOR YOUR CONVENIENCE.

Most likely you chose the second column of signs. They present a more caring image. This is an often overlooked part of a practice's tangible identity. Take a tour of your office today; see if your signs communicate the image you've defined for your practice. Look in your reception window and on the counter; are there taped, handlettered warning notices? Are memos and reminders to staff scrawled and stuck to desks and walls? Has professional signage been covered over with notes and files?

OTHER WAYS TO CREATE AN IDENTITY

Use your logo and name on prescription pads, note pads, appointment cards, name tags for your staff and on a variety of advertising specialty products (pens, paper clips, coffee mugs, t-shirts, and educational materials).

AND FINALLY . . .

The image you decide upon must be nurtured through constant communication, through frequent and consistent visible impressions. The identity established through your logo and practice name is just one way of communicating that image. A key to promotional success is to reflect that image in every aspect of your practice. Use your logo and practice name as an extension of your quality medical care and your identity will become synonymous with quality.

Enhancing Personal Relationships

Chapter 6

Involving and Communicating with Staff

So you've decided to begin a promotional campaign for your practice. You're full of enthusiasm and ideas, eager to get all sorts of special activities underway—an open house, educational seminar, community speaking engagements, perhaps even an ad in your city's monthly magazine. . . .

You're sure your promotion will work. You've attended two marketing seminars, done a practice assessment, developed a marketing plan, and you've come up with some specific goals and related strategies that give you a real sense of direction.

But somehow, when each day is through, you're so overwhelmed with patient problems, practice decisions and administrative details, there's no time to work on any of those great strategies.

"I guess my plans for promoting my practice will have to wait until next week . . . or maybe next month, when I have the time," you think.

YOU ARE NOT ALONE

Like many physicians eager to begin practice marketing efforts, you've assumed you must do it all yourself. On the contrary, you are not alone. You have a well-trained, professional staff, committed to the development of your practice, eager to grow with it.

With any promotional campaign, there are certain key players who help assure its success. The physician, of course, is the cornerstone of the practice and any marketing effort. Your practice reflects your personal style, and your staff is a primary conduit. Your receptionist, nurse, assistant, technician, accounts clerk and office manager generally are knowledgeable about practice policies, services and especially patients. Staff members may have special skills of which you are unaware (photography, writing, planning events) which could be well used in promoting your practice. They often have more opportunity to become acquainted with patients, their families, their jobs, patients' likes and dislikes. They can be helpful to you in establishing a warm, personal relationship with each patient.

Patients frequently are introduced to the practice through your staff. While the patient's experience with you creates a strong and, we hope, positive impression, most often the staff has the first and last word with patients. So it's important that their manner be as friendly and upbeat as yours, if that's your style.

Your employees are dependent on you. They look to you for direction, guidance and feedback; they will often consciously or unconsciously emulate the personal "style" with which you stamp your practice. In fact, an employee who leaves a practice often will do so because she cannot adapt her style to that of the physician(s).

A physician's office staff is probably more important to the success of the practice than many people realize. In a 1986 survey by National Research Corp., the friendliness of the office staff was ranked by women (the primary selectors of health care services for the family) as the second most important factor in choosing and continuing to use a physician. (The physician's interest in, and concern about them, was the most important criterion.)

It's easy to see how integral your employees are to the ultimate success of your practice. In this chapter, we'll take a look at some ways of making them more effective, more positive and better representatives of the practice. We'll look at how you communicate with them, how they communicate with patients, and how you can influence that whole process. We'll help you get a clear picture of the right person to hire when you have a vacancy, and we'll discuss some ways of retaining top-notch personnel once you've got them on board.

HELLO AND GOODBYE

Let's look more closely at how your staff affects your practice and your patients. As we pointed out, your employees provide the first and last contact for your patients. When the receptionist answers the phone or greets a patient, she is saying something to that individual about what to expect. A phone that's answered in a harried, hurried voice, "Dr. Jones' office. Hold please," may say to the caller that the doctor will rush through his appointment in order to make time for more patients. This may be far from the truth, but the initial greeting says there's no time for friendliness, courtesy, or interest in the patient's call.

When Mr. Bates' appointment is over and you've handed the chart to your accounts clerk and bid your patient goodbye with an encouraging "Call me, Mr. Bates, if you have any problems," your clerk should exhibit the same friendly manner. If, instead, she is busy complaining to the office manager about Ms. Abbott's check being returned for insufficient funds, the positive feeling you left your patient with will evaporate. Instead he will worry, "Am I going to be the subject of conversation as soon as I walk out the door?"

THE TWO C'S—CONTINUITY AND COMMITMENT

Practice promotion consists of various types of communication designed to stimulate a response from the receiver. If you're an ob-gyn who sends a practice newsletter to patients and others in the community, you are providing them with needed health care information. You're also hoping your newsletter article discussing the need for regular breast exams will prompt women to call you for an appointment. If you're an infertility specialist advertising a seminar on new discoveries in infertility treatment, you're hoping it will stimulate registration calls.

When the calls come in, your receptionist and all of your staff should be knowledgeable and helpful, or the time, effort and dollars spent on the promotional effort may be wasted. By communicating with your staff, and setting a positive example yourself, you provide continuity between the promotion and the hoped-for results.

Given information, direction and incentives, your staff will become as committed to your short- and long-range marketing goals as you are. But it doesn't just happen. And for the effect to be lasting, it takes consistent, positive feedback from you.

Achieving your objective depends in part on your practice image. Image is partly a reflection of your personal style, and partly a conscious decision you make in determining how you want your practice to be perceived compared to others in the marketplace *(positioning)*. Your staff must understand and be committed to the image you've chosen. It's up to you to convey to them what your practice image is, or what you want it to be. Do you want to be seen as family oriented? The doctor of choice for sports and fitness medicine? A doctor who takes extra time with each patient? Whatever image you choose, you reinforce it by the manner in which you respond to patients' questions, by the services you offer, your attire, office decor and the amenities you provide. You create an impression by requiring that staff members answer the phone courteously, identifying the practice and themselves, and by not permitting overbooking. Your ads, brochure, newsletter, TV and newspaper coverage support the image you create and create continuity between you, your staff and your sought-after marketplace position.

You can gain the commitment of your employees by turning to them for ideas, suggestions and assistance before you embark on a new venture or publicity effort.

You create enthusiasm and energy by putting individual staff members in charge of certain promotion projects, and giving them praise and credit for results. This encourages them to take "ownership" in a service or event. And doesn't everyone take better care of something when it belongs to them?

GETTING YOUR STAFF INVOLVED AND ENTHUSIASTIC

Are you becoming convinced that those great marketing ideas you've come up with are realistic and achievable with the help of your staff? Involving your staff in your marketing effort will be vital to its success, because:

- It will be difficult to accomplish singlehandedly all of the tasks a promotional campaign requires.
- The more involved your staff is, the more committed they become.
- Your staff is as familiar as you are with your patients, their needs and interests (perhaps more so) and can provide helpful insight and suggestions.
- The community affiliations, family, friends and contacts each of your employees has will multiply the number of potential new patients and referral sources.
- Most importantly, your staff represents you and your practice to your patients. They must share your attitude, approach and philosophy both in person and on the phone in order that the patients you generate through promotional efforts are retained.

Here are a few ways in which to involve your staff in promotional efforts:

- Encourage key employees to make presentations to community groups or do health screenings for target groups.
- Designate a capable staff person to edit your practice newsletter.
- Solicit article ideas from your staff for your newsletter.
- Select a staff member to coordinate the planning details of your practice brochure.
- Hold health educational classes or seminars for the public, with yourself and appropriate staff members as instructors.
- Include photos and bios of staff in your reception area, in your newsletter, even in your ads.
- Select a marketing coordinator to oversee major projects, ensure assignments are made and tasks completed.
- Choose and publicize an employee of the month or quarter.
- Ask a team of one or two employees to "cruise" the office looking for ways to fix up, spruce up, brighten or otherwise make the environment more attractive to patients.

TO SEE OURSELVES AS OTHERS SEE US . . .

With your internal communication program and your external promotional campaign, you and your staff create your practice image. At this point, you may be saying to yourself, "I don't have to worry. My practice has a good image. No one complains, and I'm staying busy, so everything must be fine."

If you haven't surveyed your patients within the past 12 to 18 months, you can't be sure what they think. They may not be complaining to you; they may be just leaving or, worse, telling others about their complaints. Your current marketing efforts may be simply maintaining your patient load instead of increasing it.

St. Paul Insurance, a large medical liability underwriter, reports that the top patient complaints about doctors include these staff-related concerns:

"They never tell me what they're doing and why."
"My doctor's staff seems so inconsiderate."
"Everyone in the waiting room can hear the personal questions they ask."

Patient perception of your practice can also be influenced or affected by a new location, new services and new staff members as well as factors such as competitors. It's a good idea to survey your patients every year or so, or implement a continuing post-visit survey to spot trends, problems and opportunities in the early stages, and be certain the image you have is the one you desire.

HIRING STAFF: A TIME TO BE CHOOSY

Hiring employees is a difficult, time-consuming job in any office. In a medical practice, where staff can have such an influence on patient perceptions, the hiring process is crucial. The person hired must possess certain qualifications; he or she must get along with a variety of co-workers, as well as an assortment of patients. Most important, the employee must be courteous, knowledgeable and pleasant, especially when the patient is not.

You know what technical skills you need in each position you fill. We'd like to discuss the personality characteristics that are important in a busy medical practice—particularly a practice with a proactive marketing emphasis. Here are some of the traits many doctors find important:

- Pleasant, friendly demeanor. (How much does the person smile? If she doesn't smile much in an interview, she'll smile even less on the job.)
- Promptness. A well-run practice runs on time, but it depends on each individual arriving on time and staying on schedule in completing their tasks.
- Enthusiasm. Does the person seem truly interested in working for you? Or does she convey the impression this is "just another job?"
- Neatness in personal appearance and work.
- Intelligence. Is the applicant's language filled with grammatical errors, colloquialisms, and syntax errors? Patients expect everyone in a doctor's office to sound literate.
- Patience. Schedules will get backed up; patients will become perturbed over bills; several phone lines will ring at once. Coping serenely with these situations or at least waiting until it's "safe" to vent is an important attribute for all members of your office staff.
- Versatility. The ability and willingness to adapt to a variety of situations, tasks and people are key characteristics. You can determine versatility in part by looking at an applicant's job experience, and by questioning the individual about her experience and enjoyment in a variety of duties.

TRAINING: OFF ON THE RIGHT FOOT

Do you want your staff to have good habits, work well together, understand your goals and enhance your practice image? These traits must be indoctrinated when a new employee is hired, and continually reinforced with all staff.

For new staff members this means expectations, duties and office policies should be verbally reviewed on the first day by you or your office manager. Provide specific job requirements in writing to reinforce verbal instructions.

To properly orient a new employee, allow time on the first day for an extended discussion of job responsibilities, your expectations, the office structure, and a review of other staff and their duties. Spell out specifically how you see the practice and how you want patients and others to see it.

During a new staff member's first several weeks, be sure to set aside time to discuss questions or problems, and to reinforce positive actions with praise.

Creating a responsive and enthusiastic staff also puts demands on you, their employer. You must know what your employees want from their jobs. Studies show that there's quite a disparity between what employees want and what their employers think they want. What they want above all is interesting work, followed by appreciation for work done, a feeling of being "in" on office affairs, job security and good pay. Interestingly, most employers think pay is the most important criteria to their staff, and employers put appreciation for work done at the bottom of the list.

Staff satisfaction, as well as your own, also depends on your knowledge and understanding of your employees' responsibilities. Ask questions, and if you're not satisfied with the answers, or if the answers are vague, persist. Doctors who are unfamiliar with office affairs may find themselves confronting unpleasant surprises in office management, finances, patient relations and other vital areas.

CREATE PARTICIPATION WITH INFORMATION

If you want your staff to be committed to your marketing and promotional efforts, they must understand each project and its purpose. In other words, don't just tell your staff you're planning to start a practice newsletter. Explain why you think it will be helpful to patients and the practice (i.e., it will provide information and education, and it will help generate and retain patients). Explain who your target audience is, what the newsletter will contain, and what you hope to accomplish with it.

Then (here's where the involvement comes in) ask your staff for their ideas, suggestions and comments—positive and negative. Ask for suggestions for the newsletter name. Have a contest with a prize for the winner. Jot the ideas down, or ask one of your staff to take notes.

When you've gotten your employees involved, get them committed. It's not a good idea at the outset to ask for a volunteer editor; such a move may be interpreted as "the doctor gets the idea and we get the work." Instead, tell them you want to feature a staff member in every issue, and you'd like them to select the first staff person to be highlighted. (This is not a good move if you're planning to fire or lay off a staff member. They could pick that person!) Or ask each person to submit an idea for a story.

Updating your staff and soliciting their input and involvement in your marketing efforts should become a regular part of your staff meetings. However, a directive requiring participation will defeat your goal of enthusiastic involvement. Rather, create an atmosphere in which your staff wants to be a part of the creativity of marketing and promotion. You'll know your staff is committed to your promotion program when they take a proprietary interest in the progress and results.

THE STAFF MEETING

Any group of office workers is just that—a group of individuals sharing office space—unless they have a common objective and they are all working together to achieve it.

In a medical practice, your primary goal is to provide high quality medical care to your patients. Among your marketing/promotion objectives may be retention of current patients and an increase in the number of new patients you see.

But have you communicated this clearly to your staff? Have you told them *how* you hope to achieve these marketing objectives, and what their role is in the process? Do you emphasize the importance of a continued flow of new patients to the success of the practice, and their jobs? And do you provide regular updates, with opportunities for feedback and interaction? Staff meetings are a perfect forum for this. Yet a surprisingly large number of active medical practices have no formal mechanism for communicating with staff on a regular basis.

How you conduct your staff meeting, when and how often it's held, agenda topics and other variables depend on your practice and your personal style. Following is how one large multispecialty group practice handles staff meetings.

Meetings are held weekly at noon. Luncheon is ordered for all employees at practice expense. (It's a benefit as well as an incentive to get employees to attend the meetings on time.) An agenda is prepared before the meeting, and everyone has an opportunity to list items for discussion.

The meeting is conducted, not by the doctors, but by the office manager. In fact, unless the physicians have an agenda item, they do not attend the meeting, in order to encourage free-flowing discussion and resolution of problems between the staff and the office manager. (We do not necessarily recommend the doctor-less approach, although it works well for this particular practice.)

Only topics that affect the practice in general or most of the staff are brought up for discussion. Those that can be resolved by one or two people are handled outside of the staff meeting, although results may be reported in the meeting.

Assignments and dates are made for all items requiring action; this assures that something doesn't get "discussed to death" or forgotten in the shuffle of business.

Of course, this format may not be ideal for your practice. Only you and your staff can determine the appropriate frequency, time, place and structure for your meetings. But the following guidelines may help:

1. Solicit agenda items from all staff prior to the meeting. Everyone should have an opportunity to include important, practice-related matters for discussion or action. Distribute the agenda in advance. A sample agenda is found in Figure 6-1.

2. Always start promptly at the announced time. This prevents stragglers from delaying or disrupting the meeting. Eventually, as they discover the meetings won't wait for them, latecomers will begin arriving on time.

3. Discuss agenda items in order, keeping discussion to the matter at hand. If a new item or subject is brought up out of order, defer it to the end. If there's no time in the meeting for the new topic, save it for the next meeting, or deal with it separately if it's urgent or affecting patient care.

4. Assign an action, person responsible and due date for each agenda item.

5. Have someone take notes during the meeting, to assure that responsibilities, actions, and resolution of problems are recorded. You can distribute the minutes at the next meeting, or reserve them for use by the physician and office manager.

6. Make time during each meeting to pass on praise from patients and to acknowledge extra effort, a situation handled well, a job well done.

7. Allow time to explain new techniques, products or services you'll be using, and

FIGURE 6-1 A Sample Staff Meeting Agenda

---

1. Call to order

2. Old business:
   - Report on success of evening hours
   - Surgery schedule change
   - Handling of prescription refill calls

3. New business:
   - New computer
   - Dr. Jones' upcoming CME conference
   - Parenting classes: tasks and assignments

4. Office environment
   - Lunch room clean-up responsibilities
   - Allowable bulletin board material

5. Kudos
   - Marcy for her handling of Mrs. Pain
   - Dr. Jones for staying on schedule

6. Marketing
   - Report on Channel 6 interview
   - Newsletter: ideas for next issue
   - Linda K's Little Tots Preschool screening

7. A word from Dr. Jones

8. Adjourn

---

to discuss promotional efforts and results. Seek feedback and ideas from your staff.

Why Staff Meetings Are Important. Staff meetings are too often viewed by both staff and physician as dull, time-consuming and non-essential. They can be if they are not planned well. On the other hand, well-run staff meetings:

- provide a forum for communication
- ensure understanding of practice goals
- clarify employee roles and responsibilities
- permit sharing of information and ideas
- help dispel myths and rumors
- allow cooperative problem solving.

TEAM BUILDING

You have the makings of a team with your staff, but you must coalesce them, create an attitude that "we're in this together for the benefit of patients, the practice and, ultimately, each other."

It doesn't take much to create a team identity and promote your practice at the same time. Some ideas: name tags with the practice logo imprinted, and the employee's name in easy-to-read type; uniforms that look professional (and stay that way throughout a busy day); personalized business cards for every member of the staff.

You also build your team by:

- Assigning a project to a group of employees and letting them work together to achieve results.
- Including them in your promotional material—brochure, ads, newsletters, etc.
- Listening with interest to their opinions and comments, soliciting them when it's appropriate, and implementing their ideas whenever possible.
- Developing a job description for every position. A job description helps clarify responsibilities and duties, and prevents the "not my job" reaction to unpleasant assignments. (You achieve this by incorporating some open-endedness in every job description, i.e., "other duties as assigned.").
- Praising (and occasionally rewarding) cooperative efforts, particularly those that occur without your request or direction.
- Showing interest in their personal lives (within reason) as well as their work performance.

Group Incentives and Acknowledgments. You encourage teamwork when you notice and reward cooperative efforts. Group incentives can include:

- Cash or prize bonuses for practice promotion efforts by staff (for example, generating the most inquiries or appointments among friends, family, neighbors).

- Movie tickets or restaurant gift certificate on completion of a big project by staff.
- A make-your-own sundae party on Friday afternoon at the end of an especially productive week.
- Photo of all your staff framed and hung in your reception area, and perhaps appearing in an issue of your practice newsletter.
- Special mention of your staff in referring physician thank-you letters, patient thank-yous, your newsletter and brochure, and media publicity, as appropriate. By frequent reference to your staff with patients, the public and other physicians, you let them know you truly can't get along without them. And that's a great incentive to continued teamwork!

Individual Incentives and Acknowledgements. It's good to notice and reward standout performance by individual staff members as well. Here are some ideas:

- A simple "Thank you. You did great."
- A written commendation letter with a copy to the individual, one for the bulletin board and one in his/her personnel file.
- Mention outstanding performance in your practice newsletter.
- Occasionally select an "Employee of the Day" for out-of-the ordinary performance. Post the individual's name and photo on the bulletin board in your reception area.
- Give the employee a bud vase of flowers, a gift certificate for lunch or dinner for two at a favorite restaurant, or a jar of nuts or candy.
- A Thank-You-Gram.
- A full- or half-day off with pay.
- Provide opportunities for personal and professional growth. Your practice and patients will benefit as well as your staff member.
- Paid attendance at a continuing education program or conference that will upgrade skills. (Be sure to provide time in staff meetings for employees to report on what they have learned from professional seminars.)
- Payment of annual membership dues for professional associations to which they belong, and perhaps even monthly meeting fees.

Any of these group or individual incentives can be used to show appreciation and/or encourage your staff to participate in promoting your practice—by handing out their business cards and talking about the practice in a positive fashion with friends and acquaintances; by informing you of opportunities for practice promotion—a health fair at their child's school or a new physician who is a potential referral source. The more you make them feel an important part of the practice, the more they'll contribute to its growth.

BRAINSTORM!

Brainstorm sessions can be fun and productive if they're well-planned and well-moderated. Plan a brainstorming session once or twice a year to generate new promotion ideas for your practice, to solve problems creatively, and to spark enthusiasm.

Hold the session at a time and place where you'll be undisturbed for several hours. A weekend may be best—perhaps Saturday morning. Bring rolls, coffee and juice if you get an early start, or sandwiches if it's midday.

For a successful, creative session:

- Have a moderator—yourself, your office manager, your marketing coordinator or someone who can keep things on track.
- Maintain a sense of order and flow to the session and get your staff involved by soliciting from them in advance the areas they'd like to address, topics they'd like to brainstorm, practice problems that have resisted resolution.
- Limit the topics you wish to cover to two or three, depending on the complexity and the amount of time available.
- List the ideas on a flip chart. This will help stimulate further ideas. Also, the flip chart pages can be used as "notes" from the meeting and transcribed for distribution and action afterward.
- Every idea has merit, no matter how wild, or impossible. Discourage negativism from participants.
- Encourage discussion with specific, targeted questions when an idea seems to stimulate a reaction from one or more members of the group.
- Remember that the purpose of this session is to stimulate creativity and innovation.

A brainstorming session can be fun, productive and helpful for solving practice problems or providing new ways of looking at old situations. Be sure that you sift through the many ideas you and your staff come up with and categorize them according to their potential. Here are suggested categories for brainstorm ideas:

- Excellent. Investigate and implement immediately.
- Great potential, needs refinement and clarification. Assign to appropriate employee(s) to investigate and report back.
- Not usable now, but perhaps in the future. File with tickler date for review.
- Great idea but impossible to implement. Save to get things started in next brainstorming session.

Then, be sure to take the workable ideas and implement them or assign them to someone to research and put in place.

SELECTING A MARKETING COORDINATOR

Unless your practice and staff are minuscule, or you're super-human, it will be necessary to designate someone to coordinate much of the internal and external marketing in your office.

The marketing coordinator in most practices is generally not a separate, full-time position, but rather an add-on to existing duties for a capable, personable and responsible member of your staff. The individual may be the receptionist, secretary or office manager. These are some of the responsibilities you may wish to discuss with and assign the marketing coordinator:

- Delegating duties for specific marketing efforts. For instance, if you're holding an open house, the marketing coordinator may assign staff members to carry out certain tasks for the event.
- Establishing and circulating an agenda in advance of staff meetings.
- Coordinating production of the practice newsletter.
- Assisting with publicity and media contacts.
- Serving as liaison between staff and physician for communicating marketing ideas, patient problems, etc.
- Overseeing or assigning coordination of patient surveys.
- Ensuring immediate resolution or attention to staff and patient problems and issues.
- Coordinating due dates for advertising material such as Yellow Pages, local newspaper ads, etc.

Characteristics of a Staff Marketing Coordinator. What characteristics should a marketing coordinator possess? Here are some suggestions:

- Outgoing personality
- Attention to detail
- Well-liked and respected by co-workers
- Awareness of "the big picture" in the practice, able to coordinate long-range and short-term needs
- Patient oriented
- Stable (preferably familiar with your practice through at least 9 to 12 months' employment)
- Desire to grow with the practice
- Leadership capability

It's important that your marketing coordinator be current with your plans, programs, services, media contact, etc. To assure that you keep him or her up to date, consider a weekly meeting to review current tasks, assignments and questions. This meeting need take no more than 30 minutes, but it will save you hours of review and perhaps confusion or miscommunication.

COMMUNICATION TECHNIQUES

Communication, as we have stressed, is the heart of practice marketing and promotion. In truth, promotion is communication, employing various approaches and media directed at a variety of audiences.

Nowhere is communication more important than with your staff. We've already explained how to structure a staff meeting. Here are other means of communicating with staff:

- Written memo to all staff.
- Personalized memo or letter to individual staff members needing information, incentive, praise, feedback, instruction.
- One-on-one meeting. Face-to-face communication is helpful for serious matters such as policy infractions affecting patient care, or to personally thank, an employee for an outstanding job. (Of course, be sure to publicly praise the staff member as well, either verbally or in writing.)
- Brief thank-you or "keep up the good work" note inserted in individual paycheck envelopes as appropriate.
- Small group meeting with employees involved in a specific project or who work together (i.e., billing/insurance/Medicare). The meeting can be held before the workday starts, during lunch or at the end of the day (just keep it brief, and expect to pay overtime for employees going over 8 or 40 hours).

THE TELEPHONE

Dr. Case, an ophthalmologist, was very pleased with his promotional campaign. He began with an ad that appeared regularly in a local publication for parents; it explained the importance of children's eye exams. He also suggested a feature story to the daily newspaper's medical editor on the kinds of eye problems in children that may not be diagnosed during a school vision screening, such as strabismus and amblyopia. He created an informational pamphlet on how to recognize these two eye problems and distributed them to pediatricians and family physicians. Through persistent but polite contact with a TV reporter, he was able to get a story on the evening news on the importance of eye exams for children under six, as part of the station's week-long "Back to School" series on children's health.

A number of his patients reported having seen the ad, article or TV spot, and Dr. Case was delighted. But he was mystified that his appointment schedule seemed to reflect no change.

He happened to be at the front desk one day when he overheard this conversation:

"Doctor's office."
"Is he injured? . . . Well, that doesn't sound like an emergency. We couldn't get you in at that time for a month or more. . . ."
"No, he's going to a convention next week."
"What article? A TV program. I don't know anything about that. You must be thinking of another doctor."
"Yeah, sure. Bye now."

When he questioned his receptionist, he learned that the caller had seen the article and the TV news segment, and suspected her four-year-old might have strabismus. She wanted to make an appointment as soon as possible, preferably in the early morning, but the receptionist told her the early morning schedule was fully booked. The uncooperative receptionist not only didn't try to schedule the mother for another time, she literally sent the potential patient to another ophthalmologist.

Dr. Case made several errors in staff communication, and his receptionist compounded them with her less-than-helpful telephone response.

- Dr. Case did not communicate with his staff before or after his successful media efforts. They knew little or nothing of the ad or article, and had not seen the TV news coverage, even though he had made a videotape of it.
- He did not review with his staff the type of calls or medical problems that might result from the publicity. Although he was willing to come in early or stay late in order to accommodate these callers, he had not informed his staff of this.
- He had never discussed basic telephone etiquette with his staff, simply assuming they knew how to answer the phone and handle calls properly and promptly.

The telephone is *always* an important tool in a medical practice. During a promotional campaign, the telephone is crucial, because a campaign's success is often measured in part by the ringing of the phone. The telephone becomes the first *personal* contact for potential patients. If not handled pleasantly and informatively, it may be the last contact.

Following are guidelines that might be helpful for your staff, and Figure 6-2 is a self-test that your staff can take.

Creating a Positive Telephone Image. Never underestimate your importance. People's lives and health, plus the future of the practice, depend on how well you do your job:

- Answer a ringing phone within three rings.
- Identify both the practice and yourself. People like to know to whom they're speaking.
- Ask the caller's name, and use it in conversation.
- Never leave callers on indefinite hold. Come back on the line after 30 to 60 seconds and let them know how much longer it will be, or offer to have someone call them back.
- Even if there are several lines ringing at once, always give callers a chance to respond before putting them on hold.
- Don't leave the phone unattended. It's the lifeline of the practice—and sometimes a life-saving line for patients.
- Speak with *friendly authority*. When there's a smile on your face, it will carry through in your voice. When your voice is calm, confident and courteous, it will reassure worried, anxious, even angry callers.
- Listen carefully. The closer you listen, the easier it will be to sort out the really important facts. Soon you'll be able to hear what's unsaid—such as frustration in a patient's voice—and help people when they really need it.
- Know the doctor's schedule. Get in the habit of asking, "Where will you be today?" Eventually the doctor will tell you his/her schedule every morning before you ask.

FIGURE 6-2 A Telephone Self Test for Your Staff

Test Your Telephone Habits

	Always	Usually	Seldom
1. Before leaving my phone, I leave word where I am going and when I'll be back.			
2. I answer phones promptly, before the second ring.			
3. I identify myself at the beginning of a conversation whether I am answering or placing a call.			
4. I speak directly into the telephone, clearly, naturally and pleasantly.			
5. I try to personalize my conversation by using the caller's name at every opportunity.			
6. I try to be helpful when taking calls for others.			
7. When taking messages, I note all essential information and double check it if necessary.			
8. If it is necessary for me to put someone on hold for more than a minute, I offer to return the call.			
9. I thank the party for calling.			
10. I return all calls promptly, or let callers know approximately when someone will call them back.			
11. I treat all messages as important, prioritizing them if necessary.			
12. I record all medically related telephone discussions with patients in their chart.			

SCORING:

Give yourself four points for every "always," 2 points for every "usually" and no points for "seldom."

48 points: Super! Your telephone personality is a winner!

37–26: Try incorporating some of the suggestions on the previous page and everyone will want to talk to **you**!

25 or less: Remember how you like to be treated on a business call – then practice doing the same for patients who call the office. Take a deep breath and SMILE before picking up the phone!

- Develop a "hot line" list to keep track of symptoms or complaints that the doctor wants to know about immediately.
- Avoid technical expressions and medical jargon.
- Make the caller feel you're truly interested in helping him or her. (You are, aren't you?)
- If the caller asks about or mentions something you're unfamiliar with, find out. Be helpful and informative; that's what you're there for.

- Follow through with all promises and requests for information.
- Apologize for errors or delays.
- Treat callers as you would wish to be treated.

Remember, every call is important to the person on the other end of the line.

AND FINALLY . . .

Providing high quality medical care to your patients is the goal of every good physician. There's a personal and professional satisfaction you gain from healing body as well as mind and soul. When you can focus on your patients' physical and emotional needs, the healing and recovery process comes easier. And when your staff shares your goal—when everyone tries separately and as a team to assure satisfied patients—the goal is easily achieved. We've seen it happen. We know of practices in which the staff willingly works on evenings and weekends for a special event or seminar. This staff constantly comes up with new ideas for improving patient satisfaction, and continually strives to meet the high standards set by the physicians. The patients return surveys with pleased comments about individual staff members and the overall atmosphere of the practice. We even know of practices where former patients serve as volunteers, working in the office at a variety of tasks, such as counseling others about to undergo surgical procedures.

How do you ensure patient satisfaction? By enhancing staff motivation and involvement. Remember these guidelines:

1. Increase or clarify your expectations. Don't assume your goals are your staff's goals. Be specific regarding what you want or expect your employees to do.
2. Let employees know how they're doing. Let them know if they're achieving your expectations, and if not, what they can do to reach your standards. Be objective, yet positive, in giving feedback.
3. Assume employees want to do well. Focus on instructing, not laying blame.
4. Reward good performance with verbal or written praise, or a tangible reward. Know what each of your employees responds to.
5. Build confidence and self-esteem. It improves productivity.
6. Invite participation and discussion.
7. Set an example. Your staff takes their cue from you.

A successful practice is the sum of its parts. The physician provides the medical diagnosis, treatment and advice, but he or she also creates the image of the practice. It may be warm and homey and personal or it may be elegant and formal. Whatever your chosen image, your staff must reflect it. Don't depend on luck and assume they'll know what impression you want your patients and the public to have. Tell them informally and formally—in staff meetings, in hallway conversations, in your attire, in your office decor, in how you respond to your patients. The consistent impression you create will build and grow, and you and your practice will be remembered for it.

BIBLIOGRAPHY

Jensen and Miklovic: Consumers Cite Physician Interest as Most Important Factor in Selection. *Modern Healthcare* 1986; January 17.

Smith: Personal Touches Pay Sales Dividends. *The Business Journal* 1987; 7, (49).

Improve Your Practice With Public Relations. *Physician's Management* 1987; January: 122.

Building and Maintaining Your Practice. Washington, D.C., American Society of Internal Medicine, April 1983.

Hospital Guest Relations Report, Washington, D.C., St. Anthony Publications, 1987; 2, (8).

Chapter 7

Communicating with Patients

Nowhere is communication more important than in the practice of medicine, where a fine line exists between wellness and illness, life and death, compliance and noncompliance. Your patients can't follow your instructions if they don't understand them. Unfortunately, miscommunication too often takes place among you, your staff and your patients when the assumption is made that a message has not only been heard, but comprehended.

In this chapter we'll take a look at patient communication—interpersonal as well as printed and audiovisual. We'll discuss how you can improve patient trust and compliance through effective communication. And we'll explain ways to use patient educational material to enhance the patient's perception of value and quality from their visit to your practice.

I KNOW YOU THINK YOU UNDERSTAND
WHAT YOU THOUGHT YOU HEARD ME SAY . . .

Like many professionals, physicians often get caught up in using jargon that patients may find foreign and intimidating. Thus a well-intentioned message vital to good medical care is heard but not accurately interpreted.

Your patient's background also may affect understanding of your message. It's important to consider your patient's educational level, his or her socioeconomic status, religious beliefs, cultural and ethnic background, and age, and frame your message, words and even physical stance accordingly.

FEEDBACK

You may tell a newly diagnosed patient everything she needs to know about diabetes mellitis, her diet and other important aspects of treatment. Your patient may nod her head understandingly. But did your message get through?

You need to be sure your patients comprehend the diagnoses, instructions and information you give them. Patients should be made aware that they are the most important part of the treatment process, that without their full cooperation and understanding your efforts to help them are futile. You can only provide them with the information, instruction and medication. Unless they follow through, success will be limited.

PERCEPTIONS OF QUALITY TIME

Communication involves more than talking. It's the stance of your body, the tilt of your head, the attention you give your patient. To enhance verbal communication and increase the quality of the time you spend with each patient, incorporate interactive skills with your spoken message. For instance:

- Touching the patient in a comforting, non-clinical manner (a pat on the hand, a touch on the shoulder) can soothe and relax the individual as well as make you appear less intimidating and more human. You seem more relaxed; therefore the patient perceives you as more attentive, concerned.
- Eye contact with the patient shows him he has your undivided attention. It demonstrates a sincere interest in his specific problem. Try to avoid writing on charts or talking to staff during patient-physician interaction. Give your patient your full attention.
- Try to sit on the patient's level or lower to avoid towering over him, which is an intimidating, removed position. Lean toward your patient. This posture will draw you closer to the patient not only physically, but also on an emotional level.
- Never allow your time with the patient to be interrupted unless it's an absolute emergency. Even a brief visit will seem longer to the patient if your attention is focused, concerned and uninterrupted.

Here are some examples of the above techniques as they were actually tested in patient/physician interactions:

Scenario 1. The physician enters the exam room where the patient is already draped. Wearing a white coat, the physician stands over the patient who is lying on the table and immediately asks what the problem is. Several times during the 15-minute visit the nurse interrupts the physician requesting that he take phone calls.

Scenario 2. The physician enters the exam room where the patient is seated in a chair. The doctor continues standing and reads the chart before finally acknowledging the presence of the patient with a "Good afternoon, Mrs. Jones." He immediately asks what is wrong and then leaves to answer a phone call while the nurse drapes the patient.

Scenario 3. The physician enters the room where the patient is seated. He pulls up a chair and inquires how the patient is doing, how the family is, and other general questions. He then inquires about the present complaints and listens as the patient describes the problem. He is careful to keep the patient on track but conveys concern as he directs the conversation. The physician then informs the patient about the exam procedure he is about to begin before calling the nurse to drape the patient. After the encounter, when the patient is dressed in street clothes, he solicits follow-up questions and makes certain that the patient understands the diagnosis and treatment before providing her some informational material and saying good-bye.

In the last scenario, the physician actually spent the least amount of time with the patient, yet the patient was satisfied with the encounter. Effective communication techniques save time and convey quality.

A major benefit of effective communication may be a decreased incidence of legal challenges. When patients have good relationships with their doctors and accept some responsibility for their treatment, they may be less likely to initiate legal proceedings if the expected outcome isn't achieved. Irwin Press, PhD, concluded in his 1984 report, "The Predisposition to File Claims: The Patient's Perspective," that it is the patient's perception of his medical care that determines whether he will file a lawsuit—not the presence of injury.

Communication, we have seen, can definitely influence a patient's perception of quality.

Donald Fager, vice president of a New York malpractice insurer, is quoted in the April 18, 1988 issue of *Medical Economics* as saying, "A lot of claims are brought because the doctor didn't have a good relationship with the patient." Adds an anesthesiologist, "Physicians' lack of rapport with patients and patients' consequent lack of trust in them are big contributors to the malpractice crisis." One in five doctors regards good communication with patients as essential to avoiding legal claims.

It goes without saying that accurate documentation is a very important facet of communication. Keep your records organized, readable and legible. Include in your records all information given to the patient and what educational material was utilized. Note the patient's level of comprehension in the document. This will give a clear picture of the patient to anyone who may need access to the patient's chart, especially new employees.

COMMUNICATION = EDUCATION

As mentioned earlier, providing written or audiovisual material enhances verbal communication, patient trust and compliance. The doctor's office is a setting many people find stressful. Your patients do not make an appointment with you, as a rule, if they are healthy and have no problems. And even if they have scheduled a routine checkup, they worry that you may find something wrong.

As you are explaining a diagnosis, treatment, medication, exercise or diet routine, the individual may still be fretting about a statement you made several minutes ago. When you ask him if he understands, your patient may say yes, embarrassed to admit that he does not understand or that he is troubled by what you have told him. Not wanting to appear ignorant, he remains silent. So you forge ahead with your explanation, unaware of his anxiety and that he's not hearing you.

This scenario can have serious consequences. It can result in increased stress for the patient and more time spent by you or your staff on the telephone reviewing your diagnosis or instructions.

When you provide patients with tangible reinforcement of your instructions in written materials, the chances of misunderstanding, miscommunication, and even potential malpractice liability are reduced. You also create conditions that help assure greater patient satisfaction and finally, you provide a tangible reminder of your practice. This visible reinforcement helps create an impression of value in the patient's mind and may even help justify the fee charged. These are important considerations in today's era of consumer awareness and concern for value.

STUDY CONFIRMS COMMUNICATION NEED

A study was conducted in 1984 by one of the authors of this book, Stephen W. Brown, along with Teresa Swartz, both professors of marketing at Arizona State University. Nearly 1,000 adults were interviewed; their responses confirmed the impact of patient communication and education on the likelihood of malpractice suits occurring. Our study revealed that dissatisfaction with medical care is frequently the result of a discrepancy between the patient's expectations and the actual outcome of the medical problem. We learned also that individuals *likely to sue believed that physicians tend to do a poor job of explaining health problems; these individuals also expressed the need for more and better information.*

In a more recent study, the same researchers gathered data from 12 primary care physicians from around the country and over 1,000 of their patients. In evaluating the quality of the services provided by the physicians, significant gaps were uncovered in the patients' and physicians' perceptions of quality.

We believe that one way to lessen the likelihood of dissatisfaction and the potential for litigation is to improve both the quality and quantity of time spent with the patient and others involved in the situation. The more informed they are, the more likely they are to have realistic expectations concerning the medical treatment and resulting outcomes.

We also believe that doctors need to become more sensitive and empathetic when dealing with their patients. As our society becomes increasingly complex, and the marketing of professional services enters increasingly competitive environments, concern with consumer satisfaction or dissatisfaction will become even more pronounced.

Our conclusion was corroborated by a 1985 report by the President's Commission for the Study of Ethical Problems in Medicine and Biomedical and Behavioral Research. According to the report, "Physicians should discuss medical care with their patients more openly in order to create a meaningful system of informed consent in the health field."

Let us then look at how medical practitioners can implement a patient education program that meets the needs and wishes of both the consumer and the physician, and at the same time improves the delivery of health care.

THE VALUE OF EDUCATIONAL MATERIALS

When someone explains to you how to do something you've never done before—whether it's cooking the Thanksgiving turkey, changing a flat tire, or suturing a wound—the verbal instructions you're given can be bewildering. The terminology used to explain the process is new; you're also focusing on trying to retain the steps in the procedure. You may be concentrating so intently on listening that you don't assimilate everything you're told. As a result, what you hear may as well sound like this:

"Take the frammis and open it with a widget. Insert it into the barroon and hold it with a gelspur until you've located the gimcrack. Then remove the aniatrilly with a finossio, add a dollophisk and a plim and let it set for 20 minutes."

At times what you're explaining to a patient may sound the same. It is for this reason that tangible, visible and/or audible reinforcement is necessary for your patients, and for you.

Reinforcement. There's also the time gap to be reckoned with. A patient may understand your instructions in the office, but by the time he has arrived home, he has either forgotten vital information, or become confused about timing, dosage or quantity. Other factors may also affect retention of instructions. For instance, suppose you have just diagnosed an acute lumbar strain. After telling the patient about the proper use of muscle relaxants, you begin a discussion of the benefits of heat and flexion exercise. You briefly explain how and when the heat is to be applied and then demonstrate the proper way to do the exercise. Meanwhile your patient is doubled over in pain. How much will be retained? Not much, unless you reinforce these instructions with written materials he can refer to later when the pain lessens.

A Tangible Reminder. When you give your patients a pamphlet on prolapsed uterus, or the possible side effects of an antidepressant, you're giving them more than information. You're giving them a tangible reminder that you want them to be well-informed, that you and your staff care about their health and well-being. The material you provide reminds patients that you are a concerned professional who has their best interests at heart.

However, this tangible reminder is not only ineffective, but may be detrimental, if it is the *only* component of your patient education effort. Printed materials, videotapes and audiocassettes cannot substitute for your interactive, personal communication with the patient; they must *complement* it.

In a sense, patient education materials can help resolve "Post Purchase Cognitive Dissonance," or buyer uncertainty or remorse that occurs after a product or service has been purchased. The tangible reminder you offer can help to heighten consumer certainty of the appropriateness of their choice of health care provider. By providing helpful information, by placing a follow-up phone call to inquire about the well-being of a sick or post-surgical patient, by communicating through a newsletter, you enhance patient satisfaction.

Figure 7-1 contains examples of some educational pieces created by a hand surgery practice.

Clarification of Complicated Information. When a patient misunderstands information or instructions, the result may be confusion, fear, and occasionally anger toward the physician. Take the example of the young woman who comes to you for a routine checkup. She is already apprehensive because the annual checkup is not high on her list of favorite occasions.

Suppose you find a breast lump that appears to be a benign cyst. You sit down with the patient and describe the possibilities, recommending a mammogram "just to check it out." You've done a good job explaining the situation, but the patient hears only the word "lump." And all she is thinking is "cancer." She says that she understands, but in reality, she hasn't heard a word you've said. She is afraid, confused, angry.

She needs a better system of communication from you and your staff.

A better communication technique would be to supplement your verbal explanation with a short video on breast lumps, their diagnosis and treatment. Not only would this be informative, it would give the young woman time to relax, collect her thoughts, and formulate more detailed questions. Then, upon meeting with the patient after she has seen the video, you could go over your finding and answer her questions. She would be calmer, more willing to schedule the mammogram and follow up on your diagnosis.

Another example of the necessity of better explanation is in the use of diagnostic testing. It may seem reasonable to you that a 45-year-old man experiencing exertional chest pain should have a thallium scan, but to the patient, the mere mention of this test is a condemnation to life as a cardiac patient. All your verbal reassurance will not dispel his fear of the test and its potential outcome. A better approach (one that's been proven in hospital cardiac units) is to have the patient view a short video, then read an easy-to-understand pamphlet on the test. The combination of the three modes of communication—verbal, visual and print—will save countless hours of anxiety for the patient and phone calls and questions directed at the physician.

Another obvious benefit of using supportive educational materials is that it can be shared with the families of your patients. How often have you spent a great deal of time explaining something to a patient, only to have the family on the phone later that evening asking about your diagnosis, the recommended treatment, wondering why it's necessary and what it will accomplish? Sending home information with the patient, or sharing it with the family in the office, sets aside many unnecessary questions. It also helps assure patient compliance by involving the family in the treatment—for

FIGURE 7-1 Patient Education Brochures
A series of brochures, each addressing a different topic, helps to reinforce verbal information and instructions for this hand surgery practice. Developed by Indiana Center for Surgery and Rehabilitation of the Hand.

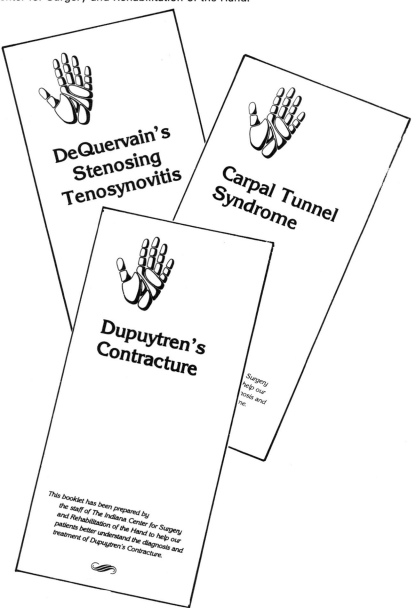

example, with a newly diagnosed Type II diabetic, for whom diet, medication and exercise are key components of treatment. Reinforcement via the family can make the difference in the outcome.

It is also very helpful to schedule a call to the patient several days after the office visit to see if there are any questions you can answer and to reinforce the return visit. At this time you (or a member of your staff) can reiterate to the patient and his family the importance of reviewing the material you've sent home.

Videotapes, audiocassettes and educational pamphlets also are valuable in making patient expectations more realistic regarding outcome or results to be expected from the treatment, therapy or medication you've prescribed. Misinformation your patients hear from family, friends or the media about a procedure or medication may elevate their expectations to an unrealistic level. The "over-promising" by some less-than-ethical practitioners through advertising and media publicity creates images or hopes that simply can't be met.

Your patients, having heard and believed these lofty claims, come to you expecting an instant cure, a perfect appearance, complete wellness and health. Despite your verbal clarification, your patient may yet hold fast to these "impossible dreams." Seeing the truth in black and white or on the video screen helps to re-introduce reality.

There's another point to be made about educational materials for your patients. When you or one of your staff takes a patient into your health education library and seats her in front of a VCR to watch a videotape on breast self-examination, you emphasize the value you place on this information. You are telling your patient you feel it is important enough for her to know about breast self-exam for you to have invested time and money in acquiring educational materials on the topic.

You further emphasize the importance of the information when you or a staff member demonstrates breast self-exam to the patient using a model you've purchased, and when you hand her an instructional pamphlet that reinforces what she saw and heard in the office. With all of these efforts, you increase the chances that the patient will comply with your instructions to perform BSE monthly. You convey that as her physician, you're concerned about her health and welfare. You've made her feel that she's gained a great deal during the 30 to 45 minutes she may have spent in your office, although only part of that time was spent directly with you.

Assuming the rest of her encounter is as positive, you not only retain her as a patient, you probably enhance the probability that she will refer others to you. And most important, you've performed your responsibilities as a medical professional in a most thorough, effective and ethical manner.

HEALTH EDUCATION MATERIALS:
OPTIONS AVAILABLE

Not long ago, patient education material meant a printed handout. Period. And frequently, that pamphlet was written in dry, dusty language with a heavy sprinkling of medical jargon. Interesting? Hardly. Did patients read it? Not as often as doctors liked to believe.

As physicians began to realize the benefits of educational material to themselves and their staffs as well as to their patients, and as the types of information technology have multiplied, more and more educational options have become available.

In addition, there is a growing awareness that different people respond to different approaches. Some people prefer to augment verbal instructions with something in writing which they can read at their leisure. Some retain information better when they view a videotape in the physician's office; still others comprehend better when the physician demonstrates using a model or diagrams. And all patients understand and retain a difficult explanation best when a combination of these educational approaches is used.

The types of health education materials available to the medical practice include:

Printed handouts. Pharmaceutical firms, health care agencies and businesses provide printed materials on topics ranging from specific diseases and diagnoses such as diabetes, osteoporosis, testicular cancer, to self-help subjects like how to reduce stress. Medical specialty organizations such as the American Academy of Plastic Surgery, the Arthritis Foundation, and American Cancer Society; and firms such as the Channing L. Bete Company offer an assortment of brochures, booklets and print pieces free or at a relatively low cost. Some hospitals provide educational booklets as a service to their medical staff.

Some of these materials can be ordered imprinted with your practice name, address, telephone number and logo for a small additional charge; others leave a space on which this information can be stamped.

For some medical practices, the information that's contained in these pre-printed pieces may be too generic, or they may offer advice that's contrary to your philosophy. Thus many doctors choose to develop their own educational material. The format selected may range from a simple typewritten page to a slick four-color brochure. Either way, the content reiterates precisely what the physician verbally tells his/her patients, and that's one of the greatest advantages to "doing it yourself."

Models. Cardiologists, obstetricians, ophthalmologists, orthopedic surgeons and many other specialists find it very helpful to have an anatomical model on which they can point out function, anomalies, procedures, etc.

This demonstrative educational process is often more meaningful to the patient, especially when a procedure or physical process is involved.

Videotape. This is the generation that has been incubated, bred, educated and entertained on television, so it's no wonder that the video library has become so commonplace and so effective in many medical practices. Many patients respond well to information they gain from the television screen because it is the way in which they are accustomed to learning. Some medical practices allow patients to check out a videotape on a certain topic, watch it at home when it's convenient, then bring or mail it back to the office. We know of one doctor who makes his own videotapes: he sets up the videocamera, sits in a chair and videotapes himself answering the questions that patients ask most frequently in his practice. Each videotape covers a different topic. This approach offers the advantage of credibility and familiarity—"That's *my* doctor telling me this, so it must be true." And it's an inexpensive way to keep an up-to-date supply of topics on hand as well. Then too, there's the added advantage of being able to add to or modify the tape as new information, drugs or treatments become available. Finally, when used correctly, it can make better use of your time.

Audiocassette. Books on tape have become a real hit with busy executives; why not use educational programs on audiocassette as an alternative resource for your patients who may be more inclined to learn from this technique? Cassette tapes are compact and relatively inexpensive, as are cassette players. In addition, almost everyone has a cassette player in their home or in their car, or both, making it convenient and easy for patients to listen to a health-oriented tape on the way to work, in the evening or on the weekend.

Diagrams and posters. Posters, printed illustrations and other materials can be very helpful resources for physicians, particularly those who must frequently demonstrate a surgical procedure, a malfunction or abnormality. Several companies print large, colorful wall-size posters that can be framed or simply hung on the wall. These posters may illustrate disorders like cataracts, cholesterol build-up in the arteries, or processes such as the growth of the fetus in the womb. Posters are valuable as wall decor in examining rooms: the patients study and learn from them while waiting for the doctor; and the doctor can refer to the poster when explaining a problem or process.

In addition to posters in a variety of sizes, simple black and white illustrations are also available. These show organs, body structures or systems, and abnormalities or disorders. The physician uses these printed pieces to sketch a procedure, demonstrate a process or a unique condition to a patient. The patient then is given the illustration to take home.

DEVELOPING YOUR HEALTH EDUCATION LIBRARY

OBTAINING MATERIAL

As explained earlier, existing patient education material can be obtained from a variety of sources. Some of this information is available free; most of it has some charge associated with it. Even if you think you want to develop your own educational material, it's a good idea to check with commercial suppliers or non-profit sources for samples of what they offer. You may find that something commercially available is precisely what you need and can be purchased for far less than it would cost you to create and print yourself.

These are some of the sources to check for educational material:

- Medical specialty societies (American Academy of Family Physicians; American College of Orthopedic Surgeons, etc.)
- Local, state, national medical associations or organizations
- Vendors (medical equipment suppliers, etc.)
- Pharmaceutical firms
- Hospitals and hospital chains
- Commercial publishers (Channing L. Bete Co., Whittle Publications, etc.)
- Non-profit associations (National Society for the Prevention of Blindness, Muscular Dystrophy Association, etc.)

PROVIDING SPACE

How serious is your commitment to providing a complete educational experience for your patients?

Some physicians devote a separate room in their practice to their "Patient Education Library." That's commitment! However, an education library need not take a great deal of space. A physician we worked with has a small room adjacent to (and visible from) his reception area. The room—no bigger than six feet by eight feet—contains a VCR, a TV, a few comfortable chairs and a selection of brochures on medical topics and services he offers. This is where patients and family members are taken prior to a surgical procedure to see a video about the procedure, and where a variety of informational videotapes are available for patient viewing.

VIDEO VIEWING ROOM

For certain people, learning occurs best when it occurs visually. It is for such patients as these that you may wish to establish a video viewing room stocked with a selection of appropriate videotapes. To ensure that your patients get the information they need, have your staff take them to the video room before or after you've examined them. The staff person should insert the tape and start the machine, perhaps with a few explanatory words about what the patient will see and why it's important. It's helpful also to "close" the educational experience by having a staff member or yourself review some of the points made and answer questions that may have arisen as a result of what was seen.

RECEPTION AREA CENTER

If you don't have space for a dedicated patient education room, consider creative alternatives. How about setting up a corner of your reception area with helpful books, magazines, pamphlets, cassettes and videotapes? You may wish to have a listing of cassette and videotape titles in the patient education area, rather than the tapes themselves, and have people request the title they wish from the reception desk. In that way, some control can be maintained over where the tapes go and who uses them. The important thing is to let your patients know in as many ways as appropriate that you want them to be informed about their health, their medications, their diet and their fitness, as well as the services you provide to help them maintain health and fitness.

If you set up a patient education corner in your reception area, be sure to stock it with a plentiful supply of pamphlets, handouts and health-maintenance material they may take with them. A small sign in this area should encourage patients and visitors to help themselves to printed material, and to ask you or your nurse if they have questions about something they read or hear. You might even put a supply of forms for patients to fill out to request specific information or to ask non-personal questions they may be hesitant to ask face-to-face. Have a sealed box into which the questions can be dropped. Such questions can then be answered via a typewritten hand-out or in your practice newsletter.

EXAM ROOM HANDOUT FILE SYSTEM

Frequently, it is when you are examining a patient, discussing a medical history or medical problem, that the need becomes evident for the patient to have additional information. How convenient and well-planned it would be if you had immediately accessible in each exam room a complete selection of educational handouts. Then it would be a simple matter of selecting the appropriate pamphlet from a file drawer and handing it to the patient at the time the topic comes up. In this way, you emphasize to the patient the importance you place on his/her familiarity with the information. At the same time, you demonstrate your commitment to patient education, by ensuring that your patients have complete clarification and understanding of their medical condition, medication or a procedure that is planned or contemplated.

THE IMPORTANCE OF PHYSICIAN AND STAFF

There is more to patient education than simply the materials you select, whether they are printed, audio, or audio-visual. In truth, the most important component of the educational process is not the material nor even the message, but the deliverer of the message—the physician and his or her assistants. Your belief in, and attitude toward, the information you give your patient comes across very clearly. It is reflected not only in the content of the message itself, but in your voice tone and inflection, body language and other personal communication "tools."

In order for your patients to believe in and trust the educational information you give them, you must believe it yourself. Not only that, you must convince your patient of your belief, whether you are explaining the dangers of cigarette smoking or the need for restricted activity following surgery. It is fine to espouse the philosophies of the Epilepsy Society of America or the American Heart Association, but if you are firm in your conviction, your patients will be more apt to comply.

Additionally, your staff must also share your belief in and commitment to patient education in general as well as your specific philosophies and attitudes toward wellness and medical information. They acquire their belief and commitment through observing you and by hearing it directly from you. Earlier in this chapter and in Chapter 6, we explain how communication and feedback occur, and how you can assure the best environment and approach to positive communication. We cannot overemphasize the role you and your staff have in ensuring that your message of health maintenance and wellness is not only heard, but understood and accepted.

In addition, it is medically and legally wise to ensure that your patients understand their diagnosis, condition, symptoms, treatment, medication, and potential outcome as well as their role in influencing all of these. Patient education, therefore, is not a frill, not a luxury, but as important a component of the medical care you provide as the diagnostic tests you order and your analysis of the results.

UTILIZING HEALTH EDUCATION MATERIALS

CHOOSE THE APPROPRIATE METHOD

Not everyone responds in the same way to each communication method. Using a combination of face-to-face, visual, written and aural techniques will assure that you reach your patient, if not by one method, then by another.

CREATE A RECEPTIVE ATMOSPHERE

The atmosphere and environment in which you inform your patients will be very influential in determining how much of the information you give them is retained. We talked earlier about how important your conviction and belief is in influencing your patients. The surroundings and manner in which you communicate with them is important also. How do you think an individual will react if, following an exam, her doctor says as he heads out the door, "Oh, Mary Ann, give this patient some of those flyers on chronic bowel disease. We have a ton of them cluttering our supply room." An exaggerated example, but certainly it conveys the negative environment in which communication can take place. It's doubtful the patient would pay much attention to the material or the instructions given.

Part of creating the atmosphere is the delegation of authority that occurs when a staff member such as your nurse or technician is given responsibility for patient education. Some offices designate a staff member to provide follow-up information, verbally or through printed, video or audio materials, when the physician has completed his exam and instructions. If this is your choice, it is important to stress to your patients the knowledge, expertise and reliability of the staff member. Reversing or denigrating instructions or information given by a staff member denigrates your authority as well. (It's wise to periodically review with staff members any routine instructions and post-surgical information. Instruct those charged with formal patient education responsibilities to bring unique situations or questions to you before responding to patients.) It's also a good idea to emphasize to all members of your staff—from receptionist to billing clerk— their informal roles as patient educators. You should also point out any limitations or restrictions regarding what they may say or instructions they may give.

If a room or area is to be set aside for education, be sure that it is well stocked with books, pamphlets and brochures, video and audio tapes. The equipment must all be in good working condition, and the room well-lit, with comfortable seating and table(s) if needed. Have writing implements and paper available for jotting notes or questions. Headphones for the VCR or audiocassettes keep disruption of other patients to a minimum.

If a room or area is not feasible, it's still possible and necessary to create a receptive atmosphere for patient education. Take the patient into your office when extended or complex instructions are necessary. This relocation to a less clinical, yet still professional setting emphasizes the significance of the information you are giving. It also may tend to reduce the stress imposed by the exam room, and make the patient more likely to hear and comprehend what you have to say.

When giving verbal instructions, your full attention should be on the task at hand. Don't record notes in the chart at the same time. Gain and maintain eye contact. Touch your patient—on the shoulder or the arm— to gain confidence and establish a professional intimacy.

COMMUNICATE ON THE PATIENT'S LEVEL

Physically and in several other ways, there are *levels* on which patients should be addressed for most effective communication and comprehension.

Get on the same level as your patient. If your patient is seated, sit down at his/her level. This physical approximation creates a sense of equality, and makes the individual more willing to accept your message.

Use language your patient will understand. Usually you can listen to your patient and determine his language and communication skills. Watch for signs of understanding or confusion as you explain something—a nod of the head, a look of puzzlement. Ask occasionally, "Is that clear? Do you understand this process?" Such questions are especially important if instructions are being given over the telephone, where a visual check of understanding is not possible. Explain medical terms if you must use them; even simple words like "refraction" are not in the everyday vocabulary of most individuals. It's safer to assume that clarification or explanation is needed than it is to assume that your patient assimilated your instructions on the first breeze-through.

AND FINALLY . . .

How you communicate with your patients is as important as what you say to them. Your communication technique can keep satisifed patients coming back to your practice, or it can lead to misunderstanding and even patients who leave, never to return. Patient education is a part of the communication process; it involves a variety of techniques, materials, and approaches. Most of all, it is an ongoing process that begins when the patient walks in the door of your office (or sometimes when he calls on the telephone prior to coming in). It involves all of the practice staff as well as the physician(s), and it requires commitment and a belief in the importance of educated, informed patients. Communication and education cannot be categorized or reserved for a separate time slot; realistically, it should occur throughout the patient's appointment and with each member of the staff encountered.

When it is incorporated into the total health care experience of your patients, education intensifies learning, increases compliance, strengthens the commitment to wellness and enhances the physician-patient relationship. There are few weapons in the health care practitioner's arsenal that are as potent.

BIBLIOGRAPHY

Kleisley P: *The Advertising Physician.* Phoenix, AZ, June 1985.

Brown SW, Swartz TA: Consumer Medical Complaint Behavior: Determinants of and Alternatives to Malpractice Litigation. *Journal of Public Policy and Marketing* 1984: 85–98.

Brown SW, Swartz TA: A Gap Analysis of Professional Service Encounters. *Journal of Marketing* 1989: 62.

Malpractice and Guest Relations—Are Some Researchers Overlooking the Obvious? *Hospital Guest Relations Report* 1987: August: 1.

Paxton: Why Doctors Get Sued. *Medical Economics* 1988; April 18: 46.

Owens A: Will Defensive Medicine Really Protect You? *Medical Economics* 1988; April 18: 92.

Chapter 8

Promoting to Referral Sources

How do your patients learn about you?

Depending on your specialty, up to 75 percent of your patients may be referred to your practice by other physicians. Health care professionals in the community and your own patients make up the difference if you're in a referral-dependent specialty such as surgery.

How do you communicate with these referral sources? Do you acknowledge them, letting them know you appreciate their confidence in your skills? Do you have a formal means of reporting back to these individuals regarding the patients they send you?

Do you know who your referral sources are? Do you know their names? Do you know the medical specialties and allied health fields that predominantly refer to your practice?

You should.

In this chapter, we will look at referral sources—those you're well aware of, and individuals or groups you may never have thought of as potential referrers.

We'll discuss the effect your actions and those of your staff have on your referral sources. We'll look at things you should be doing, and those you shouldn't, in order to maintain positive referral relationships. And we'll offer a variety of ethical, professional techniques for generating referrals, for sustaining awareness of your practice and maintaining positive referral relationships.

WHO ARE YOUR REFERRAL SOURCES?

If a practice is to grow in a planned fashion, the physician(s) and staff must be familiar with referral sources, by name and by specialty or category. You must know how to communicate with them, and you should know how to find out if they are satisfied with the care you've given their patients, clients, employees or students.

But it's not enough to know who is referring to your practice. You should know what individuals or groups are not, and if they are not, why not. If your practice is to *thrive,* not simply be maintained, you must develop strategies to generate referrals from sources that could send you patients, but presently don't.

Depending on the type of practice you have and your medical specialty, you may gain patients from a variety of sources. Patients and physicians, of course, will probably constitute the largest referral groups, but it's likely there are several other referral sources for your practice . . . sources you may not have considered.

From how many of the following groups do you currently receive patients?

- Physicians (by specialty)
- Patients
- Hospitals (emergency departments, urgent care programs, nurses, public relations or marketing departments, physician referral programs)
- Schools/school nurses/counselors
- Health plans
- Businesses (occupational health nurses and physicians)
- Allied health care professionals (physical therapists, social workers, discharge planners, podiatrists, chiropractors)
- Dentists
- Social service and community agencies (American Heart Association, Cancer Society, Arthritis Foundation, etc.)
- Service personnel (hair stylists, barbers, make-up artists, health and fitness instructors, etc.)
- Insurance companies
- Rehabilitation nurses

If you are uncertain what percentage of your patients are derived from any of these groups, or if you suspect that few of your patients come from any of the categories except physicians and your own patients, it may be a good idea to begin tracking your referral sources by name, address and specialty or occupation. This file should include information about everyone who has referred patients to you in the past—such as physicians, nurses, health care professionals and agencies. You should also list local business people and professionals with referral potential including social workers, clergy, attorneys, health club managers, psychologists, etc.

Developing this list for the first time may require going through patient files to jog your memory, asking for staff input, and even going through the Yellow Pages to come up with physician and organization names. After you've developed a referral list, keeping it current will be simpler because you can track future referrals with a question on your new patient information forms. If you have an office-based computer, this tracking procedure can be programmed into the routine information gathering that takes place for every new patient. (See Chapter 13.)

If, after reviewing patient records, you find that you generate few referrals from categories other than physicians, you may wish to assess your community involvement. It's difficult for others to refer to your practice if they don't know about you. Whether you choose to engage in overt promotional techniques or not, the competitive era in which you are practicing medicine demands that you make yourself and your practice known, that you engage in give-and-take with the community you serve.

Let's assume you've reviewed the referral list above and determined that, while you're doing an adequate job of communicating with some of these groups, you could probably do better and could also increase the number of referrals from others. What then, are some of the things you might do? Following is a review of likely referral sources and appropriate promotional techniques.

PHYSICIANS

Most physicians find that patients referred by their colleagues are preferable to any others. These patients are pre-screened; they are not "doctor-shopping" or "disease-shopping."

Establishing this professional relationship generally does not require great financial expenditures (in fact, expensive gifts are frowned upon and may even be unethical). Nor does it require a great deal of paperwork or time-consuming personal or telephone contact. It is primarily a matter of courtesy and communication, of treating those who send you patients as you would wish to be treated by them when you refer patients to them.

A 1983 study by Robert Ludke, PhD, and Gary Levitz, PhD, of the University of Iowa Center for Health Service Research found that, (assuming patient management and care is equivalent) the following factors have the most influence with physicians who are actual or potential referral sources:

1. Personal knowledge of the physician and practice
2. Communication with referral physician
3. Patient preference (regarding location and other convenience or personality characteristics)
4. Satisfaction expressed by previously referred patients
5. Reciprocation

To these five factors, we would add return of the patient to the referring physician once the program of care or treatment is complete.

Let's look at each of these factors individually, and how you may or may not affect them:

Personal Knowledge. The preference by referring physicians for personal knowledge of a doctor and his or her practice implies a need to introduce yourself to your colleagues who could refer to you. In this introduction—either personal or written—provide some information about your practice specialty and services, location(s), hours and special instructions or information such as an unlisted phone number designated just for physicians. If the introduction initially takes place via letter or phone call, follow it up by a formal or informal meeting. If a regular meeting of the hospital medical staff is scheduled, seek out physicians whom you've contacted, introduce yourself and engage them in conversation. If no formal means of acquainting yourself with them is upcoming, suggest a breakfast or lunch either alone or with a mutual acquaintance.

You must be sure that your colleagues know of your medical and/or surgical skills, your competence, and your patient management technique as well as your practice location and other basics.

Communication. Communication is another factor that influences physicians to refer patients. We can't emphasize enough its importance both in introducing yourself and your practice, and as a means of assuring they are well-informed about the care you provide to patients they send you. Studies have shown that referring physicians not only *expect* communication about the patients they send you, they will terminate a relationship if it doesn't occur. They want to know your diagnosis, treatment plan or surgery recommended, and eventual outcome. This communication may take the form of a telephone call, a letter, or both. We suggest that you implement a formal means of periodic reports and/or updates on all referred patients, particularly those who are in your care for an extended treatment program. You'll find a sample referral thank-you letter in Figure 8-1.

In addition to the feedback suggested above, you may find communication techniques such as a practice newsletter beneficial in cementing relationships with potential referral sources. Some of these promotional resources are discussed later in this chapter.

Patient Preference. To a certain extent, this is an area over which you may have little direct control. A referring physician may be very pleased with your care of his patients, and wish to send an individual to you for consultation, but if the patient wants a doctor whose practice is near his home, and you're located 15 miles away, the patient's wishes will usually be respected. Or if you're a male ob-gyn, and the patient wants a female doctor, her doctor will acknowledge her preference. More and more today, patients are expressing their preference for a specific medical group or individual to their doctors when a consultation is needed, and their doctors are complying with their requests. You *can* influence patient preference, however, by becoming the physician of choice because of your office ambience, staff friendliness and courtesy, and your warmth balanced with professionalism. And if you find that a number of physicians in a particular geographic area have indicated they would direct patients your way if you were more conveniently located, it may be worthwhile to consider establishing a satellite office, or even relocating if such referrals are important to your success.

Patient Satisfaction. Patient preference can be closely tied to patient satisfaction, both directly and indirectly. When referral to a specialist is

FIGURE 8-1 Sample "Thank You for Referral" Letter

Mark R. Fanshuel, M.D.
6979 Northwest Parklane, Suite 800
Limpocquet, Georgia 30086
(404) 462-9999

ADULT OPHTHALMOLOGY   DISEASES & SURGERY OF THE EYES

November 18, 1988

Dr. Anita Marlon
922 Medical Lane
Suite 1654
Decatur, GA   30030

    Re: ANTOINE REVAIS

Dear Dr. Marlon

    I examined Antoine Revais on November 17, 1988. He is a 46
year old man who had been swimming several hours a day for the
past several days in preparation for a mini-triathalon event. He
has experienced redness and some pain in both eyes. He has been
wearing extended-wear soft contact lenses, but has not been
wearing the lenses for the past three days. He has some
persistent irritation in both eyes along with the redness, with
20/30 vision in both eyes. Examination disclosed a
conjunctivitis of the right eye with a mild amount of serious
discharge. Otherwise his eyes appeared completely normal.
    It appears that he may have a mild bacterial conjunctivitis
so I placed him on BigDrugCo. eyedrops to be taken QID in the
right eye for a period of 7 days. If he has any further problems
with his eyes he has been instructed to return.
    Dr. Marlon, I truly appreciate your referral of this
patient. I have recently established a solo ophthalmology
practice in the northwest Atlanta suburbs, and am happy to serve
any of your patients with vision problems or who require check-
ups. If I can be of any further service to you, or if you have
any questions about Mr. Revais, please do not hesitate to call
me. My physicians-only telephone line is 499-9999.

Yours truly

Mark R. Fanshuel, M.D.

MRF/amn

---

needed, as mentioned earlier, patients sometimes indicate to their doctor exactly who they wish to be referred to. This can occur when a physician's reputation is widespread, or when family or friends have indicated the high quality of care provided by a certain specialist.

Satisfied patients discuss their feelings and experiences with family, friends, neighbors and co-workers. If a physician does an excellent job of caring for and communicating with patients, these patients help raise public and professional awareness of the physician's practice by talking about it. (Conversely, if they're not pleased, they'll talk about it also, to a far greater number of people.) Not only does word get around to patients and potential patients, it gets back to other physicians as well. In fact, many doctors make it a habit of *asking* returned patients who were sent to a specialist, "What did you think of this doctor? Were you satisfied?" The answers they receive constitute a "mini-review" of the specialist, and can determine whether future patients are sent to this individual or another.

Reciprocation. You are a gastroenterologist in a multi-specialty group practice. You always call or write your referral sources regarding your diagnosis and the treatment outcome of their patients. You're active on your hospital's medical staff committees, your patients all express to you and to others satisfaction with your care. You get referrals on a regular basis from three family practice specialists, all of whom are good medical practitioners. One of them is a member of your church and a good golfing buddy; another has worked with you on several committees and is a member of the Rotary Club you belong to. The third family practitioner doesn't belong to your church, is in Kiwanis, not Rotary, and plays tennis rather than golf. Since you don't see him socially or otherwise, you seldom think of doctor number three when a patient of yours needs a family doctor. In the past four months, you haven't sent him any patients.

One day in reviewing your records, you notice that referrals from this physician have dropped; in fact, you haven't gotten a patient from him in 45 days. Previously, he had sent you at least one patient every two weeks.

Do you have any doubts why this doctor has ceased referring patients to you?

Reciprocity is a key ingredient in any exchange relationship. Without reciprocity, there is no exchange; in fact, there is no relationship.

Certainly some specialists will have fewer opportunities to refer patients to specific colleagues. However, there are other ethical ways besides patients for a physician to reciprocate. Reciprocation may include such activities as providing continuing education programs to doctors in specialties that could benefit from unique areas of expertise you have. It may mean sending copies of informative articles or research from your specialty journal. It may mean occasionally giving appropriate, relatively inexpensive thank-you gifts, taking a colleague to lunch or dinner, or otherwise letting him or her know you appreciate the patients referred to you.

Return of Patients. Related to reciprocity is the matter of returning patients to the referring physician or group. When you communicate with a colleague regarding your diagnosis and treatment of his or her patient, you indicate your intent to return the patient. Your attitude, type of care or treatment given, and comments to the patient regarding the referring doctor also indicate your intent to return the patient. We recommend also that you inform your patients that you will be communicating with their primary (or specialty) care physician regarding their treatment. This enhances patient satisfaction as well as physician satisfaction.

Be sure you convey to the patient that you are the medical provider only for problems in your specialty field, or for the specific condition or ailment that caused the referral. As an endocrinologist or internist, for example, once you extend your treatment of a diabetic patient beyond the diabetes and related conditions that made the family practice physician refer the patient, you tread injudiciously on primary care territory. Moreover, you ultimately risk losing not only this diabetic patient, but any future referrals from the family practitioner, and even his or her colleagues with whom your breach of referral etiquette is discussed.

DON'T TAKE YOUR REFERRAL SOURCES FOR GRANTED

The primary referral source for many physicians is other physicians. Some physicians know you and value your patient management skills. Others may not know you well nor see you frequently. Yet they will send you patients if they receive favorable reports on you from their patients, if they receive good follow-through from you, and if you maintain regular communication with them.

On the other hand, never take a referral relationship for granted. For example, if other doctors make a referral to a specific member of your group, be sure that physician sees the patient. When new associates join your group, be sure to introduce them to referring physicians.

Guidelines for Referral Physician Relationships. Developing a good relationship with your referral physicians is a form of marketing: In establishing a relationship with a colleague, analyze the needs of this important target audience, then seek ways to appropriately meet these needs.

- Contact the physician personally. Don't leave the communication task up to your staff or your nurse.
- Report back promptly to the referring physician. Let him or her know that the patient is in good hands.
- When you call a colleague, don't keep him or her waiting on the line. It shows lack of respect.
- Accommodate a referred patient promptly, even to the point of keeping places open in your appointment schedule for these patients.
- Remember that patients often report back to their original doctor. In conversation with the patient, avoid belittling any past treatments; also avoid overcharging, keeping patients waiting an excessive amount of time, or otherwise providing less than satisfactory service or care. (This goes for all of your patients, needless to say.)
- Teach your staff "referral physician etiquette." Emphasize and explain to them the value to your practice of patients referred by doctors.
- Don't be guilty of continually dumping unwanted or intractable patients just to be rid of them. You'll gain an unwanted reputation.
- Tell patients why you are referring them to another physician, and be certain they agree with the referral.
- Provide follow-up communication when you have completed treatment on a referred patient, indicating the final disposition and results.

- When a referrer calls, be sure the appropriate person (if it's not you) is available to take needed information or to provide assistance.
- Consider providing special services for referring doctors—such as a designated phone line or VIP treatment by staff for high-referring doctors.

ESTABLISHING REFERRING PHYSICIAN RELATIONSHIPS

The importance of establishing and maintaining consistent professional relationships with other physicians is obvious. But often clients of ours, particularly new or newly located physicians, want to know how to meet potential referral sources. Here are some suggestions:

1. Join hospital medical staff committees and become active on them. Volunteer to head a task force or spearhead a project. Get yourself elected committee chair.
2. Participate in medical staff events such as regular meetings, CME events, and advisory committees.
3. Join your local medical society, the state medical organization, and your local medical specialty organization, if there is one. Subscribe to their publications, which often list names and other information about new physicians and practices. Then introduce yourself to these individuals who probably have not yet created a referral network.
4. If yours is a new practice or a new office location, hold a reception or open house for your colleagues.
5. Make an effort to introduce yourself to your colleagues on a formal and informal basis in professional and social situations.
6. Send a personal letter of welcome to new doctors in your service area, on the hospital staff, and in specialty areas from which you usually derive new patients. If you're new in practice, send a letter of introduction to established doctors.
7. For group practices, send an announcement or letter to referral sources when a new physician joins the practice or when one of the group adds a specialty, gains board certification, etc. (see Figure 8-2).

MAINTAINING REFERRAL PHYSICIAN RELATIONSHIPS

Simply introducing yourself to the new internist in your medical building and the anesthesiologist who has joined your church is not enough. You must cultivate and maintain the relationship if you expect your colleagues to continue to send patients to your practice. Here are some promotional techniques for maintaining a relationship that's based on respect and reciprocity.

Communicate. Communication has been previously emphasized, both as a means of informing the referring doctor about his patient, and as a gentle reminder of your practice and services. Some communication techniques that are accepted and even expected include:

Personal call or visit. This is the preferred method for introducing yourself to a physician. Occasionally you may get a new patient from a physician you have not met, or from a new specialist who has opened a practice in your building. However you learn of this potential referral source, it is

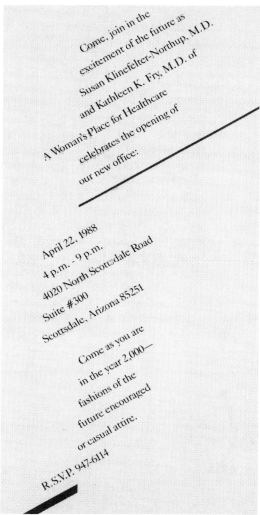

Come, join in the
excitement of the future as
Susan Klinefelter-Northup, M.D.
and Kathleen K. Fry, M.D. of
A Woman's Place for Healthcare
celebrates the opening of
our new office:

April 22, 1988
4 p.m. - 9 p.m.
4020 North Scottsdale Road
Suite #300
Scottsdale, Arizona 85251

Come as you are
in the year 2,000—
fashions of the
future encouraged
or casual attire.

R.S.V.P. 947-6114

FIGURE 8-2 Sample Open House Invitation
Holding an open house for physicians and other professional referral sources is a good
way to meet your colleagues informally.

correct to call and introduce yourself, and possibly schedule a time to meet for breakfast or lunch, or just briefly in one or the other's office. There tends to be greater confidence in a colleague with whom you've had a chance to discuss your mutual backgrounds and training. You might also call a referral physician to check on how a patient is doing after you've completed treatment and returned the individual to him or her.

Letters, cards and announcements. A friendly personal letter welcoming a new doctor, introducing yourself to established physicians, and/or thanking someone who has recently begun referring patients to you, is a good alternative when you can't immediately make the time for a personal visit. The letter shouldn't serve as a substitute for a call or visit, but it can let potential or actual referrers know you're interested in them and you appreciate their referrals. Indicate in your letter that you plan to make time in the near future to meet and introduce yourself. Group practices often find announcement cards helpful to let the professional community know when a new associate or partner has joined the practice. Nevertheless, a personal call to key referral sources should follow the card (see Figure 8-3).

The follow-up letter after you've seen a patient should be sent promptly after you have diagnosed and begun treatment, and should indicate diagnosis, course of treatment, and expected results. In the case of a serious diagnosis, or one that may generate questions from the referring physician, a phone call is recommended in addition to the letter. Some physicians

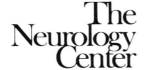

The Neurology Center

The Neurology Center
announces with pleasure the
association of

Donald H. Lussky, M.D.

and

Andrew J. Barbash, M.D.

for the practice of Clinical Neurology,
Electromyography
and Electroencephalography

Dominion Federal
Bank Building

7799 Leesburg Pike
Falls Church, VA 22043
(703) 827-4090

at its new

Northern Virginia Office.

FIGURE 8-3 New Associate Announcement Card
A card like this used to announce a new member of a practice is simple and professional and can be sent to all referral sources as well as patients.

save time by dictating the follow-up letter in the exam room with the patient present.

It's helpful medically as well as being good referral etiquette to provide periodic reports to the primary care physician on patients who require a lengthy course of treatment.

Newsletter. Some physicians, particularly specialists, can provide a real service to their referral sources by sending them needed information in newsletter format about diseases, disorders, diagnoses and treatments within their specialty. (See Chapter 12.) We know of one doctor who includes a "guest column" written by his referring colleagues in his newsletter. He gives them plenty of lead time, includes their photo, practice and biographical information, and ties the topic to issues or subjects of interest to his own audience. The physicians he asks to write the guest column are flattered and pleased.

Copies of lab/x-ray, other reports. It's good medicine and good marketing to send copies of exam results, lab or x-ray reports to the referring physician. Do the same with the primary physician even if he/she did not refer the patient. It's a good way to establish a relationship.

Other communication techniques. There are a variety of informal ways to keep communication lines open. When you come across an article in your specialty journal that you think may be helpful or of interest to one or several of your colleagues, make a copy of it and send it to them along with a brief note. Try to schedule a breakfast or lunch meeting at least weekly with one of your referral sources. Take time during professional meetings or even casual encounters to converse with a doctor who has referred a patient to you recently; let him/her know how treatment is progressing, and that you appreciate the referral. (Don't let the verbal discussion substitute for the written communication, however.)

Semi-social events. Provide opportunities to meet your referring colleagues, and for their staff to meet yours, by holding an occasional open house, holiday party or other "social" event specifically for doctors and their staff. Look for holidays or excuses to have a reception other than Christmas when schedules are crowded. For instance, how about a "Goodbye Winter, Hello Spring" affair? Or a "Have a Heart" party on or near Valentine's Day if you are a cardiologist? An orthopedic surgeon whose practice treats many skiing injuries could host a reception at the beginning of winter with the theme "It's (s)no(w) joke." You can hold your reception at your office or, if you have the budget, go all-out and have a catered affair at a hotel. Turnout would be improved, since people are less likely to see it as a business affair. Yet you'll still have a positive impact if you take a low-key approach.

Staff-to-Staff Relations. Once a physician decides to refer a patient to your practice, it's likely that your staff and the referring physician's will interact frequently in handling much of the routine follow-up communication. Therefore, "staff-to-staff etiquette" and courteous, friendly relations should be emphasized and encouraged. Give your staff opportunities to meet the office staffs of referring physicians. Some ways to do this include:

- Encourage your key staff members (nurses, technical or paraprofessionals) to schedule introductory meetings with their peers at other physician offices. A breakfast or lunch can be a good time for sharing of ideas, helpful hints and suggestions for improving relations and communication. Ultimately the referral relationship benefits. Of course, you should reimburse your staff for the expense of these meetings.
- Encourage staff members to join and become active in associations and societies for their profession. They'll have the opportunity to talk about the practice, you and your skills while strengthening referral relationships and learning about other physicians and practices where referral possibilities exist.
- Hold an open house, luncheon or reception specifically for physician office staff members. Let your staff plan the event and prepare the invitation list (although you should look it over to add names that may be forgotten).
- Offer an educational program for selected staff (nurses, technicians, etc.) of current or potential referring physicians. The program can feature a physician in your practice as guest speaker, or one of your staff may have expertise or knowledge that would benefit others. If you offer a program of this type, try to get continuing education certification for attendees. It gives your program credibility and value.
- Include individual members of physician staffs on the mailing list for your newsletter, health education materials and practice brochure. Remember, other staff members are potential referral sources themselves!
- Treat your colleagues' staff members with respect and courtesy whether on the telephone or in person. They judge your practice by the way you treat them, and they frequently pass this judgment on to their employer.
- Encourage your staff to introduce themselves to their counterparts when an errand requires a trip to a physician's office to pick up or deliver information or patient records.
- Many staff members dine in the hospital cafeteria when the office is located in a nearby medical building. If yours does so, encourage them to seek out their peers and sit with them, rather than always sitting together with co-workers from your office.
- Provide your staff opportunities to increase their professional knowledge and skills. The stronger your staff is, the more positively it reflects on you. A highly qualified staff is respected and talked about by their peers as well as yours. You and your patients will be the ultimate beneficiaries.

Most of all, it's vital that your staff knows the impact it can have on referral relationships that develop in your practice. Let members know their roles in developing and enhancing such relationships. Let them know you depend on them to be courteous, knowledgeable, friendly and helpful to other physicians, their staffs, and every patient who comes to your practice or calls on the phone.

Develop Your Professional Status. If you are to generate new patients from your colleagues, you must not only be visible, you must be perceived by them as having *professional status*. (Although the term "status" was used in the Ludke-Levitz study we cited at the beginning of this chapter, we feel a better term might be "quality," or "perception of quality" by peers.) Ludke and Levitz, in identifying the factors influencing physicians' referral decisions, found that high-, middle- and low-status (quality) physicians are most likely to refer patients to high-status physicians. You must be seen by others as a skilled physician, in whose care their patients can be trusted, and who engenders respect from other physicians.

Your professional status depends in part on the image you project. Bear in mind, we are not saying that image can substitute for skill. Nothing is further from the truth. It may be possible to initially promote a poor product or service, but it is not possible to sustain it in the marketplace. Your professional reputation must be backed up by medical ability and knowledge (see Figure 8-4).

To create awareness and enhance your status among your colleagues and the community you serve, there are a number of "visibility" techniques you can implement. All are accepted in the medical and lay community.

1. Publish papers, write letters to the editor, comments and/or articles on pertinent topics in local, state or national journals. Participate as editor or serve on the advisory board of your medical society or hospital's medical staff publication.
2. Write letters to the editor of your local newspaper.
3. Establish an area of medical expertise and become known as a local resource on the topic. Some doctors who have written books for the lay person on health and medical topics have found that even if the book isn't a best seller, just having written it gives them prestige with the public and their peers.
4. Join hospital, medical staff, and medical society committees, and become active on them. Offer your knowledge and skills. Don't just be a member, be an active participant and contributor.

Get Involved. Community involvement will enhance your image and your visibility with other physicians and potential patients while increasing public awareness of your practice and services.

1. Join and attend social and professional affairs and organizations for physicians. Get to know the members. Seek out active participation. Don't be overeager, however; enthusiasm that's perceived as excessive can turn your peers off.
2. Participate in community organizations and appropriate community events. Get elected to offices, to non-profit boards. Serve as medical advisor to agencies—such as those representing cystic fibrosis, Parkinson's, arthritis, whatever your interest is. Participate in community health fairs and events involving the medical community.
3. Volunteer to speak on medical topics to community groups, the PTA, schools, for the media. Be discriminating and become a true expert. Stay current on new findings on your selected topics (those in which you specialize or that hold a special interest for you).

FIGURE 8-4 Washington Imaging Center Case Report
This two-page clinical report is sent to referring physicians. It is educational as well as a subtle, professional marketing tool for the radiology group.

CASE
REPORT

Cervical Disc Herniation
MR Diagnosis with Clinical Correlation

John L. Sherman, M.D.

CASE #1:

Clinical Information

A 46-year-old female presented with a six-week complaint of paresthesia in the hands bilaterally. She also noted a sense of stiffness of gait. On examination there was a positive Lhermitte's sign. She made errors on joint position sense testing in both great toes. The deep tendon reflexes were diminished at the biceps but brisk bilaterally below this level. Both toes were upgoing. She underwent a course of physical therapy after which she complained of cervical pain and increased paresthesia. A CT scan without contrast was reported to show mild disc bulging, but no HNP was identified. The patient was then referred for MR evaluation of the cervical spine.

MR Evaluation

MR of the cervical spine was performed using a 5 inch surface coil. Three-millimeter thick sections were obtained with T1-weighted and dual-echo T2-weighted techniques. Oblique axial images were obtained through the intervertebral discs. A disc herniation was identified at the C5-6 level on the sagittal scans (Figs. 1A, 1B). The axial images clearly showed the central location of the herniated nucleus pulposus (HNP) and the marked focal spinal cord compression (Fig. 3).

CASE #2:

A 43-year-old female presented with neck pain, shooting pains across her left shoulder and paresthesia in her left arm.

(Discussion on reverse side)

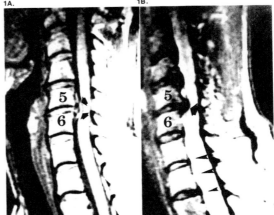

Figure 1. Central HNP at C5-6 causes marked cord compression (arrows). (A) T1-weighted image. (B) T2- weighted imaging (myelographic effect). Note bright CSF outlining spinal cord (arrowheads).

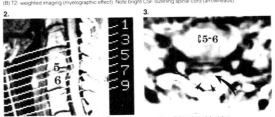

Figure 2. MR scan "localizer" shows axial scan locations arranged parallel to intervertebral disc.
Figure 3. Axial image #5 obtained through the C5-6 disc shows the central location of the HNP (arrow). Spinal cord (arrowheads) is compressed.

The following authors periodically contribute to *Case Report:*

Charles M. Citrin, M.D.   John L. Sherman. M.D.   Lawrence M. Cohen, M.D.
Bruce J. Bowen, M.D.   Howard A. Sachs, M.D.   Birgit A. Ehlers, M.D.

HOSPITALS

The hospital(s) where you are a member of the medical staff can be a good source of new patients. As with physicians and the public, you must establish yourself, become known, provide a basis for respect from the hospital staff, communicate regularly, and follow through when a referral occurs.

Here are some ways of generating referrals from your hospital:

1. Sign up with the hospital Emergency Department and Urgent Care program (if there is one) as a consultant and/or for patient referrals, if that's the procedure your hospital uses.

2. If your hospital has a Speaker's Bureau, sign up with it. Specify your topics by title, not simply by subject matter. Often the program chairperson for a group will not have a specific topic in mind for a talk, and if yours sounds particularly appealing, it can win an audience. For example, list your topic as "Seniority Can be Sexy," not "Medical Symptoms of Aging"; or "To Die For: Heart Attack Risk Factors," not "Heart Disease Facts."

3. List yourself with the Physician Referral Program, if there is one. If not, discuss with the appropriate medical staff committee the possibility of requesting that the hospital initiate one.

4. Most hospitals today sponsor health fairs, classes, seminars, and other programs for the public, and they're always seeking physicians who will participate in such programs. Let your medical staff liaison, public relations or marketing department know of your availability for such events. The hospital handles and pays for all the promotion as a rule, and your practice derives some of the benefit.

5. Let the public relations department know you're available as a medical expert anytime the media contacts them seeking a spokesperson on medical topics in your specialty.

Your hospital administrator, director of nursing, and marketing or public relations department director can be invaluable allies in generating new patients for you; let them know about your skills, interests and unique aspects of your practice.

BUSINESSES

While most physicians can't expect a large number of new patients from businesses and local industry, there is a reasonable referral potential, particularly in certain specialties. Employee physicals, on-the-job injuries, workplace health and fitness and employee assistance programs require physician involvement and can result in new patients. More and more frequently, wellness programs developed by physicians have great appeal to employers. Some promotional options to consider with businesses include the following:

1. Send an introductory letter to the occupational health nurse, medical director (if the company has one) or employee benefits department offering your ser-

vices. Suggest your availability as a speaker or to provide classes or in-service programs on topics appropriate to the employer or industry.

2. Offer your services to a company's Employee Assistance Program, either in screening employees or as a speaker or other resource.

3. Some employee publications may welcome articles or columns on workplace health and wellness issues, industrial injury prevention and similar topics. Some carry advertising, and ad rates are minimal. Advertising in these publications generates awareness and good will and may generate patients for you as well.

4. You may find it worthwhile to develop wellness, screening or work-hardening (postinjury return to work preparedness) programs for local businesses and industry. Consult with the company's human resources or employee benefits department regarding their health/medical needs in these areas, and be sure to track costs, utilization, patient compliance and results as much as possible. Employers want to know if a program is going to *cost* them or *save* them health care dollars.

5. Many smaller companies do not have a full-time medical director; they haven't the need or the budget for one. However, they may welcome the services of a qualified physician on a part-time or as-needed basis, and the patients you see on-the-job may become patients in your practice if they have no physicians of their own.

SCHOOLS

For certain specialties, schools and even day care centers can be a good source of patient referrals. Offering your services to schools can also be beneficial in heightening public awareness of your practice and increasing your image or community involvement. Consider these ideas:

1. Junior high and high schools have a variety of sports teams. The football squad may already have a team physician, but what about baseball, track, hockey, soccer, tennis or golf? Offer your services to the coaches, and even physical education teachers, in providing physicals, pre-season screenings or clinics, and on-call medical assistance during the season.

2. Science, health, home economics and similar classes in junior and high schools welcome the expertise of local physicians as speakers and class participants. Develop a specific talk or program and set up a schedule with local schools to give it to all appropriate classes or groups. Be sure to include educational handout material with your name, address and other practice information on it.

3. Schedule special clinics or services and/or practice hours geared to student health needs and schedules. Notify the schools and teachers of these programs and hours.

4. Advertise in the school newspaper. It's inexpensive, and besides creating good will, can generate patients, particularly if your ad is geared specifically to students, and not simply a version of your business card.

5. If you have expertise in an area of interest or concern to adolescents and teens, offer to write a guest column in the school newspaper, or to write or edit a question/answer column on health and medical topics. Contact the newspaper's faculty advisor and/or school administrator for this.

6. Introduce yourself to the school nurse(s) and offer your services as a resource for providing or participating in screening clinics, and/or putting on classes or programs for nurses, aides and/or students.

7. Offer smoking cessation, weight or stress reduction, nutrition and diet or other classes geared to adolescents and teens. How about a class especially for teachers? Or one for parents that's sponsored and promoted by the Parent Teacher Association?

PATIENTS

We can't emphasize enough the importance of satisfied patients as a means of generating new patients and ensuring satisfied referral sources. The patient who is immediately accommodated in your schedule, who finds a pleasant, attractive office environment and friendly, welcoming staff in your office, who encounters a knowledgeable, helpful physician, and who has a generally positive experience often opens the door to future referrals. Many times, when someone has referred a patient for the first time, the referrer will seek feedback from the patient about the experience, in order to determine whether or not to send future patients. Continued positive experiences by satisfied patients can ensure a steady stream of new patients from a variety of referral sources. In addition, your own patients are vital links in the referral chain. They come in contact with a cross-section of potential referral sources, and they can provide a continued flow of new patients to your practice—*if* you and your staff have made them feel comfortable, welcome, a part of the practice, *and* given them high quality medical care.

Throughout this book, we discuss ways to generate patients and to retain them. Patients who stay with your practice are satisfied patients, and satisfied patients will tell the world about you. Be mindful as you read the strategies and ideas outlined that almost everything you do will have an impact, for better or worse, on your patients. Your goal should be to ensure that every contact anyone has with you or a member of your staff is a positive one. Furthermore, if problems arise (and they will!), it should be your goal not only to correct the problem so it does not recur, but to ensure that the dissatisfied patient is assuaged. You cannot afford even one unhappy individual in your practice (or out of it). As consumer research has shown, the dissatisfied customer will tell 11 to 20 others of his experience; the contented customer will only relate his experience to four or five others.

Because your existing patients are so important to your referral picture, we've summarized some of the "people-satisfier" strategies you'll find scattered throughout this book:

- Personal attention. Give your patients your complete attention, especially when the appointment time is limited.
- Train your staff to represent you in a positive, professional, friendly manner to your patients, on the phone, in person and everywhere else. (See Chapter 6.)
- Communicate. Patients want information on how to stay well, how to manage their family's health, the latest medical news and research. Give it to them in as many ways as you can.

- Follow up. Call patients following surgery or serious illness. "Recruit" prodigal patients back to your practice.
- Show your gratitude. Send patients who refer others a personal thank-you card or note, a small gift. Say "thank you" verbally when they come for an appointment.
- Encourage referrals from patients. Ask them to pass on copies of your practice brochure, your newsletter, health education materials. Encourage them to tell family, friends and neighbors about your practice.
- Know what your patients want and need, medically and emotionally, and try to meet these needs. Ask them; survey them; have your staff record comments, requests, problems. Then act on this information to increase patient satisfaction.

OTHER REFERRAL SOURCES

There are any number of potential referral sources in the community; every medical specialty has different possibilities. They include podiatrists, physical therapists, psychologists, social workers, discharge planners, health care agencies. The list is limitless. Reviewing referral sources in your practice should stimulate your thinking and remind you of other possibilities.

Once you've created a list of possibilities, it's important to contact them and let them know of your practice, your services, amenities, and how you can help their clients. An introductory letter and/or brochure, personal visit or phone call, your practice newsletter or educational programs described earlier in this chapter may be appropriate.

Whatever you choose to do, and whomever you direct your efforts to, it's vital that you communicate with individuals or groups who send you patients and especially, that you acknowledge the referrals.

AND FINALLY . . .

Promoting to referral sources incorporates many of the techniques you'll find throughout this book. But even if you choose not to engage in any overt promotional strategies such as newsletters, advertising or media relations, the quality of the referral relationships you develop will depend heavily on the quality and frequency of your communication with the individuals and groups who may send patients your way.

Those who refer patients to you want to feel confident about recommending others to your practice. Instill confidence in your patients and your referral sources, and you'll have a steady influx of new patients.

BIBLIOGRAPHY

Ludke RL, Levitz GS: Physicians: The Forgotten Market. *HCM Review*. Aspen Systems Corp. 1983; Fall 13–21.

Effective Public Relations

Chapter 9

Generating Effective Publicity and Dealing with the Press

"Americans are working hard to stay well. They're hungry for health, and they're hungry for medical news . . . People used to receive information about health and disease only from their physicians—but not anymore. The major sources for medical information now seem to be monthly columns in women's magazines, diet and fitness books, celebrity exercise tapes—and television. People no longer have to go to their personal physicians to discover what's good and bad for them; they can find out about it on TV . . . ."

Bruce B. Dan, MD, *JAMA* May 22, 1987

As Americans pursue their quest for fitter bodies, healthier habits and longer lives, they will continue to seek information that helps them achieve their goals. While they prefer to receive it directly from their personal physician, this isn't always possible. So they look to other sources of medical expertise—and the media is happy to oblige by interviewing doctors locally and nationally.

In this chapter, you'll learn how you can become one of their sources. You'll learn how to approach the media with ideas for articles, TV news segments, and radio interviews. You will learn what the needs of the various media are, and how to respond to them ethically and professionally. You'll learn how to develop good press relations—and why that first contact with a reporter, editor or program producer is so important if you wish to have follow-up contact. You'll learn when to use a press release and a public service announcement (PSA), how to prepare them and who to send them to.

This chapter is a *primer* in press relations. When you've completed it, you should have a full understanding of the importance of the media on health, public education, and medical issues. Your patients and the public want to learn more about how to stay healthy and physically fit; members of the media appreciate having qualified expert resources on whom they can rely; and you can meet both these needs with the proper attitude and approach to the press.

MEDIA COVERAGE: A CREDIBLE APPROACH

Media coverage is sought after by many physicians, whether it's in the form of a story on the 6 o'clock news, an article in the morning newspaper, or a radio talk show interview. It's credible, and it can yield significant results. A surgeon interviewed about a new procedure or new surgical technique generally can expect calls from interested patients, and even other physicians and health professionals. Some of the calls result in appointments.

Dan Orsborn, president of The Orsborn Group, Inc., says that media coverage "has a much more legitimate appearance than just straight advertising . . . And when the media does provide coverage, it also supplies a kind of third-person endorsement that gives the message a credibility that you couldn't possibly get through advertising."

While there's no charge for a legitimate newspaper or magazine article, the time investment to generate a single news feature can be significant. Establishing good media relations takes an ongoing effort. One feature story or television interview does not mean the media will turn to you whenever they need an expert source in your specialty. It takes continued, consistent contact.

Nevertheless, the benefits to the public, to medicine and to your practice of a well-told, factual story about a new treatment far outweigh the time and effort it may take to achieve it.

THE MEDIA'S NEEDS AND EXPECTATIONS

Journalists rely on experts of all sorts, from plumbers to PhDs. These experts provide factual information and interpretation of events.

At the same time, reporters and editors sometimes become frustrated with their sources, particularly in professions like medicine. While journalists depend on physicians as credible sources of information, they find them difficult to interview. They cite doctors' overuse of medical jargon, failure to be on time for or keep appointments, and lack of respect for the media.

Nevertheless, you can establish a good, continuing relationship with the media, based on mutual respect, when you understand what the press wants and expects from physicians and other professionals.

What the Press Wants. You are respected as a medical professional; accord the same respect to the media by recognizing and meeting their needs.

- **Deadlines.** Journalists work on strict deadlines. For daily newspapers and TV news, deadlines are tighter and occur more frequently than for a monthly magazine or weekly newspaper, but all must be observed.
- **News.** News is new or unusual, startling, current, timely and topical. An old subject that takes a new twist is also newsworthy.
- **Human interest.** A personal appeal to the emotions. There's nothing unique

about a sick child who gets well, but if the child has a rare ailment that requires very specialized treatment, and then writes and illustrates a story describing his illness—that's human interest.

- **Timeliness.** The media wants to hear about significant, unexpected occurrences as soon as they happen, and about planned events several weeks before, not the day after.

- **The personal approach.** If you suggest a story on a new procedure or treatment, be prepared with one or two patients who consent to be interviewed. Reporters want the patient's perspective.

- **Freedom from persistent calls.** When you propose an idea in writing, a follow-up call is appropriate. If you are turned down, thank the reporter politely; don't try to persuade him to change his mind. But don't hesitate to contact the reporter again with another idea.

What the Media Expects. The press relies on people who are knowledgeable in a certain field or on a certain subject. They attempt to check facts and verify the background, experience and expertise of sources, although time doesn't always permit this. So reporters and editors have certain expectations of interview subjects:

- Accuracy in the data you provide them. If a physician tells them 15 percent of the population suffers from a particular disorder, the reporter usually will accept that figure as accurate.

- Complete information. Don't come to an interview unprepared, with only half the background information you need.

- News, not self-promotion. If you convince the media to cover a topic or event which is nothing more than a promotion for your practice, not only is the story likely never to appear, but you probably won't be called again by that reporter.

- Prompt response. Often, when a reporter calls back for additional information, he or she is on deadline. Respond immediately to the request, or arrange for one of your staff to handle the call if you can't.

- Direct contact with you, not a go-between. It's fine to have a member of your staff or a public relations consultant handle the scheduling of an interview or a simple nonmedical follow-up question, but don't substitute a staff member or even a partner for an interview unless you've cleared it with the reporter. Reporters prefer to get information directly from you.

A Case Study. The dangers of prolonged exposure to the sun have been heavily covered in the media. So Dr. Eli, a dermatologist, knew it would be fruitless to propose such a feature to the *Hometown Herald* medical reporter.

But he had a unique angle. In a brief letter to the reporter, he explained that some people develop mole-like "markers" for malignant melanoma. If these suspicious moles are found and removed early, he wrote, the melanoma danger decreases.

He described a patient in his practice who was willing to be interviewed. The reporter liked the idea, and the resulting feature appeared in the "Lifestyle" section.

A TV reporter then picked up the story for a weekly health tip series.

Because of the newspaper article and the dermatologist's credentials, the local talk radio station scheduled a program on skin cancer.

YOU, YOUR STAFF AND THE MEDIA

A successful media relationship depends on your practice staff as well as you. Here's why:

- You will need assistance in generating ideas, preparing press releases, and contacting reporter or editors.
- Your staff can help in responding to a media request for information.
- A full understanding of media needs and ethics, the current "hot" medical topics and the preferences of individual reporters will alert your staff to story ideas within the practice.

An ophthalmologist we know did cataract surgery on a 90-year old patient, who casually commented to the receptionist, "Now I'll be able to read my blueprints." She learned that he was renovating his late grandfather's 200-year-old homestead, a historic landmark, and passed this information on to the doctor. A call to a reporter resulted in a feature story on the patient's renovation plans, and included an interview with the physician about the advantage of cataract surgery at any age.

KNOW YOUR LOCAL PRESS

Developing a good relationship with reporters and editors in your community is important, but it's not always as simple as picking up the phone and introducing yourself. While there's a burgeoning public interest in health and medical information, there also are a growing number of physicians, health care professionals and their public relations consultants besieging the press with news releases, "urgent" letters and phone calls. The medical reporter for a major daily newspaper told us with a laugh about the huge quantity of promotional material thinly disguised as news that he receives—and tosses, unused—each day. No wonder the press tends to be skeptical. And no wonder they return to the same reliable, accessible sources again and again when they need information or comment.

When you understand the needs of the various media, the responsibilities and needs of individuals in the press and how best to communicate with them, you improve your chances of getting legitimate coverage. Even if you decide to hire a public relations consultant, you should know the media in your area and etiquette for dealing with them.

Television. Television is a primary source of news and information for many Americans. After hearing about a medical treatment or discovery on television, they often will turn to their personal physician for additional details.

Television offers several opportunities for physicians who wish to share their medical knowledge with the public. Many news programs are aired throughout the day from early morning to midnight, and most have at least one medical or health-related feature.

In addition to news programming, television also has public service, interview, and locally produced programs on health and medical topics. But television is visual; be prepared to do more than talk. Demonstrate a procedure or show an anatomical model of an organ when discussing a disease or disorder; have slides with before/after views; show graphs, charts or illustrations. TV editors and reporters hate the "talking head"—the on-camera interview without action or visual back-up. Even the former White House deputy press secretary acknowledges the need for visual images if the President of the United States is to get coverage on the networks: "We knew very quickly that the rule was 'no pictures, no television piece,' no matter how important our news was," Larry Speakes wrote in his book *Speaking Out.* If you can't demonstrate something on camera, be prepared to provide videotape or suggest something active that can be filmed as background for your interview.

Twice a year during "ratings" periods, TV news directors focus heavily on multi-part series that will grab viewer attention, and health and medical topics are always favorites. If you have a good idea for a health series, propose it well in advance of the ratings period (spring and fall). Be aware that "slow news days" such as Sundays or holidays also offer an opportunity to get coverage if you have a good visual idea. (Slow news days also are minimal crew days for the news department, so it may not have a crew available for your story, even if it's a good one. In that case, suggest it for another day.)

These are the people you should know at each TV station in your area:

Assignment Editor: The person who plans and schedules the day's story assignments for the team of reporters. The assignment editor is usually your initial contact for a story idea, unless the station has a health/medical reporter.

Health or Medical Reporter or Editor: Most larger city stations have a reporter assigned to health and medical topics. Get to know these individuals and develop a professional relationship with them. Keep medical reporters informed of new information, research and developments in your specialty, even if there's no immediate potential for an interview or story for you. Send articles from your professional journals (if they're written in layman's language), the *American Medical News* and other publications. Suggest a local angle when possible.

News Editor: Generally doesn't get involved hands-on in day-to-day assignments, but oversees the overall news function. Might be the person to talk with if you have a major health care feature or series to propose.

News or Interview Program Producers: For non-prime-time news programs or interview programs (such as early morning or midday), the producer often is responsible for scheduling interviews.

Public Affairs Director: If you are sponsoring a free public event, you may be able to get free air time via public service announcements (covered later in this chapter). Meet with the station's public affairs director when delivering your PSA script or audio or videotape. Check with each station's public affairs director to learn how far in advance and in what form they prefer to receive PSA material.

Community Calendar Editor: This person will list your event in the station's community calendar listing.

Health Program Host, Producer or Scheduling Coordinator: If the station has a locally produced health program, the contact person may be the host, but more often it will be the producer or a scheduling coordinator who handles the job of scheduling interviews and guests.

Cable Television. There may be opportunities with the public access channel of the cable television company in your community. You'll need to talk with the public access director for specifics. In addition, cable programs like Cable News Network and Lifetime, the "lifestyle" network, consistently seek interesting health-related stories to meet the demand for a cross-section of topics and geographic areas. Also, cable viewers tend to be more educated, higher-income audiences.

Radio Stations. With its varied formats such as classical, soft rock, big band, and talk, radio is a targeted medium. The audience for a particular format tends to fit a defined demographic description. Radio also presents a wealth of public education opportunities to physicians who are willing to familiarize themselves with the programs available, such as news, interview and public service—and the people who coordinate them. See guidelines below for being "the perfect talk show guest."

These are the individuals you should get to know on your local radio stations:

- News Director
- Talk or interview program producers and hosts
- Public affairs directors
- Community calendar editor

In a major metropolitan area where there are many stations to choose from, select those whose format appeals to your target audience. For instance, if you are a pediatrician, your target audience is the parents of your patients, who probably listen to soft rock, 50's and 60's oldies, talk or news stations. To be certain, contact stations you're interested in and ask them for their audience demographics.

Your greatest opportunity for radio coverage may lie with all-talk or all news stations. Most have 18 to 24 hours to fill each day. These include interview programs featuring experts on an assortment of topics and a call-in audience; short telephone interviews as "fillers"; news programs in which feature material is included. To determine options available in your area, it's best to listen to the stations you may be interested in, particularly those with a format that appeals to your target audience.

THE PERFECT TALK SHOW GUEST

Talk shows are excellent media outlets for physicians. They provide listeners and viewers in-depth information on medical topics, and they give you a chance to expand on important health care issues. But be prepared: landing a guest spot on a talk show requires doing your homework.

1. If you want to promote an event you're sponsoring, you need a news angle. Don't expect that because you advertise on a station, you'll automatically get news coverage. The news and advertising departments are separate. Contact the host or producer of the program you're interested in at least four to six weeks in advance of the event.
2. Talk shows producers like *immediacy* in topics aired, so if an important medical/health care topic hits the news, and you have expertise in it, contact producers about providing a local viewpoint.
3. Talk shows are targeted to specific audiences. Know the audience and pitch your topic accordingly.
4. Find an angle or "hook" that hasn't been overdone or isn't too commercial. If you're a dermatologist and the first big summer holiday is coming up, suggest a program on how to protect children against the sun. If you're an allergist and pollen season is around the corner, suggest a review of allergens, how to avoid them, and how to cope when you can't.
5. If you get an acceptance for a talk show appearance, provide the host and/or producer with:
   Brief bio or resume
   Fact sheet on your topic
   Press release if appropriate
   Brief cover letter
   List of suggested questions and/or topics to cover
6. On the air, strive for a conversational tone. Be professional, yet warm and friendly. Use humor, human interest and examples to make your point. Be brief.
7. Send thank-you notes to producer and host after the show, mentioning any comments you received from patients or the public.

Newspaper. Newspaper is the media of choice for timely topics and those best told in depth. It's the appropriate medium for developing human interest features or photo opportunities, because the reporter or photographer has the space to explore details, emotions, and events.

Newspapers are an appropriate source for announcing coming events such as a practice-sponsored class on first aid for new parents. However, don't expect major coverage for such an event unless you can find a unique news or feature angle. In major dailies you'll be lucky to get a calendar listing or a single paragraph in the "health/medical" column. Small community papers and weeklies often will provide more coverage for these events.

It's a good idea to contact the feature or medical reporter or other editorial staff member two to three weeks in advance of a special event or other unusual story. That gives the reporter time to schedule an interview; if he/she is not interested, it gives you time to contact someone else. It sometimes takes several calls and letters plus a great deal of follow-up before an editor or reporter commits to an educational feature.

These are the staff persons with whom you should become familiar at a newspaper:

Health/Medical Reporters and Editors: Most urban daily newspapers now have a medical reporter who will be a primary contact for you in most cases. Get to know this person, but don't make a pest of yourself. Reporters tell tales of overly persistent doctors trying to push non-stories. Ask the reporter what kind of story he/she is seeking, and how you can help meet the newspaper's needs for health and medical features.

Feature or "Lifestyle" Editors/Reporters: Often a "soft" medical story—one that's more human interest or feature-oriented—will be bumped to the feature desk.

City Editor/News Editor: For straight news that affects all or a large number of the residents of your area.

Calendar Editor: For advance listings of special events, classes, etc.

Human Interest and/or Health Columnists (Local, not syndicated): They are particularly interested in unusual medical cases, dramatic or unique patient stories.

Editor/Managing Editor: These individuals will be appropriate contacts for small weekly or monthly newspapers. They may be the *only* contact for such publications.

Magazines. Some larger cities have magazines that use health and medical features. There also are national magazines targeted to specific industries, age groups or interests. You may be able to interest the editor in a feature if you have a very unique angle.

For example, you're a cardiologist who has a very high compliance record with your hypertensive patients. Your secret? A written contract you've developed that addresses the specific health problems each individual patient faces. Such a feature would require documented evidence of success and two or three patients as case studies. And it would probably require you to tell the magazine's readers how they could apply the concept you've developed to their own health problems.

Since magazines usually have a long lead time prior to publication—two to six months—a magazine story must be somewhat timeless. If your goal is extensive advance coverage relating to a specific major event, then contact the magazine's editor or managing editor well in advance. Six to twelve months is not unrealistic. For a simple listing in the magazine's calendar section, two month's notice is sufficient.

National publications receive hundreds of "queries," or article suggestions, each week from professional writers. If you're seeking national recognition, you must have a story that's significant yet specific.

Placing a story with a magazine is not a simple matter, but it is achievable if you have a legitimate news or feature idea with broad appeal to the publication's audience. There are two different ways to go about it.

You can contact a freelance writer. They are skilled at presenting and writing a story that has merit. Your hospital's public relations staff or local media society should be able to suggest good writers who are familiar with the medical field. A freelance writer will only work with you if he or she sees potential in your article proposal. In dealing with a writer, discuss terms up front. Most prefer to remain independent, proposing a health care feature (if they see merit in it) to a magazine in the form of a query letter to the editor and, if the idea is accepted, receiving payment from the publication after submitting the article. They are not contracted to you in any way if this is the approach taken. On the other hand, if you hire a public relations consultant or firm to act as your agent for the publication, they will present a detailed concept (again via a query letter) to the magazine but generally will not write the actual story if it is accepted. The fee you pay a public relations firm or consultant for presenting your health care feature idea may be hourly or a flat rate, and you pay the fee whether the query idea is accepted by the publication or not. (Note: presenting an idea does not guarantee that it will be placed. And even when an editor accepts a proposal, it may be six to twelve months, or more, before the piece appears in print.)

Instead, you can contact the magazine directly, via a query or pitch letter to the editor or managing editor. If the editor is interested in the idea, a staff writer or freelancer will be assigned to the article. You pay no fee to the magazine or the writer.

NOTE: Be wary of publications that require payment for an "article" on you, your practice or a service you offer. In essence, this is paid advertising, not editorial copy, and while distribution of these publications may be broad, readership may be minimal. If you're considering paying for an article in such a publication, talk to some of the individuals in previous issues and ask what kind of response they got for their dollars spent. If you're paying for this type of editorial-advertising, it's important that you get a return on your investment.

Other Sources. Think small as well as big when it comes to generating press coverage for your practice. Publications like church bulletins, employee newsletters and small weekly newspapers may not have a large circulation, but they have a loyal, targeted readership. If you have a link to the group, you may generate more interest and attention than you could from coverage in the daily newspaper.

MAKING CONTACT

Physicians who practice in small towns or rural areas are fortunate in one sense: it is easier in these areas to introduce yourself personally to the media. They often welcome stories, interviews and news or feature ideas.

In urban areas with competitive media, getting to know the editors and reporters is not just a question of making an appointment to meet them. They're likely to turn you down unless you have a hot news item or a truly unusual human interest angle.

Instead, introduce yourself in a personal letter in which you outline your experience, medical training, expertise and specialized knowledge. Include a brief biography of a page or less. Offer to provide background information, local comment, assistance with locating medical information or data, when needed. It's helpful if you have a legitimate news or feature suggestion in the introductory letter; it starts you off on the right foot, even if you don't sell the idea right away.

After you've introduced yourself, your goal is to keep your name before reporters, editors and producers by presenting well-thought-out ideas and information so they will think of you when they need an expert in your specialty area. Consider sending copies of articles with new findings in your specialty and current research from medical publications such as the *American Medical News, JAMA, New England Journal of Medicine* and others. Medical reporters appreciate information they don't have access to, especially when it's accompanied by an idea for a local angle. It's also a good idea to include the media on your newsletter mailing list (see Figure 9-1).

THE "HOOK"

The *hook* or angle to a news or feature story is a unique approach that convinces an editor to develop the topic. For example, let's say you're an allergy specialist who would like to present accurate information to the public about asthma. There's nothing really new about medication and

FIGURE 9-1 What Makes News?

What makes news? If you're uncertain whether your idea will be of interest to the media, ask yourself these questions:

1. Is it timely? Is it happening in the immediate future, or did it occur very recently? News is fresh, recent, unique, **new.**

2. Is it seasonal and timely in current season?

3. Does it have broad appeal? Does the topic affect a large number of people—or does it strike an emotional chord?

4. Is it unique? While the medical treatment or topic may not be, the patient's occupation or background, or the circumstances in which the injury or medical condition occurred, may be newsworthy.

---

immunotherapy as treatment, but your patients always seem startled when you recommend psychotherapy or certain forms of exercise in addition to preventive medication or injections. That's your hook: how exercise can mean respiratory and physical fitness for some asthma patients.

Or consider the physicians who opened the Texas Back Institute. Their news hook was the business opportunity in specialized back care. Remember, your angle doesn't always have to be medical. In this case, a business approach targets exactly the right audience—employers whose workers are potential patients of the Back Institute. (See Figure 9-2.)

The hook narrows and focuses the topic you propose. If you can come up with a hook, or angle, that takes the topic in a direction that no one else has, you can improve your chances of selling your idea to the media. One caution: avoid using phrases like "new" or "only" when you're trying to place a story. Telling a reporter that a procedure or treatment is brand new, or that you're "the only doctor in town" trained in a certain technique is bound to get you in trouble with your colleagues, especially when you find the physician across the street is also doing the procedure.

THE FEATURE

Seldom will a story you propose to the media qualify as true hard news. Unless you're the attending physician for a well-known celebrity with a serious medical problem, or you've had a breakthrough on a major research effort, your ideas will usually qualify as feature material.

The feature story focuses less on fact and more on emotion. This is not to say that facts are not important, only that an appeal to the senses through description is a key component of the story. Feature stories also may be less concerned with timeliness. A good feature story—say a discussion of a particular surgical procedure—will mention the date the surgery took place, but the date is not as significant as other factors surrounding the subject.

OTHER APPROACHES

For physicians and their staff, the hardest part of generating press coverage is coming up with ideas. Doctors will complain, "I just have an ordinary medical practice; I see routine problems day after day. There's no news in that."

On the contrary. It's the routine conditions that affect the largest number of people, not the exotic and unusual varieties found in textbooks and third-world countries. It's the health problems people are familiar with that they want to read about or see on television.

In addition, what seems routine to the medical professional and office staff may be newsworthy, interesting, even startling to the public.

For example, an ob-gyn specialist sees patients every day who are in various stages of pregnancy. Most of the pregnancies are routine, but

FIGURE 9-2   The Unique Angle
The "hook" or unique angle is what will interest the media in your or your subject. In this feature, the "hook" is medical care as a business opportunity. Reprinted with permission of the *Dallas Morning News.*

Physicians find gamble paying off

Plano back institute proving successful

By Joe Simnacher
Staff Writer

Dr. Stephen H. Hochschuler and Dr. Ralph F. Rashbaum thought they saw a medical need and business opportunity in specialized back care, but they weren't sure.

So when the surgeons put a rehabilitation pool in the first floor of their building — on the HCA Medical Center campus in Plano — they de-

ENTREPRENEURS

cided that if their Texas Back Institute failed, the swimming area could be ¿ome garden office space.

"It was a big risk w en we first did it," Hochschuler recalls.

Five years later, the pool is full of water and patients, busy rehabilitating their backs. The doctors not only use the building's original 14,000 square feet, but their institute now occupies a total of 50,000 square feet.

With five staff spine surgeons and two spine fellows, it is one of the largest such institutes anywhere. The two physicians think North Texas is the right place to practice medicine as a business.

Their interest in backs stemmed from their stints in the Air Force, where the two doctors saw a lot of back complaints and realized not much was known about spine problems.

"Everybody hated to deal with backs," Hochschuler said. "They hated to deal with backs, because they didn't know what do do with them, nor did we. It was just like general surgery was 100 years ago."

Hochschuler and Rashbaum met by chance at
Please see PLANO on Page 2H.

Plano back institute proving successful

Specialized clinic pays off for two Air Force buddies

Continued from Page 1H.

Sheppard Air Force Base in Wichita Falls.

Rashbaum was leaving the base exchange just as Hochschuler was entering it to buy a $60 dress uniform for the base commander's Christmas party. Rashbaum offered to sell the rookie his once-worn dress uniform for $30. The team was formed.

Hochschuler, who came to Dallas to do his residency at the University of Texas Southwestern Medical School, invited Rashbaum down to visit.

"On the weekends, I used to come here to buy bagels," Rashbaum said.

Dallas quickly moved to the top of Rashbaum's list as he searched for a site for his practice. "I decided I didn't want to live in Houston, and I knew I didn't want to go to the Northeast," Rashbaum said.

Rashbaum started his practice at the Dallas Veteran's Administration hospital. In 1978, he and Hochschuler rejoined forces, a medical association and an interest in backs that started with their military service.

The surgeons decided to establish a comprehensive back-care program — including psychology, education, rehabilitation, occupational therapy, prevention and post-rehabilitation return to normal activities.

"We cover the whole gamut," Hochschuler said. "Even though the founding physicians in this group and the main physicians in that group are spine surgeons, we probably operate on less than 10 percent of the patients we see."

To assist the surgeons in their young program, they brought in a multidisciplinary team. The institute now employs doctors, therapists, nurses and assistants.

Hochschuler said 40 percent of the Texas Back Institute's patients come from a 50- to 100-mile radius of the clinic. But individuals 'have traveled from as far away as Seoul, South Korea, for treatment.

The doctors said Dallas' entrepreneurial spirit played an important role in establishing their clinic.

"I've never lived in a place that's been more optimistic," Hochschuler said. "We're still in a recession, and most people are pretty positive. That's terrific. The East Coast doesn't have as good an attitude."

Like many others in the Dallas medical and business communities, the doctors recently took a look at the marketing side of their business.

"We didn't understand anything about marketing," Hochschuler said.

To their surprise, the institute's marketing program has actually improved the quality of medical care they offer.

The marketing program's initial effort surveyed patient's attitudes toward the institute, asking such questions as: "How long did you have to wait? Who referred you?" and "How far did you travel?"

"Medicine is a strange business," Mooney said. "The more it becomes a business, the more complex the issues get."

The controversial element of the Texas Back Institute's marketing program is its direct advertising to the public, circumventing the traditional primary-care physician's re-

something that doesn't always sit well with other doctors.

"I guarantee you, the average physician doesn't think of those things," Hochschuler said.

Dr. Vert Mooney, chairman of orthopedic surgery at UT Southwestern Medical School, said the Texas Back Institute does a good job in both practicing medicine and operating a business —

ferral.

"They're trying to get the patient who has a backache to show up . . . and those who need surgery are funneled into their care, which I guess is the American way," Mooney said. "It's offensive to the rest of the doctors who are as equally competent, but don't feel it's useful to advertise — mostly because they haven't put themselves in a pack-

age like that that can afford advertising."

But having seen the success of their program, the back institute founders said all Dallas medicine should more actively seek patients rather than reacting to lost business.

"Unlike the Cleveland Clinic and the Mayo Clinic that have marketed themselves . . . Dallas hasn't

done a thing," Hochschuler said.

Ira Korman, director of Humana Hospital Medical-City Dallas, said the Texas Back Institute is unique as a private clinic in its spine research and rehabilitation efforts. He also applauded their efforts on the business front.

"They are more in step with the times," Korman said. "It reflects the challenge of today."

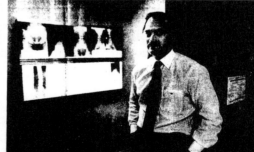

The Dallas Morning News: Juan Garcia

Stephen Hochschuler says 40 percent of the Texas Back Institute's patients come from a 50- to 100-mile radius of the clinic in Plano.

perhaps one in ten will experience some complication like diabetes, tox-emia, or multiple births.

To the public, *all* of these conditions are unusual. In fact, if he or she were to present the idea clearly and succinctly, the obstetrician might be able to persuade the local Sunday newspaper magazine supplement to do a feature on the ten most common complications of pregnancy. The obstetrician would be a source of information, and could also recommend other sources such as the American College of Obstetrics and Gynecology.

It's a good idea to meet weekly with your staff to review potential media ideas. Sometimes, the individual who will be able to pinpoint a potential story is the staff member who has the least clinical knowledge, since she will be looking at it from the non-medical point of view.

GETTING THE NEWS OUT

There are many ways to ensure that your news reaches the proper media source. Using the proper method of contact will heighten your chances that attention is paid to your news once it reaches the source.

Press Release Pointers. A press release is a brief typewritten, factual narrative about an event, individual or news item. Writing a press release is not difficult, and neither is getting it read if you follow a few guidelines. A sample press release is shown in Figure 9-3.

1. Don't write a press release unless the subject warrants it. A class you're of-fering, a promotion, a new office location may be appropriate material. As a rule, a feature story should not be developed as a press release. Major pub-lications prefer to assign their own reporters to write feature articles; it's best with small publications to contact the editor first and see if there's interest in using your proposed piece. If the answer is yes, then you can develop it in press release format.
2. Be brief. Limit most releases to one page. Reporters and editors get hundreds of pieces of mail across their desk every day. No matter how scintillating your writing style, they're not going to wade through three pages of descriptive detail of your practice open house. If the editor wants additional information, he or she will call you.
3. Include the who, what, where, when, how and why first, with other details in descending order of importance. This decreases the chance of essential infor-mation being deleted in the editing process, since articles are usually cut from the bottom up.
4. Stick to the facts. Hyperbole and outlandish statements don't belong in a press release.
5. Send press releases to specifìc names, not just titles, e.g. "Jane Doe, Assign-ment Editor, KTKV-TV," not "Assignment Desk, WBCD-TV."
6. Be sure to include the date, and the date the news can be announced (if different from the date on which it's mailed or delivered.) If the date is the same, use the words "For Immediate Release" below the date.
7. A name and telephone number of a contact person for the editor should always be included on a press release.
8. Allow ample time before an event or occurrence when mailing a release. Two

FIGURE 9-3   Sample Press Release

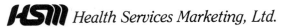

HSM *Health Services Marketing, Ltd.*

Marketing · Strategic Planning · Communications · Research

June 13, 1987

FOR IMMEDIATE RELEASE

DERMATOLOGY INSTITUTE
ANNOUNCES NEW CLINIC

A Wednesday evening clinic for persons suffering from
psoriasis has been started by the physicians of the Dermatology
Institute in Springfield.

The clinic will be held every Wednesday from 7 to 9 p.m. and
will provide diagnosis and treatment by dermatologists. In
addition, a support group will be formed if enough interest is
expressed. It will be lead by Karen Helppe, M.A., a counselor
affiliated with the Dermatology Institute. There is no charge
for the support group.

The psoriasis clinic was formed because the problems
experienced by sufferers are chronic and painful and require
ongoing treatment, according to dermatologist Jackson Clerskin,
M.D., Dermatology Institute medical director.

Appointments are requested for the clinic. For more
information, call 999-9999.

-30-

FOR MORE INFORMATION, CALL:
Ima Nerss, RN
Dermatology Institute
999-9999

6908 E. Thomas Rd., Scottsdale, Arizona 85251   (602) 947-8078
3756 LaVista Road, Suite 200   Tucker, Georgia 30084   (404) 634-6855

to three weeks in advance is not too soon for a daily or weekly publication.

9. Make your news release readable and professional. Type in upper and lower case and double-space it, being sure to check for grammatical and spelling accuracy, especially with names.

10. Don't belabor the obvious, exaggerate the facts or call something "unique" if it's not.

11. Some editors don't mind a follow-up call to confirm receipt of your press release

and to ask if there are any additional questions you can answer. Others do. The best way to find out is to get to know the editors and reporters you're dealing with. Meet them personally, if possible; perhaps the first time you do a press release, you could hand-deliver it.

12. Sometimes a fact sheet may be appropriate to include with a press release. A fact sheet is just what it says: a summary sheet outlining important facts and details pertaining to a topic. The fact sheet should be one page only, and written in bullet listings, rather than paragraph form.

The Query Letter. Often you'll have better success in generating media coverage if you send a personal letter to an individual reporter or editor. This is called a query letter, and it describes a specific story idea, and outlines why it is appropriate for coverage by the publication or station. You also should describe your own expertise, experience or interest in the topic in order to provide a reason for the reporter to use you as a source. It's a good idea to include a brief biography and perhaps a practice brochure or practice information. Your query should be a page or less. Follow it up with a phone call after a week or two.

It's important not to send the same letter or idea to more than one reporter or editor at a time. Generally, a query indicates exclusivity. If you offer the idea to several editors and more than one wants to follow up on it, you may jeopardize your relationships with the editors contacted.

A sample query letter is shown in Figure 9-4.

The News Tip Sheet. This option is available to physicians in larger communities where there are several newspapers and magazines and a variety of radio and television stations. In smaller communities, the press release or personal contact makes more sense and is more likely to get results.

The news tip sheet lists four or five different health or medical story ideas pertaining to your practice or specialty. A one-paragraph description of each idea is sufficient, but the paragraph must be written succinctly, factually and in attention-grabbing style.

Ideas in a news tip sheet should be relatively timeless in nature, because editors will hang on to the "tip sheet" for months. In fact, it's a good idea to include a cover letter the first time you send out a tip sheet, explaining what you're enclosing and encouraging the editor to hold on to it for reference when he or she needs a health care story quickly. And, of course, if something occurs nationally that relates to an item on your news tip sheet, send out an update with details on the national event so that reporters can consider localizing it. An excellent example of a national medical story that was given local treatment with a physician interview is shown in Figure 9-5.

Personal Contact. There are times when the best way to get your story publicized is to contact a reporter or editor personally via the telephone. It's most effective when the idea you wish to present is uncomplicated and can be easily explained and understood.

FIGURE 9-4 Sample Query Letter

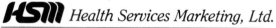 **Health Services Marketing, Ltd.**

Marketing · Strategic Planning · Communications · Research

May 28, 1988

Maybelle Smith
Cityville Business Gazette
1234 N. Central
Cityville, USA 86666

Dear Maybelle:

The Hispanic market is getting special attention all across the
country by businesses and services suddenly realizing that this
ethnic group makes up an important segment of the consuming
public.

That's true in Cityville, too, where Hispanics are more than 10
percent of the population. At Jones Medical Clinic, we are
acknowledging in several ways the need to communicate with our
Hispanic patients.

Not only are many Hispanics seen at the clinic, we also actively
seek out Hispanic patients, with screening programs at such
locations as the Francisco de Gamey Senior Center and Primavera
Casa in South Cityville. Our 20-member staff at the Jones
Medical Clinic is currently taking a Spanish class. It is taught
by two RNs to assure that medical as well as everyday language
and slang are translated.

In addition, we have translated into Spanish all the forms we
use. Since I am fluent in Spanish, it makes sense to target this
population, especially because I lived in several Latin American
countries following college graduation.

If you're interested in pursuing a story on how a physician is
targeting the hispanic market, I'd be happy to talk with you.
Please call me at 999-9999 for more information.

Sincerely,

Ivan M. Jones, M.D.

6908 E. Thomas Rd., Scottsdale, Arizona 85251 (602) 947-8078
3756 LaVista Road, Suite 200 Tucker, Georgia 30084 (404) 634-6855

Calendar Notices. Don't forget the calendar listings in newspapers,
magazines, on radio and television stations, as well as in small publications
like church bulletins, and organization newsletters for announcement of a
coming event, a class or other scheduled event. While brief, such listings
are cumulative in their effect; if you mail your notice early enough, you
can hit a variety of publications and stations.

The Press Conference. On very rare occasions, a press conference

FIGURE 9-5 Stimulate Media Interest

Articles that appear in professional publications can be used to stimulate media interest in a timely topic. A family physician or pediatrician could contact a TV or newspaper health reporter, provide them with a copy of this article, and offer to be interviewed on appropriate use of over-the-counter medication for children. The media appreciates receiving topical information to which they may otherwise not have access. From *American Medical News*, November 13, 1987.

Mothers need more education about drugs for children

Many mothers keep home medicine chests well-stocked for treating their children, but often use the drugs ineffectively and sometimes dangerously, says a U. of Michigan researcher.

"There is a tremendous need to educate mothers about which over-the-counter medicines are useful for what symptoms and about which over-the-counter medications not to use," said Marshall H. Becker, PhD, professor and associate dean at the U. of Michigan School of Public Health.

Mothers also need to be alerted to the potential danger of saving prescription drugs for reuse after they have expired, he said. Tetracycline, for example, can be toxic if used beyond its shelf life.

Dr. Becker recommends that pediatricians assume the primary role in educating mothers about using medications.

"Pediatricians nowadays are widely involved with well-care because we have a generally healthy population," he said. "It's the ideal role for pediatricians as educators; it makes the doctor's visit more worthwhile to the mothers."

IN ONE STUDY, Dr. Becker and colleagues interviewed 500 mothers about the kinds of drugs they stocked and which ones they gave to their children.

All 500 mothers reported giving their children medications. Seventy-nine percent said they would medicate their children for fever without consulting a physician. And 50% of the mothers kept seven or more categories of drugs on hand for their children.

THE STUDY CONCLUDED with a panel of six pediatricians reviewing data from interviews and scoring the mothers on their choice of drugs and how effectively the drugs were used. Overall ratings were low to moderate. The mothers got fairly high marks for the use of painkillers and low marks for the use of vitamins.

"Vitamins are the perfect example of an abused over-the-counter drug," Dr. Becker said. "There are children in parts of the country who are in trouble, who are starving, on poor diets, who may benefit from vitamin supplements. But those are rare events. The vast majority of children in this country don't need vitamin supplementation."

In addition, the pediatric panel found that the mothers often picked relatively useless over-the-counter medications to treat upset stomachs and skin rashes, but made moderately wiser choices when treating their children for headaches and cold symptoms.

Dr. Becker noted that some mothers give laxatives to their children every day in the hope that the medication will prevent constipation. Others give their children aspirin tablets daily to prevent headaches. Neither practice is necessary and both can cause health problems, he noted.

THE PEDIATRIC PANEL gave overall lower ratings to mothers of lower socioeconomic status.

"There is clear evidence from our work that the greater problems are with children of lower socioeconomic status," Dr. Becker said.

A number of forces act to influence mothers to medicate their children, he noted. Some believe they are well-informed about the use of medicines and some actually are. Others want to avoid the cost of going to a physician or hospital. Some mothers become annoyed when they take their children in to see a physician, only to be told that the child has a common cold and nothing can be done.

"Pediatricians need to be educated to talk with mothers about medicating their children and to ask mothers what medicines they have been giving to their children," Dr. Becker said.

"We need to raise everybody's consciousness about it, but it's best to get pediatricians talking about it," he said.

may be appropriate as a method of getting the word out to all the major media. However, the press conference is usually reserved for announcing a major decision or occurrence. An example of an event that might be appropriately announced through a press conference would be if a large group of ob-gyn specialists were to decide to cease obstetrical services in protest against high malpractice premiums. Or a cardiovascular specialist who plans to build an institute for the study of cardiac disease might announce it at a press conference. This gives all the media an equal opportunity to ask questions.

If you decide your announcement warrants a press conference, follow these guidelines:

1. Be aware of media deadlines and try to plan around them. Daily newspapers published in the afternoon generally must have their information prior to noon; morning papers have until 5 or 6 PM for non-latebreaking news. TV stations begin editing for their evening newscast by 3 PM. The best time for a news conference is 9:30 or 10 AM for a morning event, or 1:30 or 2 PM for one held in the afternoon.
2. Keep your notice brief and to the point. Specify in the heading that it's a press conference notice. Stick to the basic facts: what the topic of the conference will be, why it's being held, the time, date and place, and who will be present to answer media questions.
3. Send out the notice at least a week before the date set for your press conference.
4. Prepare media packets for everyone attending. The media packet should include a *fact sheet,* a *press release* covering the information you provide verbally at the press conference; *biographies* of key individuals; 5 x 7 or 8 x 10 *glossy black and white photos* of pertinent individuals, facilities or equipment under discussion at the press conference; and any related material such as journal articles that may be helpful to the media.

Public Service Announcements. Public service announcements, or PSAs, are available on a limited basis to individuals and groups holding free public events. The event should be educational and general in nature, preferably involving other community organizations and agencies as well as private practitioner(s). For instance, a seminar on radial keratotomy offered by an ophthalmologist probably would not qualify for PSA time, but a health fair by an ophthalmologist involving the local eye bank, the Society for the Prevention of Blindness and other agencies might. The purpose of the event should be public benefit.

PSAs vary in lengths of 10, 20, 30 and 60 seconds. Many radio stations will accept typewritten PSAs as long as they follow the appropriate format, but some prefer or will accept only audiotapes. It's best to check with each station. TV stations also vary; some will take written copy plus 1–3 slides; others want only ¾″ videotapes.

Be brief and to the point; there's no time for details, only the highlights such as event, place, date, and telephone number for contact. Try to repeat the telephone number (or practice name) at least once. Time your PSA by reading it aloud at the same pace as a radio announcer, then cut words as needed.

PSAs should be typed in all caps (this is the only time all caps is used for any information to the media), with the pronunciation of unusual names given phonetically in parentheses.

Specify at the beginning of each PSA how long it is. You should send at least three different PSA lengths to each station; for example, on one page you can include a 10-, 20- and 30-second PSA. Indicate the date the announcement should begin to run and when it should stop (i.e. if the event occurs on Feb. 18, you may ask that your PSA begin Feb. 11 and continue through Feb. 18.)

Be a Winner with the Press. A reporter with the Metropolitan Daily News calls you. She has received your query letter and is interested in your idea for an article discussing advantages and disadvantages of over-the-counter remedies for the common cold. She also wants some medical tips on self-care for colds. "I'd like to do a telephone interview sometime within the next few days," she says. "When would be the best time for you?"

"How about this afternoon after 5:30?" you suggest. "I'll be through with patients and will have an uninterrupted block of time. That way you'll be sure to meet your deadline."

"I appreciate that," Lois says. "But I've got an appointment scheduled already for that time. What about tomorrow?"

"I've got a full patient load tomorrow, but I could take some time during the middle of the day. I have to return patient calls at noon, but I should be done with that by 12:30. Why don't we say 12:45 just to be safe? Will that fit in with your deadline?"

"Great," Lois says. Meanwhile she's thinking, "This doctor puts his patients before me. Now that kind of doctor impresses me!"

You make arrangements for the interview and hang up. She's pleased that the interview has been so easily scheduled, and you're pleased to have gotten a response to an idea you've suggested. The toughest part is done, you think. .

Many an interview subject does a great deal of planning regarding media contact *up to the time of the interview*. Then, with the thought that an interview is simply a matter of imparting wisdom to a lay person, he or she does no further preparation. That's a mistake. You'll find a complete list of *Tips for Media Interviews* in the Appendix.

IN CONCLUSION

Press coverage can be one of the most effective components of your marketing plan. It enhances and adds credibility to your practice and to an advertising campaign, gets your patients talking about you to their family, friends, neighbors and co-workers, and is an ethical means of practice promotion. But as we've emphasized, the effect of media contact and the resulting coverage is cumulative; one phone call or one article won't create instant results.

Take advantage of the opportunity that awaits you with the media. The public wants to know how you can help them get healthy and stay that way, and reporters and editors want to hear from you.

BIBLIOGRAPHY

Dan, BB: One Minute Medicine. *JAMA* 1987; May 22: 2798.

Longsdorf R: Will a Press Agent Help or Hinder Your Image? *Private Practice* 1983; July: 20.

Speakes L, Pack R: Beat the Press. *TV Guide* 1988; May 14: 4.

Chapter 10

The Public Relations Benefits
of Community Involvement

Upon researching the conditions in women's shelters in her city, a family practice physician was appalled that no health care was available to these women and their children. Taking her healing arts to the street, she spent several hours each Saturday afternoon at a local shelter treating women and children who had been battered or abandoned.

Her efforts were picked up by the local media, which gave her extensive publicity. As a result, she was asked to speak to local civic groups about the health care plight of these broken families. Her work earned her numerous awards as well as the respect of the community.

Her family medicine practice grew because people perceived her as a compassionate, caring physician. This doctor not only demonstrated humane values while practicing good medicine, she was practicing public relations.

Public relations affects almost everyone who has contact with others. But public relations is not an all-encompassing label to hang on special events or people who make news. It is not advertising or sales. Rather, it is an attempt to align an organization's concern with the public interest. Public relations is establishing and nurturing a meaningful relationship with the public. In the medical field, this can be defined as "community involvement."

While specific definitions of public relations (PR) differ, the effective practice of good PR involves the following:

- A foundation of knowledge
- Solid judgment
- Strong communication skills
- Uncompromised professionalism
- Accurate interpretation of public needs
- Dissemination of the sought-after message to the public

According to Walt Seifer, Professor of Public Relations in the School of Journalism at Ohio State University, public relations is "doing good and making sure you get caught." Another way of saying this is "good deeds made known."

Effective public relations involves a four-part process known as the RACE approach.

- Research
- Action
- Communication
- Evaluation

Or more simply, it is planning, doing, telling and proving.

PUBLIC RELATIONS AND THE PHYSICIAN

As a physician, you are a step ahead in applying public relations principles. Your approach to the diagnosis and treatment of medical problems is based on the RACE plan.

You begin **research** by examining the patient and gathering information about his or her symptoms. Next, you determine your course of treatment, or **action.** Then you help the patient understand how to assist in the course of treatment, and what outcome may be expected, by **communication.** Finally, you **evaluate** the patient's progress to determine the success of the treatment.

In this chapter, we will discuss just what public relations is—and what it is not—and explain how to identify an opportunity for beneficial community involvement or public relations by applying the RACE approach. You'll also find detailed instructions for applying public relations techniques in planning special events, and generating public speaking engagements as well as generating print, radio and television coverage.

· First, let's review the RACE approach:

- **Research.** Determining the needs of the community and how, through your professional commitment and interest, you can assist in meeting those needs.
- **Action.** Strategies and tactics for implementing targeted public relations efforts in your community.
- **Communication.** Utilizing your staff, patients, the media and community groups to disseminate health education as well as information about you, your practice and your services.
- **Evaluation.** Assessing your public relations efforts for results. Did the strategy yield phone calls? Patients? Requests for information?

COMMUNITY AWARENESS: RESEARCH

Communities vary greatly in their mix of ages, ethnicity, occupations, income and interests. These demographic differences can have a profound impact on the success or failure of a particular public relations approach. It's a good idea, therefore, to know the demographic mix of your community or your service area, and the people you want to know about your practice or services. These are some factors you will consider:

Population. A rural area or small town will not have the same problems or needs that a more heavily populated urban area will have.

Size of the Area. The geographic size of your service area will determine how broad or narrow your approach must be, such as addressing a whole city through a newspaper article or just a community civic organization.

Age. The age breakdown of the population will guide you in determining the needs of that community. A community with a high percentage of individuals over 65, for example, will need more information on diseases of aging.

Income. A wealthier community may be interested in technological advances in elective surgery, whereas a lower income community will want to know how to make their health care dollars go farther.

Social Structure (marital status, ethnic background). This is a most important area for you in determining your public relations goals. By studying the social units in the community, you can determine appropriate topics and audiences for your speaking engagements, special events and other strategies.

Occupation. Primary trades and industries in your service area can mean a great deal to your medical practice. An employer with a large number of manual laborers will have a high percentage of back problems— a significant patient base for an orthopedic surgeon.

Small local newspapers provide an excellent source for monitoring trends and changes in the community. By reading the local weekly paper as well as the metropolitan daily, you can obtain ideas on timely subjects for speaking engagements, and decide where your services are most needed. A community's concerns, needs and values are expressed in newspaper editorials and articles. For example, let's say you have done your homework and have found the following information about your community:

1. There are four new subdivisions of moderately priced homes.
2. There are three local high schools and a junior college that offers a vocational program.
3. Four high-rise apartments for the elderly are also in the community.
4. The population is 25,000, but the 25–39 age group has experienced a 15 percent increase in the past five years.
5. An increasing number of young couples are buying and restoring homes in a formerly rundown neighborhood a mile from your practice.
6. The paper reveals concerns about a toxic waste dump, strong support for the local soccer team, and a large number of health conscious people who participate in regular exercise classes offered through the "Y." Seniors also have several active groups and senior centers.

Let's see where you can begin implementing public relations strategies that will benefit your practice:

With the abundance of high schools, there will be parents active in the PTA. Develop talks and classes on children and stress, substance abuse and teenagers, AIDS and other sexually-transmitted diseases, parental counseling, acne. For the grammar schools, speak to parents on the use and value of immunizations, common infectious problems like head lice, childhood illnesses, first-aid techniques parents should know, and other concerns of parents.

Visit elementary and junior high schools to educate youngsters about the dangers of smoking and drugs and the importance of water and bike safety.

The high-rise apartments for the elderly present opportunities for you and your staff to provide screenings for cataracts, diabetes, arthritis and many other conditions that develop with age. You can speak on vitamins and diet, stress and heart disease, exercise and osteoporosis, Alzheimer's and memory loss, and aging gracefully. Have a pharmaceutical company provide free vitamin samples, and offer educational information with your name, practice name and telephone number on it.

The young couples settling in the neighborhood near your office would probably be interested in establishing an affiliation with a physician who is so conveniently located. Perhaps you could let them know through a welcome letter about your evening and weekend hours and other services.

Every age group would welcome the opportunity to talk to a doctor first-hand—without paying for it. A multi-specialty group practice could host its own series of "Conversations with the Doctor" featuring a different specialist each week, moving the series from site to site, and always notifying the media in advance. When the newest diet book hits the bestseller lists, suggest a feature story to the local paper on fad diets. Write a letter to the editor about the hazard to the community if a toxic dump should be placed in the area.

These are just a few ideas that can be implemented once you have done research and know the community where you live and practice.

TIME FOR ACTION

A physician in the town described previously was surprised at how little effort it took to interest the newspaper in doing an article on the benefits of walking as a form of exercise, particularly for the elderly. She used one of her patients, a 76-year-old great-grandmother, as an example. The article generated positive comments from her patients, and even a few appointments from the young couples in the nearby neighborhood. A month later, the newspaper contacted the doctor again, this time for background for an article on the benefits and hazards of over-the-counter medications for treatment of aches and strains due to injury or age. The doctor provided helpful information, then suggested the reporter also talk to a pharmacist she knew. The referral solidified a developing referral relationship between the doctor and pharmacist. When the article appeared, the doctor sent thank-you notes commending the factual nature to the reporter and editor, and tacked a copy on her office bulletin board for patients to see.

Public relations begins with a commitment of time and energy. To determine how much time you can devote to your effort, the self-assessment reviewed in Chapter 3 is helpful.

Be realistic in determining your public relations commitment. Remain flexible in developing your strategies and learn to recognize and take advantage of an opportunity when one emerges, bringing your staff into the effort whenever possible. Allow time for planning, implementation and evaluation of your efforts. Your practice will not suffer, it will grow—if you utilize time and energy wisely in increasing your visibility and activity in the community. Don't just participate in a special event because it's *there*. Do it because it will yield results: new patients or requests for information.

Avenues for public relations exist everywhere. Your choices are determined by how much time you have to give, who your target audience is and what your interests and objectives are. Here are suggestions on where to get started: Join church, civic and professional organizations. Offer to speak on health issues to church groups, civic organizations, business associations, service clubs, local schools and the PTA. Hold classes and seminars on current health topics for the public and special interest groups. Encourage your staff to become active in local organizations and clubs that interest them. Write articles for the local papers. Become active in groups which share your hobbies or personal interests, such as sports, travel or the arts. Give your business card to everyone you meet. Align your medical specialty with the needs of your area, such as pediatricians with schools, orthopedists with sports injury, and gynecologists with women's health. Utilize the airwaves by offering to host a health-oriented question-and-answer format radio show. Do a segment on the local newscast about how to stop smoking and avoid weight gain.

Donate your time to an organization or agency requiring your medical knowledge. Do as Sydney Crackower, MD, of Abbeville, Louisiana does and sponsor an occasional free clinic for patients with no insurance or who are indigent. Or hold an annual free flu shot program.

Have an open house or holiday party for referring physicians, hospital surgical and emergency department nurses and other professionals, or current and potential patients. Offer tours or career talks to students, and get involved in career fairs. Hold a seminar on Alzheimer's disease for public fiduciaries, attorneys, trust officers and social workers.

Include your patients in your promotional efforts by displaying newspaper clippings and special achievements by you and your staff on a bulletin board. Have a health fair for the community and invite area pharmacies, pharmaceutical company reps and local health care agencies to participate, and possibly help sponsor it, with services and information.

Such public relations activities will enhance the community's perception of you as a doctor concerned about the health and well-being of people in the community.

PUBLIC SPEAKING: COMMUNICATING EFFECTIVELY TO THE COMMUNITY

Initiating or accepting opportunities to speak is one of the most effective ways to reach potential patients. It's the next best thing to a personal conversation because it allows people to hear you and form an impression in a face-to-face setting. Public speaking allows you to increase your community recognition and involvement. An entertaining and informative presentation by a skilled, knowledgeable speaker creates an image of professional concern, while providing relevant health information. Finally, public speaking allows you to position yourself as an expert on a particular topic—because you choose the topic(s) and the audience(s) you address.

There are unlimited occasions for physicians who are willing to speak at no charge. If you have a flair for public speaking and feel comfortable doing so, this may be one of your primary techniques for increasing your visibility in the community. If you're not comfortable with public speaking, and/or you don't do it well, you're not alone. In that case, consider taking a Dale Carnegie course or joining Toastmasters. You'll conquer your fear of public speaking while at the same time making new contacts.

Make It Memorable. In order to assure that your speaking engagement is memorable and aimed at the right group, these are steps you should take:

- Identify your target audience
- Select or refine your topic
- Define the message you want to send
- Select audiovisuals, demonstrations or other techniques to add sparkle to your talk.

First, list several groups you have identified as appropriate audiences. Write a personal letter to the president or program chairperson about your interest in being a guest speaker at no cost. Offer two or three topics with which you are comfortable, topics with a timely angle (which can be easily updated) and that would be of interest to the group. Be sure to have your staff follow up your letter with a phone call within a week or two. It can also be helpful in gathering information you can use in your talk, and making contacts for you. Be an effective delegator, but be sure to thank your staff for their help.

Below are some groups and topics you may wish to consider:

- **Rotary, Kiwanis and other civic or fraternal clubs.** Prostate problems, impotence, laser surgery in heart disease, stress reduction, cancer prevention, cosmetic surgery for men.
- **Retirement communities, senior centers, elderly housing complexes.** Nutrition and vitamin therapy, osteoporosis, exercise, incontinence, skin care, depression, hearing loss, diminished senses, arthritis and joint problems.

- **Youth groups.** Skin care, exercise, nutrition, dealing with stress, physical and emotional changes of adolescence, alternatives to drugs, teen suicide, family relationships.
- **Women's groups.** What a pelvic exam reveals, menopause, PMS, coping with the physical changes of aging, mammograms, cosmetic surgery, stress, family relationships, skin care/dermatological problems, first aid.
- **Cancer Society, Diabetes Association, Heart Association.** Specific breakthroughs, the latest news in diagnosis, technology and treatment.
- **Support groups for catastrophic illnesses.** Full explanation of the condition, the importance of maintaining contact with the person involved, ways in which the family can cope.
- **Professional groups, business organizations.** Stress reduction, nutrition, exercise, slowing down the pace, physical exams, looking your best through cosmetic surgery or dermabrasion, chemical face lifts and other nonsurgical techniques.

You can purchase current lists of organizations and their officers from the Chamber of Commerce and mailing houses. Or check the Yellow Pages under "Associations," "Senior Organizations," etc.

As you become a regular on the speaking circuit, people will begin to contact you about engagements. Then you can become more selective, choosing those groups most likely to benefit from the services of your practice as well as from the information you have to offer.

Do Your Homework. Once you've received an invitation to speak, you should do a little homework. Gather basic information about the group and its members. A contact person within the group can help you by lending insight into the demographics, experiences, values and interests of the group. The contact person can also assist with any special needs you may have regarding audiovisual equipment or handout materials.

Be sure your topics are appropriate to the audience. A group of professional women may benefit from a talk on ways to reduce the stress of career and family, or nutrition tips. Seniors may find a talk on new medications and therapies for osteoarthritis helpful, with demonstrations on how to keep joints mobile. Bring a staff member or invite a physical or occupational therapist to demonstrate some simple stretching and ROM exercises for the elderly. (An added benefit when you involve another health care professional is that you generate or enhance referral relationships.)

The elementary school Parent-Teacher Association would be a receptive group for talks dealing with the welfare of children. How about a discussion of infectious illnesses in children: how to recognize and treat them, which ones to worry about, and why doctors prescribe the treatments they do?

Your speaking engagement will have more impact—and potential for media coverage—if aligned with a timely or newsworthy medical event. When a near-drowning occurs in your community, a talk on pool safety and the value of CPR suddenly becomes very popular. People are emotionally receptive to a speech that relates to a newsmaking event or person. You will receive more questions and audience involvement. And don't forget, if you're scheduled to give a talk on a topic that's getting media attention, let the newspapers, TV news desks, and radio talk show hosts know. They may perceive you as an expert for future interviews, and may decide to cover your talk.

An example of a newsworthy event was the mammogram, biopsy and modified radical mastectomy former First Lady Nancy Reagan underwent for breast cancer. Following this type of medical news, requests for information and speakers on the subject soar. So when a medical breakthrough hits the general media; when a celebrity develops a disease, has surgery or specialized treatment; or when unusual circumstances bring an ordinary person into the healthcare spotlight, be sure you let your hospital public relations department and appropriate media outlets know if you have a special expertise on the topic. They'll be seeking physicians who can localize national news.

Visual Aids Add Sparkle. One of the best ways to get your message across and hold the interest of the audience is with visual aids. The more frequently you use these aids, the more comfortable you become with them. Here is an assortment of visual aids you may wish to use:

Handout: A printed piece that provides a brief summary and offers additional information on a specific health care topic. Be sure to include your name, address and telephone number on the handout.

Flip Charts and Boards: Use this to highlight points and to present questions to be answered in a logical format. Always concentrate on the chart first, then turn toward the audience before continuing to speak. Never speak with your back to the audience. Practice using a flip chart until you are comfortable; it's not as simple as effective speakers make it seem.

Posters and Transparencies: Add a professional touch and graphic explanation to your presentation. Use to emphasize key points. Keep the language simple and the format uncluttered.

Slides, Videos or Film: Use these to add drama and action to your presentation. Become familiar with your equipment before attempting to show slides or videos. If you are using your own audiovisual aids, you will want as professional a product as possible. This will require a small investment, but it's well worth the return. (And remember, you can often use them in your practice for patient education.)

Whatever visuals you use, you must become comfortable in manipulating the equipment as you speak so you will not distract the audience. It's best to have an assistant, if possible. A member of your staff can do this, and also help distribute handouts, collect question cards, and make certain everyone signs a guest book or mailing list for health care information. Develop an evaluation form to get audience feedback on your speaking technique, topic, visual materials, etc. (See Figure 10-1.)

Speaking Up. To be a good speaker, you must establish a bond with your audience. They must feel that you understand them. To achieve that bond, try to incorporate these suggestions into your presentation and style.

FIGURE 10-1   Speaker Evaluation Form

1. Did the topic interest you? _____ Yes _____ No

2. Was the topic relevant to you? _____ Yes _____ No

3. Please rate the speaker's presentation skills:
   ____Excellent ____Fair ____Poor

4. Would you recommend the speaker to other groups?
   _____Yes _____No

5. What other health care topics would interest you?
   _____
   _____

6. Please list other organizations of which you are a member that you feel would enjoy this or a similar presentation:
   _____

Name (Optional) _____

Address _____

- Know the major characteristics of your audience, and try to find some experience, interest or characteristic you share with them. This will establish the connection between you and your listeners early. It helps if you learn something specific about one or two individuals in the audience, and refer to it during your presentation. You become one of them.

- Vary the inflection of your voice. Make a point not only with your words, but with your voice tone, pitch and volume. Whisper to be heard. Put a smile into it. Make your speech patterns, as well as your speech, interesting.

- Be sincere. Sound committed. If you read your speech, your lack of commitment will be obvious. Use a well-fleshed outline rather than a fully spelled-out talk. Mean what you say. If you don't, your audience will know it.

- How's your timing? Do you use pauses, rich and lengthy, to draw out a point? Do you speed up to convey a sense of urgency in a phrase? Practice your timing. Use it to increase the impact of what you say.

- Use frequent examples, case studies, actual experiences to illustrate your points. People identify with descriptive situations, and they grab your meaning more quickly if you illustrate it. Collect stories from your practice, from books, magazines, newspapers, your colleagues.

- Involve your audience. Ask them questions. Ask for comments and opinions. Give them a brief form, a game, a quick quiz to complete. Use their names.

- Read. Be familiar with your community, your audience, their concerns and interests. Stay current with the news in medicine and the world at large.

- Once you've developed a good presentation, work on developing another. And another. If you become a popular speaker, you'll need variety in your topics, or soon repeat audience members will spread the word: "Oh, I've heard this one before. . . ." Adapt your talks to changes in medicine, your community, your audience. Change the stories and examples you tell. Incorporate new ones; update the old ones. Keep the pizazz in your presentation.

- Practice. And practice some more. You'll become more comfortable, and it will show. Your audience will become more comfortable with you, and that will make you a better speaker.

PUBLICITY: THE *COMMUNICATION* COMPONENT

Publicity is the most well-known aspect of public relations. Publicity broadens public knowledge and awareness and provides positive recognition about an organization or business, its people and activities. And while there are other facets of the communication phase of the RACE approach, publicity gained through media coverage is probably the most broad-based.

The potential for publicity for your speaking engagement or community action effort exists both before and after an event. But you must take the initiative. Following the guidelines described in Chapter 9, you can generate media coverage if you *actively* initiate contact with a reporter, send a press release, or call the TV news assignment desk. Be certain that you've gained approval from the co-sponsor or community group if the speaking engagement or event involves others, however. Develop a brief fact sheet and bio about yourself and your topic or event for distribution to appropriate media outlets. Mail your press release at least one to two weeks before the event, and keep it brief. One page is enough.

OTHER COMMUNICATION TECHNIQUES

You can't depend entirely on the media to get the word out about your talk, health fair, classes or seminars, sponsorship of a contest or awards, program or other promotion project. Fortunately, there are a number of other communication techniques available for making the public aware of what you're doing. For example:

Your Practice Newsletter. A practice newsletter is a well-read source of information about speaking engagements and community events you are involved in. It's even more helpful when it is distributed to a variety of audiences: patients, referral sources, health and social service agencies, community organizations, senior and/or day care centers and the media. In it you can promote all practice activities, awards and events in the newsletter before and after they occur, with comments from participants and perhaps even photos. And you should definitely send copies of the newsletter to anyone not currently on the mailing list who may be mentioned or pictured in your publication.

Employee Publications for Local Firms/Industries: Depending on the topic, editors of some employee publications welcome articles that provide health information and tips for preventing injury, illness or disease. If you're sponsoring a class for the public on first aid, or a free health screening, the editor may accept an article pointing out the benefits of knowing first aid techniques along with mention of the class. With your staff's assistance, you might even develop a series of brief health tips that could be supplied to local employee publications at regular intervals.

School Newspapers. If you can suggest a tie-in to a school activity or to student concerns, you may be able to arrange to be interviewed by a reporter for a high school newspaper.

Public Service Announcements (PSAs). A free event that's open to the public and of broad interest may be promoted by the local media through public service announcements. This topic is covered in Chapter 9.

Posters and Flyers. Fast food restaurants, day care centers, schools and other locations may be willing to distribute flyers and/or allow you to put up a poster promoting a special event if it's of interest to their students, clients or customers. You may wish to consider a co-sponsorship in order to broaden the market you reach, to have access to mailing lists, and possibly get assistance with expenses and publicity.

Direct Mail. A mailing (invitation, letter and/or flyer) to your patients, referral sources, community leaders and other target groups will help generate interest and enthusiasm in your public relations effort. Be sure to point out in your mailing the benefit to the individual(s) or group(s) of your event.

PLANNING A SPECIAL EVENT

If you decide to hold a special event, whether it's a class for parents-to-be or a reception for referral sources, you must plan ahead. The success or failure of any function, no matter how simple or elaborate, depends on planning, delegation, and follow-through. The series of steps described here may help you and your staff plan your next special event or open house.

1. Select someone from your staff to coordinate the event. Even if you're working with a public relations or marketing firm, you'll need someone in the practice to handle details, make assignments and ensure that things get done.

2. Establish your budget. You can't accomplish anything until you know what you've set aside for the event.

3. Set the date. Depending on what the event is, allow plenty of time to plan it, order, write and send invitations, make special arrangements such as catering, and arrange publicity. Three months is not too far in advance for a major function such as an open house; for a big event like a dedication of a new building, you may need four to six months.

4. Establish a timeline. Determine what needs to be done, working back from the date you've set. Figure out how much time each arrangement will require for completion, whether it's ordering VIP gifts or decorating the site.

5. Choose a location and time. If your event is not to be held at your practice, where will it be? A local hotel or reception hall? A community room of a bank? Confirm the location, date and time in writing. Then put it on your practice calendar.

6. Choose a theme. For a class, a theme is unnecessary (although you'll want to come up with a clever or intriguing title), but for a party or reception, a theme gives you something to work with for decorations and invitations.

7. Make up your guest list. Don't forget VIPs if it's that kind of event—community and political leaders, officers of local professional organizations, your colleagues, and the media.

8. Arrange for catering, flowers, rentals, etc.

9. Order invitations, or have them designed and printed.
10. Plan your advertising/publicity strategy. Will you advertise this event in the local paper and on radio? Use press releases and PSAs only? Try to schedule talk show and news program appearances that tie into your event theme? Don't forget to publicize it with your patients, if they are invited or involved.
11. Order giveaways and VIP gifts.
12. Consider details like parking, a rain date for outdoor events, guest speaker(s), a member of the clergy for an invocation if appropriate, etc.
13. Make staff assignments for the day of the event.
14. (After the event) Write thank-you letters to individuals, organizations and businesses that assisted with donations or other help. Say a special thank you—with a pizza lunch, for example—to your staff.

Here's how one family practice center in Texas used the start of the school year as the focus of a series of special events for the practice. They felt that September—when parents and teachers are concerned with check-ups, diagnosis of problems or disabilities that may hinder learning, and illness-prevention in children—would be an ideal time to increase their visibility in the small town where they were located.

First, speaking engagements by the physicians were arranged with local business groups and the PTAs of several schools. These speeches focused on the importance of complete health check-ups, the value of immunizations and how nutrition can affect academic performance. All these engagements were announced free of charge in local papers, in community service broadcasts on radio and TV, and through flyers sent home with students from the schools.

The physicians then sponsored a half-day seminar for the school nurses and aides in the community. In the seminars they presented the latest information on Reye syndrome, the use of Ritalin in attention deficit disorder, allergies and asthma in children, psychosomatic illnesses, and injuries. They offered plenty of hand-out material, and stressed the availability of the practice as a resource when a difficult problem came up.

A practice open house aimed at de-sensitizing children's attitudes toward the doctor's office was arranged for parents and children on a weeknight. Physicians gave walking tours of the facility, demonstrating equipment and allowing children to touch and look at it. The practice staff was on hand to answer questions and meet and greet youngsters and their parents. During the open house it was announced that the center would welcome children for field trips during the school year. A reporter and a photographer from the neighborhood paper attended the open house; an article and several photos ran later that week on the center and services offered. Requests for classroom field trips were so heavy the practice staff had to set aside a day each month when tours could be given without interfering with patient care.

One physician in the group wrote a letter to the editor of the sports section of the metropolitan area daily newspaper in response to an article on injuries in young soccer players. After his letter appeared, he was asked to speak to the 30 coaches of the local soccer league on prevention of injuries.

Community involvement helped this practice raise its profile, generate new patients and learn of some of the interests and concerns of the people in the town.

A Practice Open House. Consider having an open house or—if you are relocating your practice or opening a satellite office—a grand opening. A family clinic in Texas did, offering an assortment of free health tests during their week-long "public awareness" week. The response was overwhelming (see Figure 10-2).

When several South Georgia physicians opened a state-of-the-art, full service, multi-specialty clinic, it was the culmination of years of planning. The clinic offered physician services, emergency care, a diagnostic lab and radiology, and a pharmacy in one facility. The medical partners wanted their neighbors to know how comprehensive the facility really was, and the kind of people and services they would encounter when they came to the practice as patients. They felt an open house would allow them to meet a large number of people while introducing these visitors to the physicians and their staff and the pleasant, modern environment. Three months before the date they chose for the event (while the facility was still under construction) they began planning the open house, establishing a timeline as described above, ordering needed items, contacting community leaders, finalizing details and mailing invitations and notices.

A month before the date, a VIP mailing list was developed, with names of local dignitaries like the mayor and city council. These individuals received personal letters inviting them to be guests of honor. Several were asked to speak, and gifts were ordered for each.

Two weeks before the open house, invitations were sent to every household in the service area, press releases were mailed and ads scheduled in the suburban newspaper. Poster and essay contests on "The Doctor's Office of the Future" sponsored by the practice were publicized through the schools. In fact, many of the elementary school teachers made entering the essay contest a part of their class work. Physicians and RNs from the practice gave several talks on medicine in the future to classes and school groups.

They invited the high school jazz band to play during the open house and, in return, made a donation to the band's travel fund. Arrangements were made with the hospital's emergency medical service to have a display vehicle and a life flight helicopter on the premises. Physician bios, practice brochures and handouts on a variety of health care topics, from arthritis to first aid, were available. Special health screening stations were planned. Giveaways were ordered two months before the event. Ten days before,

FIGURE 10-2 Glenwood Medical Clinic Open House Invitation
An open house for the public can attract a large number of people if it's well planned
and meets the interests of the audience. This open house brought out the crowds,
then callers who became patients.

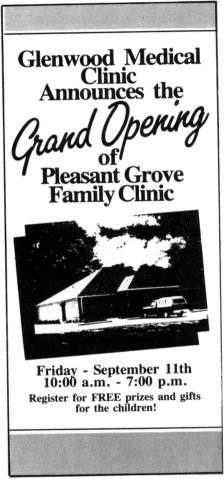

a press release and fact sheet were sent to the community newspaper, the
radio stations and the TV station. Flyers were distributed to pharmacies
and other businesses in the area.

The turnout was phenomenal. Some 900 people visited the facility. The
newspaper provided a half-page article with several photographs. Civic
leaders expressed enthusiastic support for the clinic. The huge success
resulted in an extensive mailing list for the practice, a long list of people
interested in information and classes on health and wellness, and many
appointments.

This practice was not unusual; they offered no unique services, but the physicians and staff did their homework. They were thorough in their planning and in their contacts, and the results paid off.

EVALUATION: ASSESSING RESULTS

There's no sense in spending time, money and effort on a public relations project if you don't know for certain whether it has succeeded. How do you determine success? You measure the results against the goals you've set. If you're holding an open house, your goal may be to generate 10 new patients for the practice. If within the first 30 days after the open house, 12 patients call for appointments and indicate they learned of the practice through the open house, you've succeeded.

In some cases, results may be interpreted as phone calls for information, requests for brochures or requests to be put on your newsletter mailing list. Whatever the event or promotional strategy, be sure that you know what you want to accomplish with it, and then be certain you've built in some measurement technique, even if it's simply the standard question on your new patient information sheet: "How did you hear about our practice?" Once you've built in this measurement device, then you must tally the responses on a regular basis (perhaps monthly) so you have an idea which methods have been effective and which have not. Obviously, you'll want to repeat effective strategies and modify or delete ineffective public relations efforts.

For a complete discussion of evaluation methods, see Chapter 20.

AND FINALLY . . .

The decision to devote time and energy to public relations for your practice involves the commitment of your staff as well as yourself. It involves researching your community or service area. When you take action, become involved, and begin to increase your visibility in your area, you will be perceived as a caring, concerned professional who has the public's interest and well-being at heart.

No matter what technique you choose, no matter how you choose to exhibit your civic-mindedness, you must plan ahead, and know what you want to accomplish. In the end, your efforts will be rewarded with greater patient interest in your practice and services, enhanced public image, and awareness of health care issues and, most important, a sense of personal and professional satisfaction with the role you've played.

BIBLIOGRAPHY

Seital FP: *The Practice of Public Relations,* Columbus, Ohio, Charles E. Merrill Publishing Co., 1984.

Health Care Marketing Associates: *Marketing Your Medical Practice,* The Health Care Group, 1985.

Promoting Through Printed Material

Chapter 11

The Practice Brochure:
The Publication that Talks About You

Many doctors underestimate the public's interest in health care. Your patients want to know about your medical skills, your experience and education, the people who make up your staff, the services and amenities you offer, your policies and procedures and, especially, your views on health maintenance and treatment of medical problems.

The most effective way to provide them with information about all these areas, and also create a multi-use marketing tool, is with a practice brochure. Regardless of how simple or complex the piece is, a practice brochure gives your clientele the facts about your practice and creates a communication bond. It introduces prospective patients to your practice and services (and can convince them you should be their physician).

Your objective in creating a practice brochure is to provide helpful information while reinforcing your positive image and *positioning* your practice with patients and the public. It should project your uniqueness while giving prospective patients a certain amount of factual data. And it should serve as a marketing tool for your practice. Your practice brochure should contain information that tells patients you're a careful, concerned medical practitioner, while it convinces those seeking a doctor that your medical expertise, convenience factors and philosophy of care make you a good choice.

Your brochure must be designed and written with the needs of your patients and potential patients in mind. Otherwise you may end up producing a piece that makes you feel good but is of little benefit to your practice or patients.

In this chapter, we will detail the elements of an effective practice brochure. We'll discuss how to write one your patients can understand, how to produce, distribute, and use it.

WHAT CAN A BROCHURE DO FOR YOUR PRACTICE?

A practice brochure is a visible marketing tool for your practice. If properly written and designed, it can convince people that your practice offers the kind of health care they seek, with amenities, services and convenience factors that meet their needs. It can answer common patient questions and provide necessary information about your services and basic policies. A good practice brochure can often reduce unnecessary telephone calls by 20 to 30 percent.

Your practice brochure will also be very useful to your staff. It will given them answers to questions they may have had about your practice policies and philosophy. An attractive, informative practice brochure even makes marketing "assistants" out of your patients who distribute it to friends, family, co-workers and neighbors.

Creating a practice brochure will require that you assess all your services and office policies. This is a good time to see how well you are meeting the needs of your patients, as well as how you are communicating those services to them.

The brochure can be a useful and educational marketing tool to send to new patients and new residents in your service area. It's also helpful for referring physicians to have available for patients they send to your practice.

If you're not sure exactly what you want in a brochure, it helps to get samples of others. Your local medical society or hospital public relations or marketing department may be able to show you some. Figure 11-1 shows a sample layout.

There are many uses for your practice brochure. Some we'll describe, some you'll discover. First, we'll concentrate on objectives to help you determine content, audience and distribution.

BROCHURE OBJECTIVES

There are two important elements to keep in mind when developing your practice brochure: your objectives and your audience. What do you hope to accomplish with your brochure? Here are some possibilities:

- Inform current patients about your background and your practice policies
- Educate the public about your services and philosophy of care
- Educate new patients about services, features and staff
- Present an image of you and your practice
- Promote a separate "product line" or service of your practice (See Figure 11-2 for an example of a targeted brochure.)

When you've spelled out your objectives, then determine your audience. Most likely, it will be patients as well as potential patients, giving your brochure a dual function. Large practices or those very committed to marketing may even develop two separate brochures—one specifically to inform current patients about services, policies and features of the practice, another aimed at potential patients, with more emphasis on the benefits patients derive from your approach to medical care, and less policy information.

Specialized Brochures. You may find, when you analyze your objectives, that you require an additional targeted brochure. If you have established a distinct *product line* or service within your practice—perhaps you're a urologist with an impotence program—then you may need a descriptive brochure that specifically addresses that program and the needs of its target audience. It's difficult to answer every question and address a broad patient base in one promotional piece, and it's best not to try if you have such targeted programs in your practice. (Of course, be sure to mention the specialized services in your general brochure, and refer readers to additional information that's available from your practice, even if it's only in typewritten form.)

In a specialized brochure, your focus will be somewhat different than a general practice brochure. Following is information you should include:

Audience or potential patients: Who should or could use the services you're describing?

History or overview: Describe the program you're offering. Define and describe the condition (if your program is geared to a specific medical problem), its causes, typical patients, and when treatment is recommended.

Program: What will a patient encounter when they come for a visit?

Staff: If it's a multidisciplinary program, who is involved from your staff and other practices, and what do they provide in the therapeutic realm?

Diagnosis: How is a diagnosis arrived at, and who is involved in the diagnostic process?

Treatment: Describe possible treatments or therapies

Referral: Is referral necessary? If so from whom? If not, what is the appointment or registration process?

Fees and payment policies: Is the service generally covered by insurance? Are payment plans available? What other payment terms or programs are offered?

Location and hours: Where is the service offered? When are patients seen?

THE BROCHURE AS MARKETING TOOL

Your practice brochure may be the appropriate place to alert potential patients about symptoms that may require medical attention such as eye problems in children that may indicate strabismus; warning signs of skin cancer; neurological symptoms that should be taken seriously.

By addressing these concerns here, you provide valuable health education and clarify for potential patients when a doctor visit may be appropriate. You also respond to the question of why they should consult *you*. What problems or needs exist that you can fill? And what specifically do you have to offer in services, philosophy and amenities that differs from other physicians?

Your practice brochure also can be used to inform referral sources about your practice and services. In fact, more and more medical practices are developing brochures that are designed specifically for referring physicians. Chapter 8 on marketing to referral sources contains more on this topic.

FIGURE 11-1   A Sample Practice Brochure

■ INTERIOR PANEL 1

- Services offered
- Specialty

Tell people about your practice and your medical specialty

_____
_____
_____
_____
_____
_____
_____

Explain the training a physician in your specialty must have

and describe problems and conditions for which an individual should consult you.

_____
_____
_____

What procedures or services do you offer?

List and describe your services and procedures, amenities and other helpful information.

■ INTERIOR PANEL 2

- Hours
- Appointments
- Financial information

Appointments and office hours

You want to encourage people to see you for a medical problem and for health maintenance, so be sure to emphasize accessibility and ease of making an appointment. Provide information that lets potential patients know your office is designed for **their** convenience.

Financial information

Include a brief general discussion of payment policy, Medicare and insurance reimbursement. Your goal is to stress the ease and variety of payment mechanisms, not to emphasize "cash on delivery of care."

■ INTERIOR PANEL 3

- Location(s)
- Map
- First visit/consultation information

How to get to this office

Provide easy to follow directions, landmarks or major intersections, and public transit information if appropriate. A map is often helpful.

```
┌─────────────────────┐
│                     │
│                     │
│                     │
│         MAP         │
│                     │
│                     │
└─────────────────────┘
```

Free first consultation visit

Encourage people to make an appointment for a no-charge get acquainted visit, before a medical emergency arises when they need a doctor.

4. Your brochure copy should be patient-oriented, e.g., copy should stress what **you** (the patient) will gain by seeing a doctor, why **you** will benefit by selecting this medical practice. Your brochure should project concern and warmth yet professionalism.

5. Your practice brochure is your opportunity to convince individuals that they will gain — better health, a better appearance, good medical care — by choosing your practice. Use the limited space you have within your brochure for that purpose — not to discuss the nitty-gritty details of financial requirements or office policy.

6. Copy should be friendly, readable. Think of how you would describe your practice to a friend. That's the tone to take.

■ **INTERIOR PANEL 4**

- Personal background

About you

A casual yet professional photo personalizes your brochure and tells potential patients something about you.

Describe your education, residency, specialized training and related experience.

Tell a little about yourself personally — interests, awards, community organizations you participate in, your family, hobbies, interests.

Discuss your staff, but you may wish to avoid specific names to prevent outdating your brochure should someone leave. (Or you can include staff information as an insert.)

1. Use a clear, legible typeface, preferably a serif face. **No** script faces — they're hard to read. Use a larger typeface if your patients are elderly.

■ **BACK OR MAILING PANEL**

- Return address
- Mailing label (Optional)

Your return address ⟶

The back panel can be set up as a self-mailer, although as a rule you'll probably mail your brochure in an envelope with a cover letter.

2. If only one ink color is to be used, make it black, dark grey, dark brown or possibly dark blue. Avoid red, bright green, purple or similar colors for a single-color job, particularly if there will be photos in the brochure.

■ **FRONT PANEL (COVER)**

- Headline
- Photo or illustration
- Practice name
- Practice logo

The headline should be benefit-oriented and informational

(Logo or illustration)

Ima Doctor, M.D.
Practice Name
Address
City, State, Zip

Telephone Number

3. Use a good quality stock in a subtle tone — ivory, grey, pale peach or white.

FIGURE 11-2   A Targeted Brochure
A group of specialists formed a separate service for diagnosis and treatment of attention deficit disorder, then created a brochure to spread the word to parents, teachers and other referral sources.

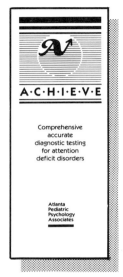

KEY POINTS TO COVER

There are a few essential items to include in a practice brochure.

Physician Credentials. Your credentials are important. You should provide information regarding your medical education and specialty training in terms the layperson will understand. It means more to your patients when you say that you have had specialized postgraduate training in eye surgery than that your fellowship was at St. Elygius University in Ophthalmic Surgical Procedures. A significant number of your patients will have no idea what a "fellowship" is or what significance it has in your training. So use the professional terminology, but then explain what it means.

Another aspect of your credentials to discuss in laymen's terms is an explanation of your medical specialty. If you're an orthopedic surgeon, take a few sentences to describe what types of medical problems you treat and what kind of surgery you do. You might say, "As an orthopedic specialist, I treat problems of the bones and joints, including those caused by accidental injury, sports wear and tear, arthritis and the aging process. Treatment may include medical or surgical solutions." An ob-gyn group might define their specialty in this manner: "The Women's Health Group specializes in health care for women, before, during and after their childbearing years."

Practice Philosophy. You should give some detail about your philosophy of medical care and your approach to patient health and wellness. This kind of information is especially helpful to today's consumers who want physicians whose attitude and beliefs about health care reflect theirs, or whose instructions are provided in a manner they will heed.

Your Staff. Chapter 6 delineates how important your staff is to your practice. Be sure you tell your patients in your brochure. It's not necessary to name staff members individually—in fact, we don't recommend it; when someone leaves, your brochure becomes dated. But you can describe their positions, their responsibilities, how they interact with patients, and how patients can and should interact with them. For instance, if your RN usually returns routine and non-emergency patient calls about medications and illnesses, you should say so in your brochure. Convey this information in a positive fashion: "To assure that you get a quick response to your questions, our nurse will call you for more information, or, frequently, to give you the answer you need."

What to Expect in an Office Visit. If your medical specialty requires a lengthy first visit, or if it requires that patients prepare in some special way, you may wish to inform them of this in your brochure, or in an insert to it. Try to keep the information general. Describe approximately how long the initial visit will take, how long to allow for completion of forms before the appointment time, what to bring in the way of medications currently being taken, immunization records, personal and family medical history, past medical records, and what procedures to expect. (Of course, it's best if you can send this information to the patient prior to the first visit.)

Office Hours and Location. Here you can describe your office hours and appointment schedule. You may not wish to go into specific detail, particularly if your practice is new or you are trying out evening or Saturday hours. If you change your hours, your brochure becomes dated and could cause disappointment in patients anticipating the possibility of an after-work or weekend appointment.

Naturally, you should include all telephone numbers that a patient may need, including answering service and emergency numbers. Be sure to explain what each of the alternative numbers is, and what message to leave if, for instance, they reach an answering service. You also should assure your patients that all calls will be returned within a specified period of time.

It's helpful to provide a simple map with a few landmarks on your brochure, even if you feel your office location is easy to find. Remember, someone who is new in town may have no idea where "Doctors Medical Building adjacent to Cityville General Hospital" is. A picture (or in this case, a map) is better than a thousand words—or a frustrated phone call from a patient 20 minutes late for his appointment saying, "I can't find your office!" Note on the map where parking is located, or where the patient can be dropped off.

Hospital Privileges. You may wish to list the hospitals where you have privileges and/or where you do all or most of your surgery. This helps patients plan if hospitalization is necessary and, in the case of prospective patients, may influence them to choose you if they have already established a relationship with a particular hospital.

Referrals and Second Opinions. Some primary care physicians or group practices describe in their brochures how and when they refer patients to other specialists and even how they handle or encourage a patient's desire for a second opinion. This kind of information helps convey your practice philosophy; it also can be reassuring to patients and would-be patients who see such up-front information as a sign of the physician's confidence and credibility.

Logo. As we discussed in Chapter 5, your practice logo belongs on all your communication materials. Incorporating your logo on your brochure helps reinforce the connection between your practice name and logo and other promotional efforts.

Office Policy. If you are doing a brochure aimed at both patients and the public, you may want to briefly mention office policies and procedures. This is not the place to go into great detail, however; save that for a less costly handout that can be changed more easily.

You might also discuss how quickly someone can expect to be seen if they are suddenly sick or injured, and how emergencies are handled.

Services, Equipment and Amenities. Don't forget to include a brief description of the range of services you offer, such as exams, office-based surgical procedures and emergency care; the equipment you have available such as lab and x-ray; and special amenities you provide such as covered parking or a patient education library. A gastroenterologist who offers fruit juices, broths and herbal teas instead of coffee shows that he/she has patients' welfare in mind. This type of thoughtfulness impresses people; refer to it in your brochure.

Insurance/Fee Policy. In this section you can give general guidelines on payment arrangements and options such as whether you accept credit cards and personal checks; whether you bill insurance or take Medicare assignment, etc. Write this portion in general terms so the information does not become obsolete after your brochure is printed.

Telephone Calls. Patients need to feel that they can reach you during the day. On the other hand, no physician can return every call immediately and still give his office patients proper treatment. Your patients will understand this if you clearly state your policy regarding how calls are handled, who will respond to them, and when patients can expect non-urgent calls to be returned.

If you have formalized these policies, (and good marketing recommends that you do), publish them in easily understood terms. Provide information on the following:

- The best times to call
- Information to have available when calling, such as symptoms and medications taken
- How to briefly describe the reason for the call
- Phone numbers to have available, such as pharmacy preferred

Research demonstrates that the more informed a patient is about your after-hours call policy, the fewer unnecessary calls you will get. For example, one practice does not phone refills to pharmacies after office hours. When patients were made aware of this, most of these calls stopped. Your brochure provides a tangible forum to instruct as well as educate your patients on issues that will make your practice life easier while assuring them a prompt response.

BROCHURE BASICS

Your brochure is a visible representation of your practice. Make sure the image your brochure conveys is the same quality image as that communicated by the rest of your practice. Would you greet your patients in jeans and a t-shirt? Don't give your printed pieces a "jeans and t-shirt" image. You're a professional; make your practice brochure professional too. Your patients expect nothing less.

Let's look at how to take the next step—writing and producing a brochure.

The Brochure Copy. You may be an excellent writer, and enjoy sitting down at the typewriter or computer to compose your practice copy. If not, someone on your staff may be a skilled writer. Otherwise, you'll need to hire a writer—either a freelance professional, or a public relations agency. You'll find copywriting tips in Chapter 16, and guidance for selecting a writer to prepare your brochure copy in Chapter 24.

No matter who you ultimately select, plan on spending an hour or two with the writer in order to convey your practice policy and philosophy of care. Then let the writer do the copy. You can offer guidelines for style (copy should be crisply written, clear and *concise,* while conveying warmth and concern). But you've hired a professional, so don't dictate the words to your writer. If you have other printed or promotional material, it will help him/her get a feel for your personal style and practice identity.

No matter who your patient audience, the tone your brochure takes should be unstuffy, friendly, non-technical. Remember that it is directed, not at your peers, but to non-medical people. Keep your patients in mind when writing or reviewing the copy for your brochure. Use the personal approach: "**You** will be called," "**You** are our first concern." Be warm, yet professional. Remember the importance of simplicity. In essence, you are translating the practice of medicine into layman's language. The generally accepted rule is to write to a seventh to ninth-grade education level.

That is not meant to insult your patient's intelligence; rather, it acknowledges the fact that most of us comprehend the printed word at this level.

Review the draft of the copy. After you make recommendations for changes and additions, the final version will be the one your graphic artist uses in developing a brochure design.

You may wish to let one or two of your staff review the copy. (Don't let them get into critiquing writing style or you'll never get the job done!) You might even ask for comments from one or two patients, or a colleague. You'll need a second opinion. You're too close to this project to be objective, so seek comments and listen to the suggestions you get (see Figure 11-3).

The Brochure Design. We recommend using a graphic artist to design a brochure layout, rather than trying to self- or staff-design this project. Following are design considerations:

Size. Will it be a standard 8½" x 11", 3-panel piece that fits in a business envelope? Or do you have a different size in mind? Consider how the brochure will be mailed—will you need to have special envelopes for an odd size? Will it fit in your office brochure racks?

Color(s). One ink color—black, blue, brown—is inexpensive, but can be drab and lack impact. Two ink colors (black plus a second contrasting color) offers variety. A four-color piece is dramatic, rich and costly.

Stock. The weight, color, quality and type of paper chosen for your brochure can have a tremendous effect on its appearance and cost.

Photos and artwork. Photos personalize a brochure; they tell readers something about you. They also add somewhat to the final cost, especially if you have to hire a photographer. But the results may be worth the expense. Illustrations can help reinforce your image and emphasize points, but custom illustration is also expensive. However, remember that anything done for your brochure can be used again in other promotional material.

Type style. Avoid ornate typefaces for your brochure. Don't mix too many faces. Select a style that's compatible with the typeface used for your name and logo. Remember that when it comes to italics and boldface, a little goes a long way; never print all the body copy in italic or boldface. Keep your patients in mind when determining type size and style. Elderly people have a hard time reading anything smaller than 11 point type, so if you have a high percentage of aging patients, use large type. (See Figure 11-4.)

A Word About the Cover. The first thing people will see is the cover of the brochure, so make it memorable. Give it a look and message that demands to be read.

The cover should contain a phrase or headline that entices the reader to open it. "The problem no one ever talked about . . . now has several solutions" was used on a brochure for an impotence program of a urology practice. The headline grabs and keeps the reader's attention. (See Figure 11-5.)

FIGURE 11-3 Sample Practice Brochure
A practice brochure should be informative while giving patients a sense of your philosophy and services.

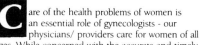

WOMEN'S HEALTH CARE ASSOCIATES

OUR SPECIALITY

Our specialty: Obstetrics, Gynecology and Infertility is a specialty of medicine requiring 4-5 additional years of study and practice beyond the granting of a medical degree. Our physicians are fully trained in all aspects of this specialty and have undergone a minimum of 8 years of formal medical training.

We perform major and minor gynecologic surgeries. Routine as well as high risk birthing is available for our obstetrical patients and we utilize the most advanced technology available for our patients. Infertility evaluations and surgery when necessary are available in our practice.

Some women choose to use their gynecologist for their primary care and we are pleased to assist you when appropriate.

GYNECOLOGIC CARE

Care of the health problems of women is an essential role of gynecologists - our physicians/ providers care for women of all ages. While concerned with the accurate and timely diagnosis and treatment of your individual problem, we also give priority to assisting women in remaining healthy through annual screening (pap smears, physical exams, mammography, breast ultrasound) examination and healthful hints on your well being.

Our practice is designed to cover the comprehensive nature of female health surgical and medical care with support and counseling needed to assist our patients during all phases of their care.

OBSTETRICAL CARE

Pregnancy is a normal, healthful process and we proceed from that premise - maternal and fetal problems can exist or occur at any time during your pregnancy.

Most problems related to pregnancy can be identified and proper steps taken to assure or improve the health of the mother and infant.

The most current obstetrical services are available to assist us in your care including full-time ultrasonography and fetal monitoring.

(In the United States 4-5% of all pregnancies will have untreatable or undiagnoseable genetic problems or birth defects.)

During your pregnancy our staff attempts to help the bonding of the couple into a family unit and prepare to accept the responsibility and joy of a new life.

FIGURE 11-4 Comparison of Typefaces and Sizes
Serif type is more appropriate for text, while sans serif offers advantages for headlines.

Serif
Bodoni

9 pt   This is an example of serif type.

10 pt   This is an example of serif type.

11 pt   This is an example of serif type.

12 pt   This is an example of serif type.

18 pt   This is an example of serif type.

24 pt   This is an example of serif type.

Sans Serif
Helvetica

9 pt   This is an example of sans serif type.

10 pt   This is an example of sans serif type.

11 pt   This is an example of sans serif type.

12 pt   This is an example of sans serif type.

18 pt   This is an example of sans serif type.

24 pt   This is an example of sans serif type.

Or start a phrase on the cover . . . and continue it inside. Use a dramatic, factual statement, such as "One million Americans will suffer heart attacks this year." Involve the reader with your cover message and design.

Printer. Selecting a good, dependable printer is the final step in producing a brochure. There usually are a number of printers from which to select; the best one for you will depend on brochure design, colors, dimensions, quantity, type of photos and other factors. Printer selection is covered in Appendix F.

Determining Quantity. How many brochures will you order? You'll need enough for at least six months to a year. When getting printing prices,

FIGURE 11-5   Brochure Headline Gets Reader Attention
A strong headline draws readers' attention and keeps them reading. From the Impotence Center of the East Valley, Mesa, Arizona.

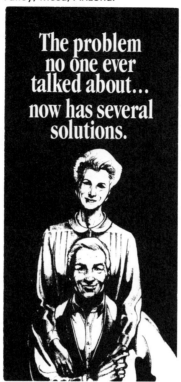

The problem
no one ever
talked about...
now has several
solutions.

ask for quotes on various quantities—i.e., 1,000, 2,500 and 5,000. That way you can determine if it's more cost-effective to have a larger number printed. (Don't have massive quantities printed, however, just because the per piece cost is lower. You have to store everything you're not using, and if you change policies, services or locations, your brochure becomes outdated.)

After reading the next section on where and how to distribute your practice brochure, you'll have a better idea of the quantity your practice needs.

As in any business decision the question arises: how much will this cost? You'll find costs are influenced not only by quantity, but by whether you use special paper, more than one color, photos or illustrations and a professional artist and writer.

A simple job can also be done by a quick-print firm rather than a full-service printer, and be typed on a good machine rather than be typeset. The difference in appearance is noticeable, of course, but each version can be effective and accomplish its goal. The final choice depends on the type of practice and patients you have, your practice needs, desired image, and budget.

Whatever you do, don't cut corners or "go cheap" thinking it will never show. A practice brochure represents you and the medical care you provide. Don't compromise that quality image to save a few dollars.

DISTRIBUTION AND USES OF YOUR PRACTICE BROCHURE

Even before it is off the press, you should have a plan for distributing and using your practice brochures. Copies should, of course, be available in your reception area, and your receptionist should give every patient a copy. Also consider a mailing to your current patients with a cover letter. Distribute brochures at speaking engagements (if permitted), special events you're involved in such as health fairs, public seminars and classes, health screenings at community sites. Finally, consider mailing them with a cover letter to lists of potential patients. The chapter on uses of direct mail offers more details.

Mail your brochure to new patients when they make an appointment. This will give them a chance to prepare for the office visit and also answer many questions they would normally have to ask your receptionist or nurses.

As indicated in Chapter 8, a brochure can also be helpful for referring physicians who must explain your services to a potential patient. Mail a few copies with a cover letter to your referral network. Or have your staff hand-deliver copies to the offices of your referring physicians.

The only thing worse than not having a practice brochure is going to the time and expense of creating one, then letting it sit in an obscure corner of your reception area (or your supply closet) collecting dust until it's out of date.

AND FINALLY . . .

A practice brochure can be one of the most important marketing tools you create for your practice. It can become an extension of the care you give your patients by expressing your concern for informing them.

It also gives satisfied patients, staff and friends something with which to "market" your practice. Developing it forces you to evaluate your office policies and practices, answer commonly asked questions and provide useful information to your patients. Make certain you develop a brochure which is consistent in writing style, design and overall quality with the image of your practice.

Your brochure is your calling card; make it say great things about you!

Chapter 12

Newsletters for Patients and Referring Physicians

HEALTH NEWS IS GOOD NEWS

Insurance companies, CPAs, attorneys and architects and now physicians have all discovered a most successful method of communicating personally and regularly with a large audience: the newsletter.

In our over-communicating society, where a constant barrage of information and advertising often makes the intended audience tune out unconsciously, people want to be kept informed and educated by the professional resources they rely on. Patients express enthusiasm for the helpful information they receive from their doctors, whether it's at the office or in their mailbox at home. And when there is no regular communication (such as a practice newsletter) they express interest in receiving one.

Professionals who refer to you (physicians in other specialties, therapists and health care agencies) also appreciate receiving information on current thinking in a specialty that may affect their patients or clients. A Florida physician discovered this when he began his referring physician newsletter several years ago. In an article in *Medical Economics,* John J. Fisher, MD, reported that "the feedback I get from physicians who receive the newsletter has been extremely positive. Several of them have stopped me in the halls of the hospital to . . . tell me how much they appreciate what I'm doing." With a referral source newsletter, you can help referring physicians and other health care professionals provide better care for their patients while also informing them about your expertise as well as the latest medical information in your field.

To many doctors, the thought of starting a newsletter—much less publishing one on a regular schedule—is overwhelming. But it need not be and, in this chapter, we'll "demystify" the process of planning, organizing, developing and actually creating a practice newsletter. We'll help you find ideas for newsletter topics right in your practice and in the material you receive every day in the mail. We'll explain how and when to use resources like graphic artists, copywriters, advertising or public relations firms, and your own staff. We'll also review options that may be appropriate for your practice and your patients, such as purchased newsletters that can be partly or completely customized in copy and graphics.

We hope that when you have completed this chapter, you'll see the benefits to your patients, potential patients and your practice—and to the medical profession in general—of an educational, informative periodic newsletter.

AN ETHICAL APPROACH

A practice newsletter offers you the chance to communicate and inform in a highly ethical manner. Health and medical information is at the top of the public's "want to know" list of topics. Naturally, your patients prefer to get this information from you, face-to-face, one-to-one, during an office visit. But they understand the limitations of your time as well as theirs. That's why they enjoy receiving written material from you, to be read at their leisure.

In a practice newsletter, you can tell your patients why they should have flu shots; if they could be candidates for radial keratotomy; or you can describe exercise to prevent back problems. You can describe the 10K race recently completed by a member of your staff, and from there discuss prevention of injuries while running; you can offer suggestions on the newest OTC medications for arthritis or gastrointestinal ailments.

One practice management firm found, during an audit of patient charts, that 20 percent of patients in the average practice need follow-up medical care of some sort. Half of these individuals can be attracted back to the practice, the consultants found. Communication and helpful information from their physician can convince these "prodigal patients" of the benefit of returning for the care they need.

The flow chart in Figure 12-1 takes you, step by step, through the process of developing and printing a practice newsletter.

THE NEWSLETTER AUDIENCE

A well-designed newsletter that's carefully planned, written and edited will do more than just introduce you. It will move people to act, to call your office for an appointment or for information about a program, class or service you discuss in your newsletter.

A practice newsletter is a legitimate way to establish or maintain a positive relationship with referring physicians and other health care providers. It's a gentle reminder to them about you, your staff and your philosophy of care. And if you develop a newsletter that's specifically for physicians, it becomes an acceptable way to inform them about new treatments, therapeutics and clinical findings in your specialty field. For referral-dependent physicians, a newsletter can be the primary promotional strategy for assuring a good professional relationship with colleagues. It's also a way of letting them know the types of cases you are interested in—the more complicated or specialized cases they can't or don't want to diagnose or treat.

Publishing a newsletter is *not* an overnight job. But it's not as time-

FIGURE 12-1 Flow Chart for Developing a Practice Newsletter

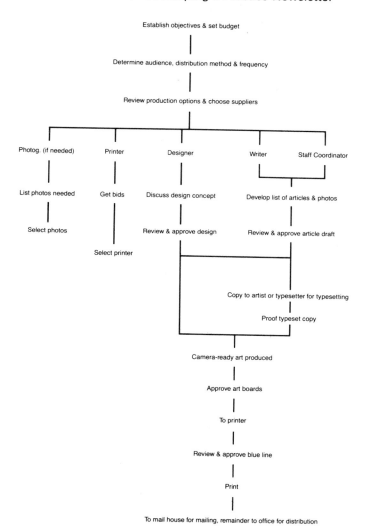

Establish objectives & set budget

Determine audience, distribution method & frequency

Review production options & choose suppliers

Photog. (if needed) | Printer | Designer | Writer | Staff Coordinator

List photos needed | Get bids | Discuss design concept | Develop list of articles & photos

Select photos | | Review & approve design | Review & approve article draft

Select printer

Copy to artist or typesetter for typesetting

Proof typeset copy

Camera-ready art produced

Approve art boards

To printer

Review & approve blue line

Print

To mail house for mailing, remainder to office for distribution

consuming or as costly as you may think, particularly if you plan ahead, and utilize all the available resources. The gynecologist who created a referral newsletter said that while gathering and composing the material for his peers "takes me a while . . . I chalk it up to keeping on my professional toes." The time for the mechanical process, he said, is "negligible. My little sheet isn't a fancy production—just two unpretentious, typed, single-spaced pages."

You don't have to do it yourself. (We cover outside resources in detail in Chapter 22. Also, much of the technical and printing information in Chapter 11 applies as well to newsletters.)

PLANNING A NEWSLETTER

Determine Your Goals. Before you begin jotting down ideas for articles, before you select an editor, before you begin looking at paper and type samples, you must decide: "What do I want to accomplish with a newsletter?"

There are many possible objectives. Look at all of them; then decide which match your needs and goals.

- Educate your patients about current health care information, your office policies, new staff
- Generate new patients
- Publicize new services
- Maintain a full appointment schedule during traditionally "slow" periods
- Keep health care professionals and agencies aware of your practice and services
- Provide health care feature ideas to the media
- Inform referring physicians of your services and new treatments in your specialty of which they may be unaware
- Retain and strengthen relationships with existing users of your service

You may have other goals as well. It's helpful to list what you wish to accomplish with your newsletter. It focuses your thinking, and makes determining your target audience and content easier.

Determine Your Audience. Depending on your objectives, your newsletter audience may be very narrow or very broad. You may decide you only want to test the water now, and therefore you'll distribute your newsletter only to your patients. If it is as well-received as most practice newsletters, you may get requests for copies from neighbors of patients, from pharmacies, senior living apartments, day care centers and other groups.

If you wish only to maintain your practice, and you are not interested in growth, you can limit your mailing list to your current patients. But if you hope to fill your scheduling book in slack periods, if you are a newly established physician seeking to attract patients, if you depend heavily on referrals from other sources and, if you are seeking to become involved in the community, you should consider expanding your newsletter distribution list.

Figure 12-2 shows possible audiences for a practice newsletter. You may think of others as well. Toward the end of the chapter we will explain how to create or acquire mailing lists that include your target market.

Establish a Budget. A newsletter can be as inexpensive or as costly as you wish and as your budget permits. The cost depends on how many copies you print, the paper stock, whether it's typed or typeset, whether you use a graphic artist or do it yourself on a desktop computer, whether

FIGURE 12-2 Possible Audiences for a Practice Newsletter

- Patients
- Patients' family members and neighbors (In each issue of your newsletter or on an office form, ask your patients to write names of others whom they feel would like to receive it.)
- New residents
- Community agencies/social service agencies (American Cancer Society, Easter Seals, etc.)
- Community leaders
- Officers of professional/civic organizations
- Health care professionals (physical and occupational therapists, private practice RNs and nurse practitioners, psychologists, dentists, etc.)
- Referring physicians
- Editors and reporters, radio/television talk or interview program hosts and producers
- Children's and adult day care centers (as appropriate)
- Senior centers; senior apartments; nursing homes
- Hospital departments
- Employees who leave on good terms
- Local employers (personnel and employee health departments; employee publication editors)
- Employee family members
- Clergy, attorneys, public fiduciaries
- Home health agencies
- Pharmacists and retail medical supply firms
- Libraries
- Schools: home economics, family living, health, social studies and science teachers; counselors; principals; PE teachers and coaches

it includes photos, whether it's one ink color or two-, three- or four-color, the method of distribution, and whether you use an outside resource such as a public relations firm, consultant, or freelance writer for all or much of the work. A simple newsletter can be done for as little as $200-$300 (excluding postage and initial design costs); a more complex, glossy publication may cost several thousand dollars or more. Lower cost, however, does not necessarily mean less impact. The effectiveness of a newsletter is determined by content, quality, professional appearance, and the audience to whom it is distributed.

Fortunately, it doesn't take a big budget to produce a newsletter that looks graphically pleasing and that carries the message you want people to receive. It will be as effective, in its own way, as the big-ticket publication with a press run of 20,000.

Following are some cost ranges for the various components of developing a newsletter. Remember that costs will vary greatly depending on the part of the country you're in, the type of service you use and other factors.

Writing: $15-75/hour. The time needed for a 4-page newsletter depends on how complete the information is you supply the writer, and how many changes you make in the copy.

Layout/Design: $25-60/hour. Once the initial design has been developed for the newsletter, each succeeding issue should follow the basic design parameters.

Printing: Printing costs depend on number of copies, paper selection, number of ink colors, whether photos are used and other variables. A quick-print firm will offer the lowest prices and is a good choice for a simple 1 or 2-color publication. But it's best to use a full-service printer for more complex jobs where a quality appearance is important.

Mailing: Mailing costs also vary widely, depending on whether you use a bulk mail rate (recommended if you're mailing 250 or more), whether the newsletter is sent in an envelope or as a self-mailer, whether there is an insert (such as a Business Reply Card) and, of course, the number to be mailed. A mailing house can review prices and options with you and recommend the most reasonable route for your practice newsletter.

Determining your newsletter budget should be a function of your overall marketing and promotion budget and the objectives and strategies laid out in your marketing plan. A point to consider in reviewing your budget is the payback. If you are an orthopedic surgeon, one new patient generated from an article on arthroscopic knee surgery may more than pay for the cost of producing an issue. That's why it's so important that you track results on every promotional strategy you implement; you will know what works (so you can do more of it) and what doesn't (so you can modify or discontinue the strategy).

Determine Frequency. How often do you want to produce a newsletter? Again, the decision will depend on who will be doing the job, how much time they and you have available, your promotion budget and even the "seasonality" of your appointment schedule. You may wish to time your newsletter publication to anticipate lighter periods in your appointment schedule. If you plan the content carefully, your newsletter can bring in calls for appointments during these periods.

A frequency of at least three times a year, and preferably quarterly, is recommended for a newsletter in order to maintain visibility.

Review Your Production Options and Select Suppliers. Producing a newsletter does not have to be a complex, time-consuming operation. With you or a designated staff member overseeing the writing and coordination, you can hire an individual or firm to handle some or all of the design and preparation of the publication.

Use a professional designer. Once you've decided to publish a newsletter, we strongly urge that you hire a professional artist to create a design that will be consistent with your practice image and style, your audience, and your existing letterhead and logo. Even if you choose to handle the production of subsequent issues internally, having a design that establishes parameters for column width, margins, typefaces, headlines and the use of photos and artwork will make your job much simpler. A graphic artist will take into account your budget as well as the time and skills of the person who will edit or coordinate the newsletter.

Hire someone to handle the job. Naturally, if you are comfortable with the idea and your budget can afford it, you can hire a marketing or public relations firm or individual to handle the whole job of producing your newsletter. A consulting firm can take it from initial design through printing. Your involvement would then include working with your consultant to plan the contents of each issue, possibly writing a column or article in each issue, reviewing copy before it is typeset, and overseeing final camera-ready art before the job goes to the printer. See Chapter 22 on working with consultants for details.

Hire a writer. You can instead hire a freelance writer to write each issue and work with a staff member who would plan and coordinate the production. The layout and paste-up of the newsletter could then be done by an independent graphic artist. (Some printers have an art department. Most quick-printers do not, but they may be able to refer you to an artist.)

Desktop publishing. Desktop publishing is becoming an increasingly common option for creating a cost-effective newsletter. You may find that one of your staff has desktop publishing capabilities on a home computer (or your office computer may have desktop publishing software). There also are desktop publishing firms that can handle your newsletter from start to finish at a very reasonable cost.

Ready-made newsletters. Finally, there are "canned" or syndicated newsletters available from a variety of sources. Some medical specialty associations have them, as do medical marketing and publishing firms. Canned newsletters will be better accepted by recipients if there is some adaptation and specific reference to you, your staff and practice. Although not preferable, an off-the-shelf newsletter is a start in establishing regular communication with patients and would-be patients.

Printing the publication. Printers generally fall into two categories: the small "quick" printers capable of handling simple jobs, and full-service printers whose emphasis is on bigger, more complex jobs. The printer you use will depend on the complexity and quantity of newsletters you need. See the Appendix for an extensive discussion of printers.

STAFF INVOLVEMENT

The decision about who will coordinate your newsletter depends on a variety of factors. Some physicians like to be closely involved in projects like this, and have the time to handle it. Others prefer to take a more distant approach, designating a staff person to act as "associate" or "assistant editor." This individual has the responsibility of coordinating each issue of the newsletter, ensuring that articles are planned, assigned and written, and photos are taken. Following the job from layout through paste-up and printing is also the assistant editor's responsibility. If outside resources are used, your assistant editor works with them.

The physician gets involved in helping plan the issue, then approving articles and final camera-ready artwork before it goes to the printer. The assistant editor and/or someone she/he assigns should carefully proofread the final typed and typeset copy for typographical errors.

In Chapter 6 we emphasized the importance of involving your staff in a project like this. It's vital for two reasons: most physicians don't have the time to spearhead a practice newsletter themselves; and your staff members will feel more a part of your practice—and therefore be more committed to it—if they are willing participants in such projects. They also may be more aware of topics and information patients want.

Here are some suggestions for involving your staff:

1. Announce the implementation of a practice newsletter at a regular staff meeting. Explain what your objectives are, how frequently you plan to publish, what kinds of articles it will contain, and what it will look like (if you know at this point). Be sure to emphasize that each issue will highlight a staff member or some aspect of staff functions, jobs and responsibilities, and that it will discuss and clarify practice policies (thus relieving some of the burden on your office staff).

2. Ask your employees to suggest names for the newsletter. You might even hold a contest, with a prize for the winning name. If you do so, establish guidelines for the name. Remember, if you hold a contest, you have to choose a winner—and if none of the names suggested are appropriate or appealing, you may be caught in an embarrassing position.

3. Involve your staff in planning each issue of the newsletter. Make the newsletter an agenda topic at each staff meeting. Ask staff for ideas for articles related to medical problems and practice questions that patients ask about.

4. Give your staff the opportunity to write articles or "guest columns" (if they have a particular specialization such as nutrition or fitness). Seek volunteers first; if no one offers, ask one of your staff to write an article. Usually, they're honored that you ask.

5. Offer incentives or small gifts for especially good ideas or extra effort related to the newsletter.

It is particularly important that you give your staff credit for their work on your newsletter by listing them on the masthead, and by highlighting them in it. In addition, stress in group and individual situations how vital each of them is in making your newsletter interesting, helpful and credible to your patients and others who receive it.

THE CONTENT QUARTET

In one week, Dr. Wyatt, a family practitioner, was asked by three different patients about the benefits of fish oil—the substance that suddenly seemed to be in all the newspapers. And the mother of a young 10-year-old boy with heel pain seemed surprised when Dr. Wyatt told her it was "growing pains" before prescribing treatment. "I thought growing pains were old-wives' tales!" she said.

During a staff meeting, the receptionist reported that a patient who arrived late had been upset that other patients were taken ahead of him. "My appointment time was before theirs," the patient complained. "How can we explain to our patients why they're not always taken in order?" the receptionist asked.

In that one week, patient questions and concerns gave Dr. Wyatt more than enough material to cover in his bimonthly newsletter. "And I thought I'd never be able to fill an issue!" he laughed.

No matter who your audience is, the primary focus and purpose of a newsletter should be education and information. That's what people want; that's what they'll read it for. The benefit of using your newsletter to enlighten readers about health and medical topics is that your publication can be recycled; past issues can be kept in the waiting room for new patients; you can take them along on speaking engagements (particularly when you're talking on a topic addressed in your newsletter); and you can use current and back issues to support information you give patients verbally.

To help you plan each issue of the newsletter, we recommend using the "content quartet" to guide you. The content quartet includes *practice information, preventive health care, self-help health tips* and *seasonal health problems.*

Practice Information. This section can be used to inform your patients about the policies and procedures of your office, particularly those you've added or changed recently, or those that seem to be generating a lot of questions or misunderstandings. Here you might want to include office hours, business and reimbursement policies and new services. You can profile staff members and their responsibilities and also answer common questions you and your staff are asked.

Self-Help Health Tips. Your patients want to know how to take care of themselves. This section gives you a chance to identify certain health problems related to your specialty (such as warning signs of cancer, or how to tell if you might be developing an ulcer), and to tell patients how they can take care of minor ailments. The more you help your patients learn about self-care and how to save unnecessary office calls or visits, the more appreciative they will be, and the more they'll utilize your services when they are needed. They'll also be more likely to recommend your practice to family, friends and co-workers who need a physician.

Preventive Health Care. This section can be used to relate important information on how to stay healthy and physically fit. Suggestions on diet, exercise and prevention of cancer and other diseases are exceptionally well received. From a marketing point of view, this section should emphasize the importance of good health while advising patients on the role of your practice in helping them to achieve that goal.

Seasonal or Timely Health Problems. Articles on seasonal health and medical problems remind patients of symptoms to watch for, how to avoid certain seasonal ailments, and when to seek treatment from you. For example, in the fall and winter you might discuss dry skin, what causes it and how to treat it, and when that itchy, scaly problem is more than just dry skin. If a politician or celebrity makes news because of some ailment or medical condition, your newsletter may be an appropriate place to discuss your approach to diagnosis and treatment of the problem, and/or to educate readers on how they can avoid it. At the start of the school year an ophthalmologist can discuss school vision tests, and what they do and don't reveal about a child's eyes. The cold and flu season lends itself to a lighthearted look at Mom's chicken soup as a remedy for congestion. You could even include your own (or a staff member's) recipe. The article could lead into a discussion of symptoms for which people should call the doctor rather than continuing to self-treat.

Besides the "Content Quartet," your newsletter also might include fun and filler items, such as healthy recipes (perhaps contributed by patients), word games and quizzes, tips for dealing with everyday life-stress, honors and awards earned by you and/or your staff, occasional humorous anecdotes, holiday features, even small items on patients with unusual vocations or hobbies, listings of health-related community events, classes, meetings, and resources.

Find out what patients would like to read about in your newsletter by asking them. When they come to your office, ask them which articles they read, which they enjoyed most, which they'd like to see more of. You can even have a short survey in your reception area along with copies of your newsletter.

You might have a section in your newsletter featuring upcoming community events that have a tie-in to a healthy lifestyle. Even if you are not a sponsor, promoting these events will position you as community-involved and concerned about your patients and the community.

Newsletters provide the opportunity to address health and medical issues that are specific to your city or geographic area. Utilize information from sources such as the *American Medical News, The Mayo Clinic Health Letter*, the *Journal of the American Medical Association* and the clinical publication for your specialty field. Be sure to attribute your source when you do this. Copyright laws require it, and quoting expert sources adds credibility to your newsletter.

With your practice newsletter, you can legitimately fulfill your patients' desire for health care and medical information; you can establish yourself as an expert in your specialty and the resource patients should turn to when they need medical help or information. You also add to your credibility as a medical practitioner when you keep your patients informed with up-to-date knowledge. A newsletter creates a sense of belonging among your patients. It keeps current patients with you and brings "lost" patients back to you. And finally, a newsletter builds employee morale by offering a forum to publicly praise and acknowledge their efforts (see Figure 12-3).

COPY THAT GETS READ

You'll find an extensive discussion on copywriting in Chapter 15, so we'll only offer a few pointers here on newsletter writing style. The most

FIGURE 12-3 Sample Newsletter

A practice newsletter can be a simple typewriten sheet or it can be more elaborate and expensive. It all depends on your time, preferred image, goals and budget. The newsletter shown here was developed by an orthopedic group for distribution to patients and referral sources. From Arizona Sports Injury and Rehabilitation Center, Mesa, Arizona.

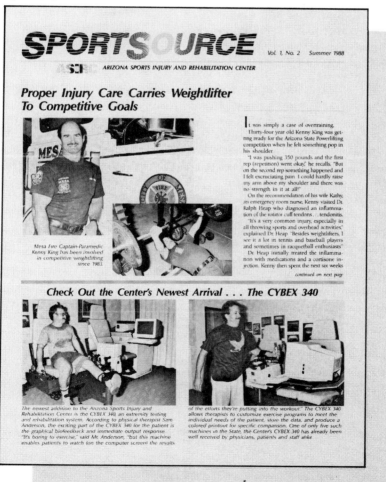

important consideration in writing copy is your audience. People are hungry for personal communication. They crave inside information; it fosters a feeling of belonging. They welcome helpful advice, wisdom and opinion. They need the comfort of authority. But they want all this in a language they understand, in terminology with which they are familiar.

Write to one person, a single reader, not to a mass audience. Consumer research continues to demonstrate the strength of the personal touch. Achieve it with large doses of YOU. Refer to each patient individually and directly—"You should know," "You will get . . ." Also get yourself and your staff involved. "I believe," "we try . . ." Write as you would to a friend.

Then cut through the fat to the meat of the subject. Waste no time setting the stage or warming up to your topic. You've got limited space; use it well. Improve your style with short sentences. Cut extra words. Reduce phrases such as "along the lines of" to one word, "like." Change "in the neighborhood of" to "about." "Since" or "because" replaces "for that reason."

Most importantly, think in terms of your readers, not yourself. Show them how they will benefit from the information you offer. Don't use your newsletter as a forum to show off your technical knowledge. Remember that your readers are lay people (unless your newsletter is specifically for referring physicians). The average person does not understand, and does not want to decipher, medical terminology. If you must use medical terms, follow them with a brief, simple explanation. A newsletter is no place for lengthy explanations about diseases, disorders, treatments or medications. Explain briefly and concisely. To make certain you've conveyed the necessary information clearly, have a non-medical person read what you've written.

Write for an audience at the seventh to ninth grade level, and use an informal, friendly style. Write as you would talk in conversation.

Finally, strive for accuracy. Double-check any names used in the newsletter; it's amazingly simple to misspell someone's name. Have someone who has not read the copy proof it for typographical errors (typos) before it goes to the typesetter or paste-up artist.

WHAT'S IN A NAME?

One of the first decisions you must make, once you've decided to publish a newsletter, is what to name it. When naming your newsletter, keep these pointers in mind:

1. Be relevant. The name should reflect your specialty, your professional field, and the purpose of the newsletter.
2. Don't be cute. You'll obscure the purpose of the newsletter, denigrate your professionalism and insult your audience.
3. Match the name with your personal and practice style. If yours is a fairly formal,

straightforward practice, your newsletter name should reflect it. "Eye Care News" would be appropriate as a newsletter name for such an office; "Eye Times" would not.

4. Keep it brief. It's easier to remember short names.

5. Remember your audience. Elderly readers will respond differently than a mostly youthful, family-oriented audience.

To get you thinking, here are some possibilities for newsletter names:

Family Practice/Ophthalmology/Dermatology Times

The Doctor's Journal

Medical News
  from the office of _____, MD

HealthTribune

HealthNews

Healthy Heart or Heart Health (from a cardiologist)

The Orthopedic/Ob-gyn, Internal Medicine Letter

Looking Good (for a dermatologist or plastic surgeon)

Good Health Gazette

Stay Well

Alive & Well

Pediatric Patter

Strides (sports medicine)

A Look In . . . (Internal Medicine)

DESIGN POINTERS

Your newsletter represents you and your practice. Be sure it has a professional appearance. Look at the format, content, typography and the weight and color of paper it is to be printed on. It may be the first, and possibly only, impression some readers get of you. Make it a good one.

Consider such elements as photos (halftones). Will you include them or not? Do you have someone on staff who is capable of taking good black and white photos? The printing cost increases slightly when photos are included. Will you need illustrations? Remember that you can't simply lift artwork or cartoons that have been printed in other publications; the material is generally copyrighted. However, art supply stores have books of "clip art" on a variety of topics that can be purchased for a reasonable amount, and reprinted. Clip art can be helpful for breaking up copy, to illustrate a particular story, and to convey a theme.

There are as many different newsletter looks or styles as there are newsletters. Your newsletter may be typewritten or typeset, and with either you have a number of graphic options. Here are the pros and cons:

Typeset or Typewritten?

Advantages of a Typeset Newsletter

1. Gives a more finished professional image.
2. Provides a greater opportunity to create visual interest by boldfacing a word, varying type size, etc.
3. Offers a wide selection of typefaces for individualized look.

Disadvantages of a Typeset Newsletter

1. Requires some graphic knowledge, or an artist to get desired look.
2. Increases production time. Depending on amount of copy, the typesetter will require two to five days turnaround time. Then additional time is required for paste-up.
3. Loses intimacy of a typewritten letter and some of its timeliness.
4. More costly.

Advantages of a Typewritten Newsletter

1. Can look more personal and timely.
2. Production costs are low, and involvement of staff in production is easier.
3. Easier to produce in-office. Stories can be typed as they are to appear on the page. Eliminates most paste-up work.
4. Corrections can be made at the last minute. Stories can be lengthened or shortened to fit without incurring additional typesetting costs.

Disadvantages of a Typewritten Newsletter

1. Type selections are limited.
2. Visually not as pleasing. Grayer, more flat look.
3. Harder to read than typeset copy, particularly long line lengths.
4. More limiting in terms of design. Varied column widths, other graphic elements can't be incorporated, or can't be incorporated as easily.
5. Can have an amateurish, or unprofessional look, particularly when done by individual(s) not skilled in layout, design and paste-up.

Regardless of which format you select, be sure to maintain a consistent design. People should be able to recognize your newsletter without seeing the name, just based on its visual "style." Don't be afraid of white space. White space sets off important stories, draws attention to photos and headlines, and increases readership.

The "Flag" or Nameplate. If you don't spend money on any other part of your newsletter, do have the nameplate (also called the "flag") professionally designed.

The "flag" or nameplate carries the name of the newsletter, the volume and issue, the date, and some reference to your office or practice so readers know who the publisher of the newsletter is.

Simplicity is far more effective than an obtrusive, overdone nameplate. Avoid ornate roman or script typefaces, obscure references or amateur drawings.

The **masthead** is a separate box usually found on an inside or back page of the newsletter. It lists information about the publisher, editor, practice location. Include your name, your practice name, address, telephone number, the editor (you or a staff member), associate editor, and any regular columnists or other contributing editorial staff. In the masthead you should mention that comments, questions, and suggestions for your publication are welcome. Also encourage readers to call if they're not on the mailing list for your newsletter and would like to be.

Consider these additional cost-saving tips:

- Use standard paper sizes, colors and weights.
- Shop and compare prices for major services such as design, typesetting and printing. But remember, too, that you usually get what you pay for.
- Enforce deadlines. Delays cost money.
- Avoid making unnecessary changes in copy, format or artwork once your newsletter has been pasted up. The time to change the copy is at first review when it's still in typewritten form, or as it's being proofed prior to paste-up.
- Check out the electronic type (desktop publishing) firms in your area. They can do both typesetting and page layout, often at very reasonable rates. Also check out desktop publishing software for use on your office computer. It has a myriad of uses besides creating newsletters. You can design forms, brochures, educational pamphlets . . . anything that will be printed can be designed with a desktop publisher.

WORKING WITH PRINTERS

The printer is bound to become an important person in your life as you begin carrying out your marketing strategies. It's important to get to know the printer (or use a designer who knows a printer very well) in order to attain the triad of price, speed and quality for your newsletter as well as other printed material.

DISTRIBUTION

Specific groups and individuals who can or should receive your newsletter are discussed earlier in this chapter. The method of distribution is something you must consider also. Will you mail it? If so, how? What other ways are there to get a newsletter into circulation?

For instance, you can hand the latest copy to individual patients when you see them for an office visit, mentioning a particular story relating to their condition or question.

You can also take newsletters along on speaking engagements and pass them to the audience, distribute them to hospitals, pharmacies, schools, grocery stores, senior centers, day care centers, fast food restaurants, dry cleaners, churches—every business that you deal with.

You can mail them to members of the media, and the president or officers of local community and civic groups.

Leave a supply at health clubs and hair salons, and offer them to local employers for their cafeteria or employee lounge.

While you should have copies of your newsletter available in your reception area and examining rooms for patients, it will be most well received if it is also mailed to patients. Have your local postmaster or post office customer service representative look at your newsletter and provide information on ways to seal and mail it.

MAILING INFORMATION

Since you'll most likely be mailing the majority of your newsletters, you or someone on your staff must become familiar with postal service regulations. Appendix G contains a discussion of some of them, and the postal service also offers pamphlets on bulk mailing. Be sure to check requirements before finalizing your newsletter, as they can affect your paper choice, size, method of mailing (envelope or self-mail), as well as your budget.

AND FINALLY . . .

Your practice newsletter is designed to help you retain patients by fostering a sense of belonging and a feeling of personal familiarity with you, your staff and practice. It's also designed to help bring patients back to your practice when they have health or medical problems. The topics you cover in your newsletter provide the "hook" to remind patients that you're available for their health care needs. And it allows you to promote your new services and techniques in an ethical, professional way. Finally, your newsletter provides a forum for building patient confidence in your experience and expertise. And when people feel confident about someone, they confidently recommend that person to others.

While you're benefiting your practice through your newsletter, you also keep your patients informed, aware and educated about their role in staying healthy and fit. As long as you are mindful of responding to your patients' needs first and foremost, your newsletter will accomplish all of your objectives and theirs too.

BIBLIOGRAPHY

Fisher, JJ: The Best Referral Booster I Ever Found *Medical Economics* 1984; February 20.

Audit the Gold Mine in Your Practice Records *Physician Marketing* 1987; April.

Chapter 13

Computers—Your Practice Promotion Ally

Dr. Blake was the newest doctor in a successful three physician surgical practice. As the most recent addition to the practice, she was interested in generating her own clientele. Dr. Blake asked Mary, the office manager, which physicians most frequently referred patients to the practice.

"We've never really analyzed it Dr. Blake," Mary said, "but I know we have it on our computer files because the patients put it on their forms when they are first seen."

"Could we get a list of our referring physicians? I'd like to send a special letter and let them know about my training and specialty interests," responded Dr. Blake.

"Well, we can sure try," said Mary. "Our system has a report generator feature that we haven't used, but it should do the job. Give me a day or so to try it out."

The next day Mary came into Dr. Blake's office with a smile and a report, "I thought it was going to be hard, but look what we have here—and it took only a little while. I had the computer program run through our patient files and count the number of referrals by each physician. Look at this! There are ten physicians who have sent us over 40 percent of the patients who've come to us through physician referrals this past year."

"That's impressive, Mary. Do we have the addresses of the physicians on this list?"

"No, but we can easily add that information to a separate file now that we've generated the list of physicians. And with the mail-merge feature I was reading about in the manual, we can send a letter to each doctor and have the system personalize the inside address and address the envelopes."

"Great, Mary. You build the file and I'll write the letter. We can send it out tomorrow."

"You know, Dr. Blake, I think we could do a lot of this kind of stuff with our computer system. We've only been using it for accounting and billing work. I see now how we could use it to build our practice."

Computers have become a part of our work, home and recreation life. A majority of physicians use some sort of computer system in their practice. Most, however, use only a limited portion of the computer capability. Significant advances in computer programs and hardware, coupled with advances that reduced computer size and cost and increased memory and processing speed, have made them powerful in identifying and communicating with important target markets (see Figure 13-1).

FIGURE 13-1 Computers in the Medical Office
A computer in a medical practice is no longer a frivolous expenditure; it's a business and marketing investment. Physicians and staff benefit from working together to get maximum use out of this practice management tool.

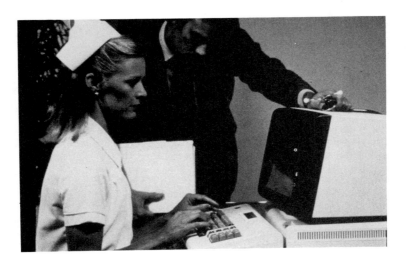

GENERATING PATIENTS WITH YOUR
COMPUTER SYSTEM

Generating patients involves identifying sources of patients (your target markets), nurturing their interest in the practice and encouraging their action to make use of your practice services. There are many ways that a computer system, effectively used, can assist in attaining these goals. One of the most powerful abilities of the computer is to organize and provide information about patients who have variously defined characteristics.

Earlier chapters have discussed the importance of identifying and encouraging use of your practice by "market segments." These segments are made up of people who can best benefit from services you currently offer or intend to provide. Further, since it's easiest to market a service to a currently satisfied patient, the information you have or can collect about that patient can become one of the most valuable assets in promoting your practice. This asset can significantly increase in value if the information you collect is coded in meaningful ways, and maintained in computer-processable form.

Let's first address the types of information the computer can analyze to identify patients whom you may wish to reach with promotions. Three important sources of information to guide your promotional activities are: patient demographics, referral sources and payment sources.

PATIENT DEMOGRAPHICS

Demographics refers to the characteristics of individuals who are, or may be, served by your practice. Examples of important demographic factors include:

Age (birth date)
Residence address and phone number
Occupation
Employer address and phone number
Sex
Race
Number in household
Name, sex and birth date of household members
Marital status
Religious preference
Insurance carriers (including HMOs and PPOs)

These factors can usually be captured on new patient registration forms, or on insurance forms for those who are already patients. This information, however, should be periodically verified with patients as several important demographic elements can change over time (e.g., employer, address, insurance carrier).

The information described above represents demographic information about the individuals and their families who have been seen in your practice. We will discuss demographics of other individuals later in this chapter.

A computer system can be very helpful in targeting promotions to selected practice demographic groups. This usually begins by identifying and quantifying current patient characteristics. For example, how many are employed by the high-tech manufacturer a half-mile away from your office? What percentage of your patients are women? What proportion are over age 65 or under 18? Physicians are often surprised at the demographics of their patients. You may find, for instance, that your patients travel a long distance for their services. Others learn there may be some geographic barrier (e.g., rivers, bridges, freeways) that tend to limit patient access to the practice.

If the practice demographics listed above are captured in computer-processed form, it should be possible to develop a practice profile that characterizes the nature of your patient base in terms of its demographics. This can lead to effective targeting of promotions to segments that are more likely to want/need the intended services. Let's say you discover that seven percent of your patients are employed by the high-tech firm mentioned above, and you are a member of a hand surgery group with in-house therapy services. You know that the type of work done by the manufacturer's employees leads to a high incidence of carpal tunnel syndrome, so it makes sense to target your patients who work for that employer, as well as other employees there, with a program offering prevention or hand therapy for carpal tunnel problems.

Another example involves a physician with a fairly successful bariatric medicine practice in a large metropolitan region. In the last several years, Dr. Shapiro has promoted his practice heavily in the various Yellow Pages directories available in his area. He spent several thousands of dollars placing in-column and display advertisements in the metropolitan directory, as well as nine suburban directories. That is, until he attended one of our practice promotion seminars and questioned one of our colleagues about his strategy. He was asked what the demographics of his patients were. More specifically, where did they live? Dr. Shapiro, somewhat embarrassed, admitted he did not know, but returned to his office determined to find out. Using his computer files, he prepared a report that listed the number and proportion of patients from each zip code. He compared this output with the zip code map of the region and found that his practice was only drawing significantly from two of the nine suburban directory areas. Based on this information, he changed his strategy and enlarged his display ads in the metropolitan area and two primary areas from which he was currently drawing patients. He also reduced his listings in the other areas to modest in-column advertisements. This resulted in significantly reduced expenditures for Yellow Pages advertising. Yet Dr. Shapiro has already seen a small increase in practice traffic resulting from the changes, including a higher concentration of patients from the suburban areas in which he expanded the size of his display ads.

Another example of the effective use of demographics and the computer concerns Dr. Dix. He is a plastic surgeon who decided to capitalize on Retin-A, the product that promised to reduce or eliminate wrinkles. Dr. Dix joined with several of his fellow plastic surgeons who feared this product could potentially reduce the need for the cosmetic surgery that was their mainstay.

However, as he studied the product and talked with some of his patients about it, he decided it could also be a vehicle to attract patients who would not benefit from Retin-A cream, but could benefit from cosmetic surgery. He decided to do a direct mail piece discussing the benefits and limitations of Retin-A, and invite readers to schedule an appointment to discuss the product at greater length. Using his computerized system, Dr. Dix extracted a list of females between the ages of 35 and 65, and prepared letters to accompany his Retin-A information pamphlet.

Dr. Dix also expanded his use of demographic information for this purpose beyond his own patient base. He contacted a local direct mail firm that maintained a computer data base of selected demographic information by zip code. He obtained a list of zip codes with the highest concentration of upper income residents. He further selected three zip codes that seemed to be the most promising, and prepared a generic form of his letter and Retin-A piece for mailing by the direct mail firm.

Both examples show how you can make excellent use of demographic information to promote patient and public interest in a medical topic.

REFERRAL SOURCES

The anecdote at the beginning of this chapter illustrates an effective way of using information about referring physicians to encourage their continued referrals. But there are other referral sources that should be systematically tapped for future business. Patients can be one of your best sources of referrals. Many physicians send patients who have referred someone to their practice a personalized "thank you" shortly after the patient is seen or scheduled for an appointment. Such a note can be kept in generic form on the computer and personalized details added where appropriate. As with previous examples, the referring patient's name and address can be easily called up from the systems to reduce the time needed to prepare the note. One physician we know builds a list on his computer system of all individuals, including physicians and other professionals, who have referred patients to him during the year. This list is created as a by-product of sending out the individual referral "thank you" notes. He then prepares a "Happy Holidays" note at the end of the year, briefly mentioning a few newsy highlights of the practice and once again thanking the individual for the confidence expressed through the referral. This list is also analyzed on the computer by selected demographics (e.g., age, sex, occupation, medical specialty if any, and residence address) to determine the type of individuals most supportive of his practice.

PAYMENT SOURCES

Who pays the bill, how much and when, are important questions where the practice's viability is concerned. The computer should be able to identify each insurance company and health plan. To carry it a bit further, physicians can do what businesses have long done, which is to quantify revenue sources for each product line. This is accomplished by first having the system identify the 10 to 20 CPT or ICD-9 codes that produce the most revenue for the practice. With those identified, the amount of revenue produced by each source for each of the coded services can be prepared. If there are several physicians in the practice, this can, of course, be expanded by developing the same kind of report for each physician as well as for the practice in aggregate. The system can and should be able to develop a list of aged accounts receivables by revenue sources to evaluate which carriers are providing payment on a timely (or untimely) basis. This is particularly helpful for health plans and can dictate a physician's choice as to whether to continue involvement in a health plan or to seek other arrangements.

Involvement in a health plan may appear to be an outstanding way of developing and/or retaining patients, but often a payment source review suggests that limited reimbursement, coupled with late payment, does not provide a surplus from this clientele.

OTHER DIRECT MAIL APPROACHES

The computer system with an automated patient data base should also allow the easy preparation of personalized mailings to patients or their family members who may benefit from a new service, or information about a new associate or more convenient location.

With an automated patient data base, your computer specialist will be able to prepare lists of new patients, patients with particular maladies, or those belonging to a certain age group with a potential need for your services. As an example, the ABC Dermatology Clinic was considering offering an acne clinic during evenings for teenagers. The plan was to charge only a modest fee, but attract teenagers who could benefit from more continual and direct treatment than the usual practice approach. The clinic prepared a report from its patient data base that listed the names, addresses and parents' names of all individuals beween 11 and 17 years of age. There were more than 600 individuals who fell within this age bracket, so it seemed reasonable to establish such an evening service for teenagers. Many of this target audience had already been patients of the practice, but many more were family members of older patients. The clinic prepared two personalized letters, one to the identified children, and one to their parents, promoting the clinic. The letter featured the clinic's understanding and care of teenagers' skin problems and included a practice brochure. Use of the computer allowed the practice to:

1. Identify the potential audience for the clinic idea.
2. Identify individuals who could most benefit from the intended service.
3. Produce the letter prepared by the practice in a form that could be personalized for each individual.
4. Prepare address labels for mailing.
5. Prepare a list of who received the letter so follow-up analysis could be performed to determine the value of this promotional effort.

The practice computer system entered the names and the salutatory opening of the letter as they were being produced. The staff folded the letters, stuffed the envelopes, and applied the computer-prepared labels to the envelopes. The computer was thus an important ingredient for a highly targeted direct mail campaign promoting a new service.

INFORMATION YOU NEED—A BY-PRODUCT OF OTHER OPERATIONS

Most of the assistance available from your computer for practice promotion purposes should be obtained as a by-product of other standard processes performed to manage the practice business. That is, the data you need to perform promotion and communication activities should be gathered, for the most part, for other purposes. The promotional activities should operate on that data using special software functions of the system.

The example at the beginning of the chapter of Dr. Blake, the surgeon, is again relevant here. You'll recall that the referring physicians' names were gathered as part of the patient registration process. This information became a part of the automated patient file, which could then be extracted according to chosen parameters, using a report writing or data base management portion of the system's software. The report could very likely be developed by simply identifying the name of the file containing the information, the name of the variable sought (e.g., referring physician) and the time period for which the data should be extracted—one year, for example. Using these parameters, the system would search the files, compile a list of names meeting the established criteria and print them out. Mary also asked the system to count how many patients were referred by each physician, and compute a percentage of the total of patients referred by physicians during the last year. She was able to have the system sort the list of physicians in descending order by the number of referrals, an indication of how much each physician was supporting the practice. A partial sample (with fictitious physician names) is given as Figure 13-2.

What else could Dr. Blake have asked for on the report? How about the specialty of each referring physician? To obtain this, and perhaps summarize the data by physician specialty, we would need to capture that

FIGURE 13-2 Sample Referring Physician Report

Bigtown Surgical Associates, Inc.
Report for Dr. Linda Lewiston
July 1–July 31, 1988

Referring Physician	Patients Referred	Previous Month
Blakemore, L.	8	9
Kozakile, M.	8	7
Ames, T.	6	7
Boxes, R.	5	5
Nielsen, X	4	6
Brown, J.	2	7
Gordon, N.	2	2
Laney, N.	0	6

information on the patient registration form (for it's highly unlikely that it would be accurate if we relied upon the patient data), or record and input the data ourselves. This entire report is only possible because referring physician information *is* captured.

WHAT YOUR COMPUTER SYSTEM SHOULD BE ABLE TO DO

Before we address other practice promotion strategies you could employ using your practice computer system, let's talk about what you would need to perform these activities (see Figure 13-3). A computer system has four important components for our purposes:

FIGURE 13-3 Personal Computer System for Practice Management and Promotion

A basic computer system for a medical practice will consist of these components: central processing unit with hard drive and/or floppy disk drive; keyboard; video monitor; and a printer capable of creating letter-quality (or near-letter quality) documents. Basic software should include practice management, word processing, data base and electronic spreadsheet.

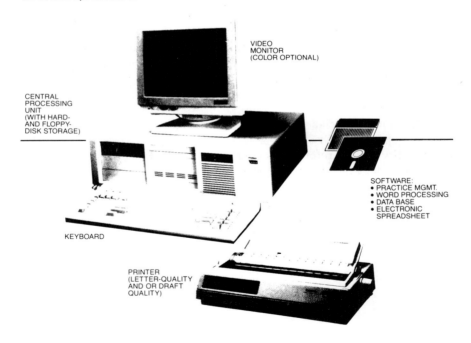

- The hardware, or computer equipment
- The software: the programs that make the hardware work
- The information (data about your practice and patients)
- Someone in your practice who understands the system sufficiently to prepare and maintain the information stored on it, and who can develop the documents or video screen output for practice use.

All four of these elements are necessary and must be obtained or prepared so they can work together. We have already addressed the information needed for practice promotion purposes, now let's concentrate on the hardware, software and personnel requirements.

COMPUTER EQUIPMENT (HARDWARE)

The computer systems employed for practice management are generally of three types: the free-standing microcomputer, the network system of microcomputers, or the minicomputer supporting several terminal stations.

Microcomputers, sometimes known as personal computers, or desktop computers, are the smallest and least expensive computer systems available. Systems appropriate for practice management range in price from $2,000 to $10,000 and are usually small enough to put on a table or desk top. These computer systems can support (as an option) the storage of a large amount of data that can be retrieved very quickly through the availability of auxiliary storage media (flexible disks, known as *floppy disks,* and hard disks). A system normally includes a video screen, a keyboard for input and some type of printing device for hard copy output.

Several microcomputer systems may be networked by coaxial cable so they operate independently or share information from a common data base (provided software you select allows it). These systems are more expensive. Networks can be convenient if you need to share a lot of information among different users or different offices (see Figure 13-4).

The multi-terminal minicomputer system looks and operates much like the networked microcomputer system. The difference is that each input/ output station (video screen and keyboard) does not have independent processing capabilities, but rather provides input to and develops output from one central computer system. Today, the multi-terminal minicomputer system compares favorably in price with the networked microcomputer systems. It is the form generally provided by vendors of practice management systems who also sell the computer programs (software).

All three types of hardware systems could support the practice promotion activities we have been discussing if sufficient internal memory is acquired to provide the storage and rapid access of information about patients in the practice.

Because much of the promotional work that will be accomplished requires preparation of hard copy output, the hardware should include both draft-quality (dot matrix) and letter-quality printers (see Figure 13-5).

FIGURE 13-4 Diagram of Networked Microcomputer System
The multiterminal computer system links individual stations with a central computer system. It's the type of system often provided by practice management computer vendors.

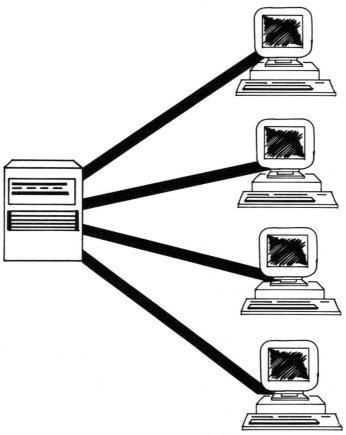

Letter-quality printers will be particularly important since much of the computer output should be personalized and professional looking. You may be generating computer letters, but they should not look like computer letters.

Quality printers today are available from a few hundred dollars to a few thousand dollars for the more flexible laser printers. Your choice of printer depends upon the volume of output expected and the sophistication of intended output. If there are plans to prepare brochures and newsletters with these systems, then laser printers with desktop publishing capabilities should be considered. If low to medium volume is expected, and most of it of a correspondence nature, then carbon ribbon impact printers are

FIGURE 13-5 Comparison of Dot Matrix and Letter-Quality Printing
The difference in printer capabilities can be seen in samples shown here. Documents created by dot matrix printers, while greatly improved over earlier versions, usually can be instantly identified as "computer generated" by the pattern of dots that makes up the print. A daisy-wheel printer creates letter-quality documents that look typewriter generated; however, daisy wheel printers cannot create graphics and cannot be used for desktop publishing. Laser printers create letter-quality documents and work with desktop publishing software but are more expensive than dot matrix or daisy-wheel printers.

```
        SAMPLE LETTER QUALITY PRINTING


Mr. Jan Swink is a very delightful 55 year
old male patient of mine who underwent a
flexible signoidoscopy during his annual
physical exam on Sept. 15, 1988.    I am
concerned about a 2-3 cm red sessile polyp
at approximately 28 cm.    It was oozing
somewhat at this time.

I have informed Mr. Swink of what I found
and asked him to call your office as soon as
possible to schedule a more extensive
colonoscope and removal of this polyp.

I appreciate your seeing Mr. Swink, and
value the care you give my patients.

Sincerely
```

```
    SAMPLE DOT MATRIX PRINTING


Mr. Jan Swink is a very delightful 55 year old male patient of
mine who underwent a flexible sigmoidoscopy during his annual
physical exam on Sept. 15, 1988.  I am concerned about a 2-3 cm
red sessile polyp at approximately 28 cm.  It was oozing somewhat
at this time.

I have informed Mr. Swink of what I found and asked him to call
your office as soon as possible to schedule a more extensive
colonoscope and removal of this polyp.

I appreciate your seeing Mr. Swink, and value the care you give
my patients.

Sincerely
```

probably satisfactory. In either event, it is probably useful to obtain a dual bin sheet feeder to allow convenient output on letterhead paper. Printers should also be capable of printing mailing labels, as well as continuous form documents (e.g., insurance forms).

SOFTWARE

Computer software refers to the programs that provide the hardware with directions to accept the input, process the information and produce the documents. The real power of computer systems today is very much related to the sophistication and ease of use (user-friendliness) of the software. As with computer hardware, there are a variety of choices and approaches for practice promotion activities.

To produce the kind of practice promotion recommendations discussed here generally requires a system that captures information about patients and practice activities on an ongoing basis. It is usually preferable, therefore, to choose a system that is capable of handling patient billing and accounts receivable activities while creating a data base of patient information.

It's also important that the system have data base management capabilities that allow the user to select subsets of patient information from the data base according to predefined criteria, and organize them for subsequent storage or output. The system should also support word processing activities to generate documents such as letters or labels prepared for the identified subsets. The word processing function is also helpful for other communication activities, such as newsletters, brochures and patient information handouts.

Other software elements that expand the system's ability to enhance promotion activities include medical records stored as part of the patient data base, an appointment and scheduling system, and statistical analysis programs. While these activities may not seem related to practice promotion, they are. They ultimately result in satisfied patients, who are your greatest source of new patients.

It is most advantageous if all the software is "integrated." That is, all the program modules should work together to allow information transfer from one module to the other without the need to physically re-enter the information. There are a number of vendors who provide integrated software, many of which run on microcomputer systems.

For practices not prepared to purchase these more costly, fully integrated systems, it is possible to begin with a patient billing and accounts receivable system capable of developing output in standard format. This may be organized by separate data base management software which, in turn, interfaces with a word processing system for merging of selected data into the desired correspondence.

To support practice promotion activities, a patient billing and accounts receivable module should generally capture and store the following information:

- Diagnosis code
- Procedure code(s)

- Service date(s)
- Service location
- Service provider identification
- Method of payment
- Amount of payment
- Date of payment

Information necessary for insurance carriers and third party payers will include the date of onset of the treated episode, information about hospitalization, an indication of whether the treatment resulted from an accident or illness, information about any previous or subsequent disability, and an indication of whether the problem was related to the individual's employment.

The computer system should be able to generate a bill for the patient at the time of the encounter. The system should also accept input about patient billing and accounts receivable from a variety of forms including a superbill, governmental claims forms, and the universal health insurance claim form.

An important consideration in acquiring hardware and software for practice promotion support is the need for both flexibility and growth. A computer system of any kind should have at least a two-fold growth potential at the time it is initially installed. Further, it should be flexible enough to accept and process a variety of software so that you can adapt as new advancements become available. It is most risky to commit to a system that has the ability to process only one or a few types of software, or to acquire software that operates on only one computer system.

Word Processing. Word processing software allows the creation and editing, formatting, storing and printing of text. (This book was written and edited using word processing software, for example.) A word processing software package can be purchased separately, or sometimes integrated within practice management software systems. Word processing software can be effective for enhancing practice productivity. It has been seen to increase productivity, compared with typewriters, from 50 to 400 percent in office use.

Desktop Publishing. Desktop publishing has become highly sophisticated recently with the advent of special software and laser printers. It is now possible to develop entire promotional brochures, newsletters, and even certain forms of advertisements with the use of these systems (see Figure 13-6).

The software necessary to drive these systems is easily acquired and runs on most medium-sized micro-computer systems. Effective generation of quality documents, however, requires a laser printer with sufficient internal memory to store the images and produce them with the clarity of typesetting.

Desktop publishing systems are capable of producing an extraordinarily

FIGURE 13-6 Sample Desktop Published Document
This newsletter for referral sources and patients was developed by an orthopedic surgeon using his computer and a desktop publishing program. Even the illustration of the total hip replacement was created using desktop publishing software. Developed by Stuart C. Kozinn, MD, The Institute for Bone and Joint Disorders, Phoenix, Arizona.

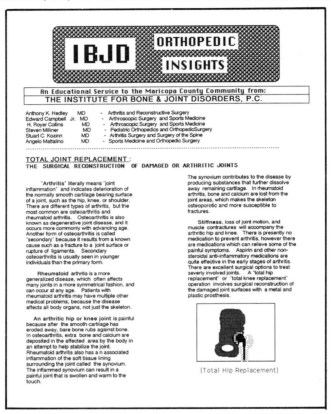

wide variety of type fonts and sizes. They can reproduce photographs and create graphic designs that seem to be professionally drawn. It is entirely possible to prepare a practice brochure, patient newsletters and flyers, educational updates to referring physicians, and other similar materials with desktop publishing systems today.

Most such systems require one to two weeks of training for an individual to become sufficiently versed in it to produce good quality printed material. For the practice engaging in the production of a variety of communication brochures, newsletters and other promotional items, however, this learning curve and the expense of a desktop publishing system quickly amortize as a good alternative to paying others to prepare materials. It may be wise to have external creative counsel initially establish the format for brochures and newsletters. The result will be a more professional publication, as your practice office staff probably does not have these capabilities.

However, once the original designs are completed, the staff and physicians in the practice should be capable of handling the ongoing adjustments to these documents.

MEDICAL RECORD SOFTWARE

Medical record software adds the important ability to segment and identify subsets of your patient population by their illness and/or treatment characteristics. This can be used for follow-up communication, monitoring patient progress and promotion of new services targeted to these specific groups.

Medical record software typically includes dictionaries that allow for parallel multiple coding of diagnoses, a list of usual and customary medications used in the practice, and lists of practice-specific procedural instructions that may be given or sent to patients. An important element of the medical record system is the ability to include historical background on patients with dates that will incorporate and organize data about the patient's personal and family medical history, hospitalization(s), immunizations, laboratory and therapy results, and surgical activity. Some systems will allow the inclusion of free text to capture narrative information gained during patient encounters for subsequent review, and formulation of a more completely documented record in computer-supported form.

PERSONNEL

Computer software should be selected so that it is easily operable by the office manager and/or secretarial staff. This is generally not a problem for traditional practice management functions such as billing, accounts receivables and even appointment scheduling. However, if the system is to be effectively used for promotional purposes, someone must be designated who understands (or will learn) the system well enough to extract information from it in the desired manner, and prepare the printed documents for use. In many cases this may be the doctor's secretary or office manager. In other cases, it may be necessary to hire a full-time programmer.

One internist reported in *Medical Economics* that his hiring of a full-time computer programmer allowed him to replace a practice secretary. The ultimate result was that, after a few years, the computer system was doing the work of three secretaries while at the same time improving relationships with patients, staff and his colleagues. His programmer created a software package for the system that assumed many of the routine secretarial chores such as composing and typing informational memos, return-to-work letters, and patient reminders about follow-up visits. The office staff had only to add the necessary information to one of the many personalized form letters stored in the computer and direct the printing of hard copy as needed.

Thus, as the computer hardware assists by converting and storing patient and practice information in a usable form, and the software is acquired to extract the information and produce the desired output, someone in the practice must take on the task of assuring that these functions are performed adequately and efficiently.

With the basic elements of your practice computer system outlined, we will turn our attention now to computer support of strategies for retaining patients.

KEEPING YOUR PATIENTS VIA COMPUTER

Throughout this book, we've emphasized that retaining patients is as important as generating new patients. Here again, a flexible computer-based system can be of help. Consider Drs. Embry and Fino, two surgeons who were interested in learning how their patients felt about their office environment, the way they were treated by physicians and staff, and the outcomes of their procedures. Dr. Fino's wife taught statistics at a local community college and impressed upon her husband how important a "random" sample was for the survey results to be generalized to the total patient population. "You can either go through your patient files manually," Mrs. Fino said, "or have your system select a "random sample" of your active patient files."

The surgeons wisely selected the second option and the computer, using a random number generator, selected 250 patient names and addresses. They had the computer prepare mailing labels, and also used it to personalize letters prepared as a transmittal document for their survey. The questionnaire and the cover letter were mailed to the selected patients. One hundred and two usable responses were returned.

As the surveys were coming back, the doctors once again consulted with Mrs. Fino, asking, "How should we go about summarizing these results?" She said, "Once again, you have a choice. You can hand-tally them, or we can acquire a simple statistical analysis program that will compute the frequencies of each response and also provide us with cross tabulation analysis, permitting us to focus on attitudes and perceptions of patients with certain characteristics."

Following Mrs. Fino's advice, the physicians acquired a simple statistical program and loaded it on their personal computer system. Their office manager entered the data from the surveys in computer-processed form and tallied the results.

In this instance the computer was effectively used to generate the sample, distribute the survey instruments and summarize the results.

The computer can generate information to identify patients who should be advised of the need for follow-up visits. Lists of patients with medical problems or disorders suggesting a need for return visits can be developed if medical record software is incorporated into the system. For example, Dr. Grant, a family practitioner, prepares a quarterly list of his hypertensive patients along with information about their last visit. Those who have not been seen during the quarter are sent a note reminding them to take their medicine (if appropriate), and suggesting they call for a follow-up appointment. Also, patients who have not been seen for extended periods of time (six to nine months), can usually be identified and their names and addresses produced for follow-up notes encouraging them to call and schedule an appointment.

Another physician uses his computer to provide him with a list of patients seen during office hours each day, and the medications or treatments prescribed for each patient. He keeps this printout by his home phone at night to be prepared for any late night phone calls. The same list is then given to his office staff the next day for telephone follow-up with the patients to see if the medication has been taken and appears to be working.

EXAM ROOM USE

Some physicians have extended the use of the computer system to their patient interaction in the exam/consulting room. This usually involves installing a personal computer in the exam room, or a video screen and keyboard linked to a computer. With these systems the physician or his/her nurse is able to call up automated medical records for the patient, and record observations, treatments and prescriptions ordered during the visit. While not currently widespread, this activity is increasing.

Incorporating the computer into the patient dialogue offers great promise in that a significant amount of information can be conveniently captured, and the patient's history effectively reviewed, during the examination and discussion. As with most activities of promise, however, there is risk. Patient satisfaction is strongly linked to a patient's perception that the doctor has identified and dealt with their concerns in a manner communicating warmth and interest. The risk is that the computer may become an obstacle in that process. The physician could be viewed as being more concerned with the computer (with technology) than with the patient.

Studies to date have shown mixed patient satisfaction results when the computer was used during the exam/consultation process. However, physicians who were able to use the computer as a resource in a way that maintained the integrity of the personal, consultative process were generally viewed positively by patients.

As an extension of this activity, a computer can be used to calculate important values while the physician spends time interpreting the results with patients. For example, the patient of one physician asked how he could figure his HDL cholesterol rating so quickly. It had taken this patient's former physician about 15 minutes to do it using pencil and paper. This physician, of course, used a computer to perform the calculation, and spent the time discussing the dangers and remedies of high cholesterol rather than performing arithmetic computations.

Another physician reported in a *Medical Economics* article the experience of a middle-aged patient who had been attending the physician's lectures on curbing alcohol consumption. The physician gave the patient a computer printout listing his elevated SGPT values along with an indication of possible liver malfunction. This printout in black and white had the desired impact: the patient cut back his drinking and took a more continued concern in his liver functions.

The same physician reports positive experiences with patients who were able to study printouts describing medical results of lab tests, and comparing their values with high and low limits. Providing this information in a comparative form to patients, with normal as well as abnormal results, allows them to monitor their own progress and to establish goals with regard to vital health indicators. Improved compliance and better health maintenance are the hoped-for results. Thus both the patient and the physician win.

MISSED APPOINTMENTS

Missed appointments by patients are both troublesome and irritating to the practice. Patients who have missed an appointment should be contacted immediately to determine the problem and reschedule another soon. Not much more can be done about the infrequent or "explained" no-show. However, with certain patients, a pattern can evolve that requires other action. The computer can become part of the solution by keeping track and providing a report listing all patients who have missed appointments in the last week, month or quarter. The report can indicate the number of appointments each patient has missed. This can be useful in contacting the individuals to determine whether there is a chronic problem (e.g., disorientation, memory lapse, lack of transportation) with which the practice can assist. Such assistance can make a very positive impression on the patient who would see the physician as someone who goes beyond the call of duty to help.

Some patients, however, abuse the convenience offered by the scheduled appointment. In such cases, stronger action may be needed. Missed appointments represent lost income as well as inconvenience to other patients. One physician prepared such lists and found that several of the individuals who had repeatedly missed appointments were members of a health plan he had contracted with. He gave the list of missed appointments to the plan administrator, and requested that the issue be addressed with the patients.

NEW PATIENTS

New patients offer a unique and important opportunity to build practice loyalty. The direct mail promotional support available from a computer system may be helpful in accomplishing that goal. Dr. Crawforde is an ophthalmologist who is doing little to promote his practice, other than relying upon word-of-mouth referrals. One week he asked his office manager to print out a list of new patients seen that month. He was a little surprised to find 36 new individuals in his practice. He then asked for another report listing these individuals along with the procedures he performed. Recognizing an opportunity, he dictated a letter which his office manager put on the computer system to be personalized with the names and addresses of each individual. The letter expressed appreciation for the confidence these patients had in the doctor's practice, wished them well, and invited them to have their friends come in if they had vision problems. The doctor personally penned a brief note at the bottom encouraging these new patients to contact him if any problems or questions arose, and/or mentioning a follow-up visit if it had been scheduled.

The patient response was so positive that the doctor now has his office manager prepare this report and personalized letters weekly for all new patients seen.

THE COMPUTER: YOUR PRACTICE ALLY

Computer systems can be a valuable asset in identifying patient segments who may be receptive to targeted promotional activities. The computer is also helpful in preparing promotional materials and supporting effective patient interaction activities. There are many forms of practice computer systems today that can be employed for these purposes. In addition, micro-computer systems using data base management languages, word processing languages, perhaps even electronic spread sheet languages (e.g., Lotus, MultiMate), can support the development of patient data bases and the generation of documents for special purposes. Effective use of computer systems for practice promotion purposes will require ongoing attention in order to create and maintain the patient data base, output reports and correspondence, and develop programs to select sub-segments of the patient data base for special promotional purposes. But the results are worth it, in terms of opportunities to increase patient satisfaction, enhance compliance, increase office productivity, and improve communications with patients, potential patients and referral sources.

Building Your Practice Through
Ethical Advertising

Chapter 14

Making Your Media Mix Work for You

Earlier in this book we said that "one Yellow Pages ad does not a marketing program make." Just as a good marketing program consists of a combination of promotional strategies, the most effective advertising campaign will consist of a combination of media. This is known as the "media mix."

The combination of media you utilize is a crucial decision, because a carefully selected mix helps you reach a broader spectrum of your target audience(s) and ensures a wiser expenditure of your advertising budget. A good selection of media also creates reinforcement and strengthening of the message and image of each individual component.

The mix is also important because media costs—the actual charges for newspaper advertising, a radio spot, a television commercial—may well represent the largest single expenditure in your advertising budget. Unfortunately, it is impossible to *guarantee* that a certain media mix will produce the results you seek for your practice. Much of the decision-making in selecting a media mix is based on a combination of experience and judgment, liberally laced with instinct.

However, through research and the information gained in this chapter about how to use research data, you'll be able to make an informed, educated judgment that will give you a better chance for positive results.

THE ELEMENTS OF THE MEDIA MIX

Let's review the types of advertising you may consider in your media mix:

- Yellow Pages
- Television (local, network and cable)
- Radio
- Newspaper (dailies, weeklies, and specialty newspapers)
- Magazines and journals (general and special interest, professional, trade)
- Direct mail
- Advertising specialties (giveaway items)
- Outdoor (billboards)

- Transit (bus, taxi, etc.)
- Miscellaneous and "goodwill" advertising (e.g. symphony program, football scoreboard, etc.)

Here are some of the benefits gained from having a media mix strategy:

1. It's usually difficult to reach everybody in your target audience(s) through one medium.
2. Repeat exposure in multiple media has an overall effect that is greater than the sum of the individual parts.
3. You avoid putting all your eggs (advertising dollars) in one basket.
4. You can emphasize the various strengths of your practice to appropriate markets by utilizing the unique advantages and audiences of different media.

SELECTING YOUR ADVERTISING MEDIA

Selection of the appropriate media for your medical practice and your promotional plan will depend on a number of criteria (see Figure 14-1). But the most important factors to be considered are the objectives of your advertising program, the characteristics of each medium and the audience profile for each, and the cost to produce and place the ad in each medium. In addition, you must evaluate the message you want to convey. It may be necessary to use a variety of media in order to assure that the various aspects of your message—demonstration, explanation, complex information—are properly communicated.

BUDGETARY REALITIES

The first step in creating a media mix that's right for your practice and promotion objectives is to determine the media that will reach the indi-

FIGURE 14-1   Advertising How-To's

---

1. Advertise to meet a need, not because the competition is doing it. Don't be reactive; be proactive.

2. Make your advertising *intrusive*. It doesn't have to be obnoxious or flamboyant, but it must be noticed. It must be seen or heard, or it's not doing its job.

3. Budget appropriately. Allocate enough to get the job done. If you don't have enough money, accumulate several weeks or months' worth until you do.

4. Invest in advertising for the long-term. There's no quick fix. Don't expect short-term results.

5. Build in measurement at every level—requests for information, phone calls, appointments, surgeries or treatments as a result of the appointments.

6. Have a plan and a strategy for your advertising campaign. Know who you're talking to and what you're talking about.

7. Train your staff to respond to your ad campaign. Be sure they know when and where your ad(s) is/are running, and what the ad says or offers.

---

viduals or groups whom you want to hear or see your message. Equally important is the question of which media will help rather than detract from your professional image.

The limitations of your budget will require streamlining the list of effective media so that your advertising is both frequent and regular, since few medical advertisers can afford to be in all the media that promise results. For most physicians whose promotion budgets are not unlimited, Yellow Pages, newspaper, radio and direct mail are the primary choices; these media enhance and reinforce one another.

With a more generous advertising budget, you can add television, magazine and perhaps even outdoor advertising to your media mix and thereby ensure excellent recognition in your market.

But realistically, you may very well have to start with a single medium and build on that as funds become available. The addition of a second medium always increases audience reach, enabling you to get your message to more people and to reinforce it to those people who are exposed to it through both media.

The key principle to remember is that adding a second medium to your mix produces two reinforcing advantages: you reach more people and you reach them more often. And of course, recognition and retention is enhanced when an ad for your colo-rectal screening program is heard on the radio, for example, and then your ad appears in the newspaper, offering a free brochure on colon cancer.

THREE KEY OBJECTIVES

A media schedule requires two decisions: how often to advertise and when to advertise. To decide how often to advertise, you must know the reach and frequency of a given medium.

Reach is the number or percentage of the audience who are (or whom you want to be) exposed to at least one of your ads within a given period. With the broadcast media, reach is normally based on a four-week time frame. With print, it is based on the effective life span of a given issue of the publication. For example, the reach for a weekly magazine like *Newsweek* is based on total circulation plus its "passalong" rate, or readers other than the subscriber or purchaser. *Newsweek* is read by about six people, a figure much higher than for daily newspapers.

Frequency refers to the average number of times individuals are exposed to a message. Frequency is much higher for newspapers, radio and television, where ads may appear daily. Yellow Pages, magazines and billboards have poorer frequency. A frequency of three is considered ideal.

The relationship between reach and frequency is called Gross Rating Points (GRP), calculated by multiplying reach by frequency. Suppose you want to reach 60 percent of your target audience over the next four weeks. With a frequency of three, your GRP objective would be 60 times three, or 180.

To achieve your desired advertising goal, you must also consider the timing of advertising exposures, also called continuity. Continuity is how your advertising is scheduled or "spaced" over a given time period. It can be a constant pattern, with advertising consistent year-round; it can be concentrated during certain months or seasons of the year; or it can be intermittent throughout the year (also called flighting or pulsing, a concept explained later in this chapter).

PLAN AHEAD

Frequency is a measure of the intensity of your plan, and is governed to some extent by the medium and your budget. Continuity, on the other hand, is something you can control. For example, if you advertise in a weekly publication, you are limited in frequency to an ad once a week. But if you advertise every week, every other week, or the last two weeks of the month, you have established a regular pattern and have achieved continuity.

One effective way to plan for and maintain continuity is through the regular use of monthly and quarterly planning sheets. Such forms are similar to accounting sheets and are used for listing your planned advertising expenditures. They provide a means of visualizing the impact and intensity of your media campaign.

The monthly planning sheet (Figure 14-2) is laid out like a calendar, with the days of the week listed horizontally across the top. The left-hand vertical column lists the media you are scheduled to use during the month. In the squares representing each day of the month, the amount spent on advertising in a given medium is indicated. The right-hand vertical column lists projected and actual expenditures for each medium for a one-week period. Finally, the form lists projected and actual media outlays for the month.

The quarterly planning sheet lists months horizontally across the top, media employed in the left-hand vertical column, production and placement costs in the right vertical columns, and monthly totals horizontally across the bottom. Expenditures by media per week are tallied on the resulting grid.

Production Costs. As you distribute the amounts you plan to spend on your chosen media, it's important to include production costs—the amount it will cost you to have a print ad written, designed and brought to camera-ready art; the cost of hiring talent and taping a radio or television spot—in your overall budget. The amount you set aside for production depends on how you intend to have your ads produced and on the media selected.

Production for TV spots is normally more expensive than for other media. Even utilizing a television station for production can be expensive, since you are billed for camera and studio time as well as the use of any

FIGURE 14-2 Monthly and Quarterly Planning Sheets

Monthly Planning Sheet

MEDIA	Sun	Mon	Tues	Wed	Thurs	Fri	Sat	Actual	Projected
	1	2	3	4	5	6	7		
TRIBUNE		125			125			250	250
HERALD									
SHOPPER				80				80	100
KMAA									
	8	9	10	11	12	13	14		
TRIBUNE		125			125			250	250
HERALD									
SHOPPER							150	150	150
KMAA									
	15	16	17	18	19	20	21		
TRIBUNE		125			125			250	250
HERALD									
SHOPPER									
KMAA									
	22	23	24	25	26	27	28		
TRIBUNE							250	250	250
HERALD							250	250	250
SHOPPER				80				80	100
KMAA									

FEB 19 81
month   TOTALS $1560 $1600

QUARTERLY PLANNING SHEET

	MEDIA	JAN	FEB	MAR	PROJECTIONS MEDIA	PRODUCTION
1st Week	TRIBUNE	240	250		590	
	HERALD					80
	SHOPPER	80	80	80	240	
	KMAA					10
2nd Week	TRIBUNE		250		250	—
	HERALD	150	150	150	450	—
	SHOPPER	200		150	350	—
	KMAA	300		300	600	—
3rd Week	TRIBUNE	350	250	350	950	—
	HERALD					—
	SHOPPER					—
	KMAA					—
4th Week	TRIBUNE					—
	HERALD	250	250	250	750	—
	SHOPPER	80	80	80	240	—
	KMAA					—
5th Week	TRIBUNE	250	250	250	750	—
	HERALD					—
	SHOPPER					—
	KMAA	300		200	500	—
	TOTALS	$2300	$1560	$1810	$5670	$90

special techniques. In addition, a professional-quality television spot usually requires the use of professional talent.

Production charges for direct mail pieces vary according to the type of piece you devise. A simple letter is relatively inexpensive; but mailing costs can add up, and if the letter is poorly done, the lack of response can make it a very expensive promotional effort. If you are planning a printed piece, you'll need to consider printing costs, paper stock, the use of color and photos, folding and design costs.

Whenever you utilize outside vendors (as opposed to the in-house services offered by radio, television, newspaper, Yellow Pages, etc.), be sure to solicit bids from several sources. If most of your production involves outside sources, you should set aside as much as 25 percent of your total budget for this expense. The remaining 75 percent can be allocated for purchasing advertising space and/or time. If, on the other hand, you are relying on in-house art/production departments to develop your ads, you can usually plan on as little as five to ten percent of your budget for production.

Planning for Effectiveness. As you build your ad schedule, be sure to look carefully at the big picture. It's not enough to simply divide your budget into 52 equal weekly outlays. It's essential to plan your media mix and schedule so your advertising is heaviest just before and during the traditionally slow periods when you need additional patients. It goes without saying that you should avoid a heavy advertising schedule when you don't need more business, or when you will be on vacation or attending continuing education seminars.

It's also important to consider any public relations efforts you plan to undertake during a specific time period. Effective public relations builds business; it's wise to take into account expected results from a PR campaign when building a media schedule, since you may not need as heavy an ad campaign. Next to not having enough business, the worst situation is having to turn patients away after spending good money to attract them to your practice. At the same time, you may need to advertise certain special events you are sponsoring; you can't rely totally on press releases, talk show interviews and other "free" promotion. You may wish to schedule an advertising campaign to coincide with or precede a PR campaign in order to gain the reinforcement advertising provides.

The quarterly form should serve as your master planning sheet, your means of laying out the big picture. The monthly form helps you take a close look at where your advertising budget actually goes.

Traffic and Recap Sheets. To help you plan your media mix, it's helpful to know what your advertising has accomplished during the previous month(s). We've stressed the importance of asking your new patients how they learned about your practice; this information can be transferred to a traffic sheet that tells you exactly how many patients resulted from each of your promotional efforts. You'll find a detailed discussion of how to develop a traffic sheet in Chapter 20 on monitoring advertising and public relations efforts.

At the end of the month, the traffic sheet totals should be transferred to a monthly recap sheet (explained in Chapter 20) that covers all your promotional efforts and indicates how many calls resulted. With this recap sheet, you can determine which strategies are most effective for the time and money you invest.

Make Your Mix Effective. If your advertising promotion efforts seem sparse when spread out over an entire month, "flighting" or "pulsing" may help you achieve greater continuity. These are options to continuous advertising, or the consistent scheduling of ads without schedule variations.

Flighting refers to the use of periodic "waves" of advertising interspersed with periods of relative inactivity. The premise behind flighting is that advertising's effectiveness is cumulative: the longer and more intense a campaign, the more response it delivers. To get the benefit of this cumulative effect, the advertiser who cannot afford to inundate the media year round, month in, month out, advertises in abbreviated bursts instead, with perhaps two weeks of steady advertising followed by two weeks with no ads. The effectiveness of an ad campaign does not diminish immediately after it stops. By allowing a campaign to run intermittently, the advertiser gains the effect of continuity, and at considerable savings.

Pulsing works on the same principle as flighting, and is merely a combination of flighting and continuous advertising. The advertising schedule is continuous, but it is supplemented and reinforced by intermittent bursts or "pulses" of heavier advertising.

Most advertisers use flights of two to six weeks, followed by a two- to three-week hiatus before the next flight. So long as the time between flights is no more than three weeks, the effect of continuity is maintained.

Large vs. Small: Size Isn't Everything. At this point, you should also consider the size of your print media ads. Is it better to run many small ads or just a few large ones? The answer to this question depends in part on whether you are using supporting media to bolster your print campaign.

Large ads offer the advantage of attention through dominance. And studies indicate that large ads do bring in more inquiries. However, the additional inquiries are not in proportion to the increased cost. If a quarter page ad generates 33 responses, a half-page will generate about 60, and a full-page about 100. Doubling the space does not double the number of inquiries.

The size of your ad should also be related to what you have to say. A small ad doesn't leave much room for anything but basics like your name and phone number. If you want to establish an image solely through your print ads, it is probably best, at least initially, to use larger ads. On the other hand, if your media mix is strong, smaller print ads might very effectively accomplish their reinforcing function.

You don't really have to be a big advertiser to be successful. A good rule of thumb is to buy the size necessary to make your message attractive, readable, and understandable—and then run it as frequently as you can, with support from other media if possible.

Saturation Through Repetition. Repetition is a necessary component of a successful advertising campaign. Long after you've tired of seeing the same ad, there still are many in your target market who have never seen it, or who have seen it only once and have not yet acted on it. Your message must saturate the market in order to become firmly implanted in the reader's mind.

If repetition bothers you, remember that you have been pondering the ad, analyzing and comparing it for weeks or even months before the public was exposed to it. You've been involved with it from conception through production. Don't underexpose your audience to the message you've so carefully developed.

Remember too that the public is bombarded with information to the point that only a percentage of it can be retained—only that which is hammered home repeatedly. In service professions like medicine, an ad may go unnoticed by a consumer until he or she wants or needs the service you offer. Then the individual will look for your message. You are not only saving the considerable time and expense of developing new ads, but you are also employing sound marketing strategy when you allow repetition to work for you.

Repeating your ad makes it easier to buy media packages. You simply turn your ad over to your media representatives, schedule according to your media plan, and let the reps handle it. You can concentrate on providing medical care to your patients, knowing that your ad campaign is running as planned. You'll receive tear sheets of your print ads and affidavits from the broadcast media assuring you that your ads ran as specified.

ALTERNATING MEDIA

If you are using more than one medium, heavy advertising periods in each should complement one another (see Figure 14-3). If magazine is used every other month, for example, radio flights can be used in alternate months. Alternating media usage keeps your message in front of your targeted audience at all times without straining your budget.

Alternating media is also a good way to determine which medium is working hardest and pulling best for you. Testing advertising effectiveness is something few small advertisers give the attention it deserves. Often a physician will know her practice has experienced an increase in patients, but she doesn't know what to attribute it to. Was it the radio spots, or the newspaper ad? Did more people respond to the ad that quoted price, or the one that appealed to the importance of regular checkups? To ensure that your marketing and promotion campaign is on track and to build a thriving practice, you must know how effective every component and every medium has been in all your advertising endeavors.

National advertisers invest substantial sums in testing advertising results, and you need to do the same on a smaller scale. It isn't even necessary to invest anything (other than the cost of the ad) to determine results. Chapter 20 explores some of the methods available to evaluate your promotional program.

One way to test the effectiveness of various print media is through coupons. An ad coupon in one publication can be a slightly different size, or coded with a non-existent "Dept. G" in the return address to differentiate it from another ad. Another technique that can be used in both print and broadcast media is to ask respondents to request a specific staffer when calling. By varying names according to the media, results are made obvious. Of course, one of the most frequently used measuring devices is the new patient information form that asks how the patient learned of your practice. Or you can simply ask your staff to query new patients when they call for an appointment or arrive for their first visit. (Be sure they also record the responses!)

The important thing is to tabulate the results, whichever method you use, and adjust your next media plan accordingly. If you do this, each successive campaign will become less subjective and more effective.

By translating your results into percentages, they become even more obvious. If 44 percent of your responses come from investing 60 percent of your budget in radio, while the remaining 56 percent come from a 40 percent investment in newspaper advertising, you will want to devote a larger share of your media mix to newspaper advertising during the following month or two—and then track those results to be certain they are relatively consistent.

A WORD ABOUT SPECIALTY ADVERTISING

Your media mix may include a component that few people tend to think of as an advertising strategy: advertising specialty items. The impact of a single imprinted refrigerator magnet might seem inconsequential. Yet magnets and other specialty items have a valid place in practice promotion.

Specialty items have a long lifespan as an advertising vehicle and can effectively complement other media efforts. They also can be used to generate a response for tracking. ("Call or write to receive your free first aid kit.") Imprinted with your practice name, address and phone number, they are welcome gifts to patients, employees, the audience at a speaking engagement and other special events. For instance, a rheumatologist speaking to an arthritis association could give out rubber jar openers imprinted with his practice name. A dermatologist may give a pocket mirror; an ophthalmologist, a magnifying glass.

Specialty items should not be considered a stand-alone strategy. Give careful consideration to the audience, their needs, your specialty and the image the item conveys when you select it. And be sure to allow plenty of time when ordering ad specialties; it can take up to four months to receive your order (see Figure 14-4).

FIGURE 14-3 Media Comparison Chart

MEDIA	ADVANTAGES	DISADVANTAGES
Radio	High demographic selectivity, low cost for production, time. Exceptional drive-time reach. Non-seasonal, flexible, personal. Audience loyal to station, air personality. Mobility, immediacy.	Clutter of competing advertisers. Fragmented audiences, fleeting message. One-dimensional.
Television	Dynamic, personalized approach. Mass-market and select-market appeal. Repetition, prestige media, image enhancement. Credible, authoritative. Highly cost-efficient for local market saturation. High impact.	Initially expensive (production and time costs). Short life of commercial message. Advertising clutter. Viewers can zap commercials on home-taped programs. Careful selection of time/program buy a must.
Cable TV	Varied programming reach. Rapidly growing medium, great local capabilities. Flexible commercial length. Upscale, younger audiences, many with children. Very targeted. Relatively low cost.	Appeal is to narrowly defined audience. Research unrefined. Short commercial message life. Evaluation of message result difficult. Proper program, time selection a must.
Yellow Pages	Near-universal circulation. Consumer convenience. Regional editions, all seasons. Consumer approval of professional advertising. Long message life. Provides complete information on practice features, benefits. Receptive audience.	Highly competitive. Poor ad reproduction, design limitations, closing date confusion with multiple regional/suburban directories. Can be costly. Wasted circulation.
Magazines	Targeted marketing. Quality reproduction. Long message life. Pass along readership. Image builder. Believability. High reader involvement. Upscale readership. Good environment for healthcare advertisers.	Long lead time, competitive clutter. High cost. Lack of immediacy, flexibility. Wasted circulation.

FIGURE 14-3 Continued

MEDIA	ADVANTAGES	DISADVANTAGES
Newspapers	Immediacy. Credibility, authority of message. Space for extensive copy. Mass medium with broad demographics. High concentration of upscale, upper income, educated adults. Flexibility, short lead time. Easy to reach local communities with suburban/zoned editions.	Can be costly. Low pass-along readership. Editorial content can be unsophisticated, lack prestige in suburban/small publications. Short life span. Poor reproduction.
Shoppers	Inexpensive. Relatively long shelf life. Multiple readership. Receptive audience. Consumer convenience.	Discount image. Poor reproduction, printing quality. Competitive clutter. Possible medical code restrictions.
Outdoor	80% market saturation. Geographically targeted. Sustained presence. High visibility, high coverage, high frequency. Good support medium. Cost per thousand low. Flexible packages available.	High out-of-pocket costs. Limited copy length. Limited recall. Audience research unreliable. Fleeting medium. Public concern over esthetics.
Direct Mail	Very targeted. Personalized message. Flexible medium. Copy, message can be as long as needed. No publication deadlines to wait for or miss. Speedy medium.	Mailing list selection must be precise, can be time-consuming. Can be costly. Competitive clutter. "Junk mail" image for poorly packaged piece.

AND FINALLY . . .

Constant vigilance is essential if your monitoring program is going to produce continuous improvements in your media mix. Revision is the name of the game: your media mix should be in a continuous state of becoming.

Initially you should plan your media mix by factoring in your budgetary limitations, your practice goals and targeted markets, the image you want to convey, and the information you have collected on the various media. But later plans should be based on your monitoring efforts as well.

Don't ever assume you have found the perfect media combination. The public, the media and your practice and services are in a constant state of change. So the media mix for every advertising campaign must be based on the sum total of available information.

Planning will gradually become easier, but it must never become static or routine. If you make your choices wisely each month, you'll protect

FIGURE 14-4 Tips for Purchasing Advertising Specialities

These guidelines may be helpful to you in purchasing your advertising items:

1. Imprinting quality is directly related to the quality of the artwork you send to the printer. It's best to provide original artwork to assure a clean final product.

2. Keep your message brief, simple and uncluttered.

3. Consider the texture of the item you want imprinted and the intricacy of your imprinted message/logo/design.

4. Most specialty items come with a one-color imprint. Other colors can often be added for an additional charge.

5. Some products can't be imprinted. Check this before ordering.

6. Be sure to allow time for production of artwork (if you don't already have it), production of the specialty item, and shipping when you're determining the date by which you need an item. Also don't forget there will be a "set-up" charge, plus tax and shipping in the total cost of your order.

your investment and guarantee a sound return. If you don't, your efforts and your money will be wasted.

BIBLIOGRAPHY

Kotler P: *Principles of Marketing*. Englewood Cliffs, NJ, Prentice Hall, Inc., 1986.

Lusch RF and VN: *Principles of Marketing*. Boston, Kent Publishing Co., 1987.

Chapter 15

Effective Copywriting

Words. They shatter, shriek, enlighten, stimulate and persuade. Words *communicate*.

No matter how impressive the photos, graphics, sound effects and other elements in a promotional approach, ultimately it is words that drive the listener or reader to action. Not just any words, but the right words linked together in a way that involves and compels the individual to action.

The purpose of this chapter is to familiarize you with the rules of good copywriting, because even if you don't write your own, you must be able to recognize copy that's written well (or poorly) by the person or firm you hire to do it. Through examples presented, you'll see how copywriting rules have been effectively applied in health care promotion. And possibly, you'll get some ideas for your next communication effort, whether it's a practice brochure, a radio spot or a newsletter article.

TO WRITE OR NOT

One of the first decisions you must make is whether you will write your own copy or turn the task over to a professional. Lacking the skill themselves or in a member of their staff, many physicians opt to use the services of a freelance or independent copywriter, and others use an agency to develop their public relations or advertising theme and copy.

Unless you have a flair for writing, a better than average command of the English language and knowledge of basic copywriting mechanics and style, as well as the time to do it, you're better off hiring a skilled copywriter. On the other hand, if you or someone on your staff enjoys writing and has the time for the challenge of developing your own copy, then give it a try.

ADVERTISING, ETHICS AND YOU

The words you use to promote your practice are the most important element in your copy. Since a prerequisite of good advertising and promotion is believability, any discussion of copywriting should begin with an awareness of ethical considerations. Nothing can promote your practice better than words, and nothing can get you in trouble faster.

When the 1977 Supreme Court decision struck down the legal profession's ban on advertising, the national, state and local associations of most professions (including medicine) revised their codes of conduct concerning advertising. Some associations, however, are still very restrictive, limiting the right to mention guarantees, discounts, endorsements or testimonials, free consultations, enticements such as free screenings, and comparative, sensational or self-aggrandizing advertising. Others simply prohibit false or misleading claims, which is a fundamental rule of the Federal Trade Commission as well.

Your right as a physician to communicate to your patients and the public about your medical services and philosophy is basic and inalienable, but with that right comes responsibility. Needless to say, it is imperative that you and everyone in your practice be able to fulfill all promises, overt or implied, made in any promotional effort you undertake. It is crucial that you possess and maintain at optimum standards the medical skills, technology and knowledge you offer to the public. It is imperative that you examine copy thoroughly to be sure it complies with the codes, regulations and laws of your local medical society or state medical association.

Unfortunately, it's often easier to talk about truth than to accomplish it, especially when conflicting codes and "legalese" complicate the issue. For our purposes, however, the issue boils down to the difference between truth and deception or puffery. Puffery is exaggeration of good qualities in order to affect people's purchasing decisions. Puffery might be considered minor deception, while distortions and untruths would qualify as major deceptions. Either type of deception is particularly inappropriate in the health care field, where people are making life-affecting decisions based on what they read, see and hear. As Mathew Daynard of the Federal Trade Commission's Bureau of Consumer Protection points out, "The consequences of false or misleading claims are more dire in the case of medical advertising, so we must use a tougher reasonable basis for substantiation of claim than we might for someone advertising a bar of soap."

If you have a promotional message that you believe may be questionable for any reason, consult your attorney, and possibly your local medical society or state medical association, before using it. Avoid the nebulous area between truth and puffery in your copy.

Your Colleagues May Judge You. Only you can judge the climate in your community regarding physician acceptance of peers who engage in the more overt forms of practice promotion, especially advertising. Your medical association may have very clearcut requirements regarding the form and content of physician advertising and advertising copy, and you may be adhering to those guidelines to the letter. Yet in the surgery locker room, in the physicians' lounge, at the quarterly medical staff meeting, you and other doctors who engage in the more overt forms of marketing communication may be the topic of conversation (not all of it polite). Not only might your colleagues talk about you disdainfully, they may even limit or cut off your patient referrals.

It is possible, and wise as well, to minimize the potential for "physician backlash" by maintaining a high awareness regarding what's considered acceptable in your community by your peers. It's also possible to lessen the impact of your advertising on your peers by the tone and wording of the copy in your ads. If you're a specialist, suggesting in your promotional copy that consumers consult their personal physician before making any health care decision lets your peers know you are not interested in stealing their patients.

Even if you're not terribly concerned about the reaction of the medical community, it's wise to be aware of the potential for reaction to your marketing communication efforts in general and the message or approach you use specifically. We would advise that initially you take a more subtle approach in your ad copy if you are uncertain how other physicians will respond. You can always strengthen the approach as time passes and your colleagues begin to accept to your promotional efforts—and perhaps even adapt some themselves.

THE FOUR R'S OF EFFECTIVE ADVERTISING

Before turning to specific copywriting techniques, let's review the four "Rs" of effective advertising. (They also apply to other forms of promotion as well.) Every word you use to promote your practice should be chosen with these elements in mind.

Reach. Whom do you want your message to reach? Target your words to that specific group. If you don't know your audience, your words will float lifelessly in a bland alphabet soup.

Readership. Copywriting is an exercise in strategy as well as creativity. Once you know your audience, you must find the best media to reach that target market efficiently and with impact. Know the audience and the vehicle that will carry your message before you write a word.

Retention. This is the number of people who remember your message after seeing or hearing it. You'll achieve high retention if your copy is meaningful and to the point, and if your words exert an emotional pull on the reader or listener. Your message must satisfy audience wants or needs, and must match their values and beliefs.

Results. The only factor that justifies your promotional investment is getting results. If you have defined your audience correctly, if you have selected your media accurately, if you have carefully matched your message to the needs of your audience, your campaign will pay off with the results you seek.

Be Clear and Simple: Be Understood.

"In communication, as in architecture, less is more. You have to sharpen your message to cut into the mind. You have to jettison the

ambiguities, simplify the message, and then simplify it some more if
you want to make a long-lasting impression."

From *Positioning: The Battle for Your Mind*
Ries and Trout, 1981

THE ART OF PROMOTIONAL COPYWRITING

Promotional copywriting is one of the most exacting forms of expression, requiring a command of the language as well as an ability to coordinate persuasive, colorful copy with music, photography, art, printing, vocal intonation and acting. It requires clarity and precision in relatively few words (see Figure 15-1).

The words used by the copywriter in medical promotion must convey empathy for the personal nature of the decision, a sympathetic tone, and an air of expertise and professionalism. For a brochure or newsletter in which explanation of a medical or technical treatment or procedure is necessary, the copy must be simple yet complete, personal yet authoritative.

The copywriter's objective is to create copy that works with the chosen medium, that talks personally to the target audience, that effectively describes and creates a positive impression of the service or product.

Research is the framework on which good copy hangs. A copywriter can't know too much about the product or service being described. If you're writing the copy, be sure you're familiar with all of the facts about your practice or service. If you utilize a professional copywriter, take the time to communicate thoroughly what your practice and services are all about. And if the copywriter doesn't seem interested in learning, find another. Remember, it is your uniqueness—the qualities that differentiate you from other physicians—that should be conveyed in all of your promotional efforts.

FIGURE 15-1 The Writer's Checklist

- Use strong verbs. Verbs make your writing vigorous. Avoid the passive voice ("It was decided" in favor of the active "We decided"). Substitute active verbs for "to be" whenever possible.
- Cut out excessive and unnecessary words. Why say "The meeting will be held" when you can say "We'll meet."
- Be specific, avoiding jargon, technical terms and pompous language. Don't say "He sustained a massive myocardial infarction resulting in mortality." Say "He had a fatal heart attack."
- Write conversationally, personally. Say "See your doctor" instead of "Consult your physician."
- Vary sentence length, fluctuating between short and medium length. Avoid very long sentences; they drag, slowing the reader. Try to limit sentences to one idea, two at the most.
- Talk to one person, not a crowd. Your message must appeal to one specific individual, not Everyman.

In developing a theme or approach to your copy, avoid duplicating a concept used by another practice in your geographic area. There's nothing wrong with adapting, modifying, or reworking something that has worked for others, but the end result must be distinctive, not an obvious copycat.

ADVERTISING COPYWRITING

Get Attention. To make your message stand out from the crowd, your copy should be provocative and memorable. If you expect your audience to respond, you must grab and keep their attention, and at the same time tell them what they need to know, relating it to their value system. This doesn't mean your words must shout or have a carnival tone. In fact, some of the most effective advertising copy whispers amid the shouts of surrounding ads. Some attention-getting techniques that are appropriate in medical promotion include *the anecdote or example; testimonials; the startling but true statement* and *the question that draws the reader into the copy,* as in "Why should I worry about breast cancer?" (see Figure 15-2).

Promote Benefits. The "first commandment" of writing effective promotional copy is "Thou shalt stress benefits, not features." A feature is a *characteristic* of your practice. A benefit is the gain or *advantage* that accrues to the person who utilizes your practice. Be aware, however, that a claim of success should not be used as a benefit; this is contrary to the AMA policy on advertising (see Appendix E).

For example, evening and Saturday hours constitute a feature; convenience is the benefit. Outpatient surgery is the feature; less time away from work is the benefit.

When you stress benefits in your copy, it answers the reader's question, "What's in it for me?"

Use Testimonials Judiciously, Effectively. Testimonials, if handled carefully and ethically, can respond to the question, "What's in it for me?" Testimonials, or personal endorsements by patients, work well simply because they are believable. They allow "real people"—your patients—to tell of their own experiences in your practice, with your procedures or services.

However, if you use testimonials, bear in mind that they must be truthful, specific, believable, varied, and directed at a specific market. Also, a testimonial works only when you have a good service or product to start with.

We emphasize at this point that if you use testimonials in your practice communications, it must be done appropriately and ethically. While not outlawing the use of testimonials, the AMA has spelled out very clearly **how** they may be used. We feel the information is important enough to reproduce it again. As indicated in the AMA policy statement on advertising:

FIGURE 15-2 The Question Headline
A question headline like the one in this ad can reflect the reader's interests or concerns, attracting her to your ad.

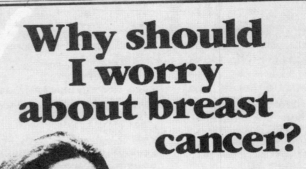

Why should I worry about breast cancer?

Ignorance won't make the facts go away. One out of every 10 women in this country will suffer from some form of breast cancer in their lifetime. Early detection is the key to CON-TROLLING THESE ODDS.

Self-examination is important; but, it is not enough. The size of a mass typically found by self-examination is three centimeters. This is approximately the size of a quarter. Studies have shown that even a tumor of this size has already been growing for 9 to 10 years. The discomforts of x-ray mammography or the fear of overexposure to radiation can no longer be a woman's excuse for relying only on breast self-examination.

Now, thanks to newer and safer technology, breast cancer CAN be detected in its earliest stages within the privacy of a physician's office. The Family Wellness Program of the Hillside Health Stop is pleased to introduce the Lintro-Scan, a totally painless, safe-breast screening procedure. Using infra-red illumination, the Lintro-Scan produces an image of the breast which can be viewed by a technician and the patient. This radiation-free procedure takes about 20 minutes to complete and has none of the discomforts normally associated with traditional x-ray mammography. Results are immediately available, another favorable feature of the Lintro-Scan. Because of its unequalled comfort and safety features, the Lintro-Scan can be used with pregnant women, women with very dense breasts and those under 35.

Ignoring breast cancer won't make it go away; only prompt diagnosis and treatment can do that. With the Lintro-Scan there's no reason to wait.

Protect yourself. Make an appointment today.

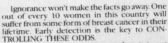

HILLSIDE HEALTH STOP
1150 Liberty Ave., Hillside
820-0202

testimonials of patients as to the physician's skill or the quality of his professional services should not be publicized. Statements relating to the quality of medical services are extremely difficult, if not impossible, to verify or measure by objective standards. Claims regarding experience, competence and the quality of physician's services may be made if they can be factually supported and if they do not imply that he has an exclusive and unique skill or remedy. A statement that a physician has cured or successfully treated a large number of cases involving a particular serious ailment may imply a certainty of result and create unjustified and misleading expectations in prospective clients.

An advertisement that meets the AMA criteria regarding testimonials is seen in Figure 15-3.

Finally, some local, state or regional medical groups may have more restrictive guidelines regarding testimonials than the AMA. It's a wise idea

FIGURE 15-3   Testimonials in Advertising
Patient testimonials are acceptable, according to the American Medical Association, if they do not attest to the doctor's medical abilities or expertise. If you have any question about a testimonial, check with your attorney and the AMA.

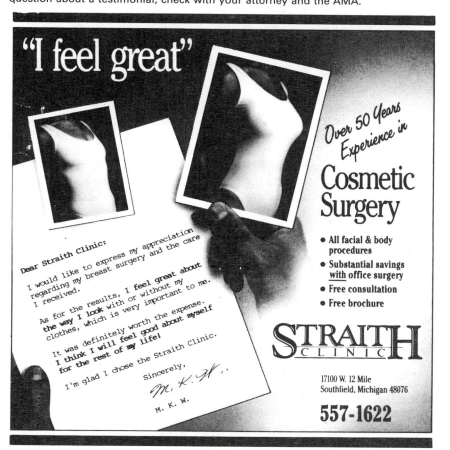

to check with your local medical society or association to be certain the use of testimonials is acceptable in your area, and what restrictions or limitations are imposed, if any.

Put Power in the Headline. How do you manage to grab attention and stress benefits at the same time? In print advertising, the most potent weapon is the headline. A good print ad begins and a bad one ends with the headline. You must get your message into the headline, because four of five readers never get beyond the headline.

Long or short, it doesn't matter. There are effective one-word headlines, and there are effective 20-word headlines (though most are going to be in the five- to seven-word range). Use active, descriptive words; cut out the flab and fat—words that sit there, doing nothing. Be precise, concise. Get to the point.

Here are examples of six of the basic types of headlines:

News:	"New Technique for Fat Reduction."
Question:	"Are You Taking Care of Your Child?"
Narrative:	"My Baby Is a WellCare Baby."
Command:	"Stop Smoking Today!"
1-2-3-Ways:	"Five Ways You Can Live a Longer Life."
How-What-Why:	"Why You Need a Family Doctor."

Avoid the label headline—the verb-less phrase such as "Family Medicine." A headline must lead the reader into the rest of the ad.

One way to capture your readers is to let them know in the headline that your message is directed at them. A neurology center in Maryland promoted its health education series on back and neck problems with an ad headlined, "You Don't Have to Take an Aching Back Lying Down." Not only was it targeted to a specific audience—people suffering from back problems—but the benefit is implied: you'll learn how to get rid of the immobilizing pain of back problems.

Headlines are further strengthened by using key words with proven pulling power—words like *you, now, free, great, save, secret,* and *warning.* The word *you* and its variations personalize your message. Be careful with words like *warning,* however; a positive approach is important in copywriting.

There are no absolute rules on what makes a headline work. Try writing several and then leave them for a day or two. You'll look at them with a fresh perspective. It also helps to study ads in newspapers and magazines. Clip those that catch your attention. Study the similarities in them; what is it about them, particularly in the headline, that made you notice them? The same elements that give any ad headline impact apply in medical advertising.

See Figure 15-4 for a final check on your headline.

Copy Consistency. After writing the headline, you should have a good idea of where to go with your body copy. You've already decided on your

FIGURE 15-4   A Headline Checklist

- Does it have immediate impact?
- Does it target your prospects?
- Does it promise a reward, a personal benefit?
- Have you used strong, forceful words, and only those words that are necessary? Have you avoided language that can be misinterpreted?
- Does the headline coordinate with the rest of the ad?

main appeal. The body copy should reinforce this appeal with specific points.

Copywriting is an exercise in balance. This is especially true of your opening sentence. An intriguing headline will grab the reader, but your first sentence must give further evidence of what the headline hints at.

Although editing down your first draft usually improves it, there's no reason to be afraid of long copy. For a complex subject, long copy may be necessary to tell the whole story. Readers will usually read to the end if their needs and values are addressed. But again, excise superfluous words.

Use everyday language, avoiding medical or technical jargon. Simple words and shorter sentences deliver your message without detracting from what you have said. But put life into your message. Colorless phrases can be just as unreadable as those that are heavy with flowery adjectives.

SOME COPY FORMATS

There are several formats you may find helpful to follow in composing ad copy. A copy format helps you compose the structure of your message, giving it direction.

The "Reason Why" Format. The "reason why" format features a reward or benefit in the headline; the body copy explains why it is true. "Reason-why" copy poses a problem and then provides a solution. The solution, of course, is to make an appointment with you. "Reason-why" is a simple, logical approach.

The "You and Me" Format. Another copy format is called "you and me," in which you speak directly to the reader in a friendly, informal tone. This approach is especially effective if you are stressing the personal service aspect of your practice. A group of California obstetricians effectively used the "you and me" approach in an ad which emphasized the teamwork between expectant mothers and the physicians and staff of the practice.

The "Understatement" Format. A third approach to copywriting is the "understatement." Understated copy is conservative in tone; it is a soft-sell, image-building approach. This format helps dispel the huckster image of hard-sell ads. In this era of increasing consumer awareness and skepticism, copy that strains credibility or shouts like a carnival salesman is less believable. An ad focusing on the individual personalities, family, hobbies and interests of the members of a group practice follows the understatement format. For instance, the Honolulu Medical Group in Hawaii features in one of its ads a photo of a physician and the headline, "Dr. Lum has hundreds of grandchildren." The copy then describes the grandchildren, parents and grandparents Dr. Lum treats in his family practice. It describes activities he enjoys, such as backpacking and astronomy. And it emphasizes expertise by pointing out that he is one of 50 specialists in the group. The close is equally strong, concluding with, "Call us. Providing the best personalized health care is something we've been doing since 1903—for families just like yours."

The "Educational" Format. Educational ads frequently involve longer copy. Avoid technical terminology, but don't avoid statistics, facts and information that gives credibility to your message. Use examples or analogies to make your meaning clear and your copy more interesting. This approach is especially effective for professionals because it projects a positive, helpful, conservative image. (An example of educational ad copy is seen in Figure 15-5.)

There are many ways to organize copy. The formats we've suggested here are a few of the more common approaches. Whatever method you choose, your copy should follow a logical sequence, flow smoothly, so that your reader easily understands the points you are making.

ASK FOR ACTION

It's surprising how many communication efforts neglect to ask the audience to take some kind of action. You must encourage the reader or listener to respond: to call for an appointment, send for a helpful brochure, visit our office today, mail this card immediately, ask about our no-charge initial consultation. With a strong headline, persuasive body copy and a call to action at the end, your ad will begin with impact, maintain interest and conclude forcefully. And that's good copywriting!

AND FINALLY . . .

Most of the suggestions offered in this chapter can be applied to writing for brochures, newsletters, direct mail pieces and other promotional techniques as well as advertising copy. For copywriting is, at the heart of it, simply a matter of good writing.

This means writing that is clear, forceful, and personal. It is not inflated with excessive language, nor full of puffed up words or technical phrases that only a physician understands. Good writing understands its audience— not thousands of readers or viewers, but one individual with his or her particular beliefs, values, interests and needs. It consists of words well-chosen to give pleasure while they inform, educate and persuade (see Figure 15-6).

FIGURE 15-5 Educational Ad Copy
One goal of health care advertising should be to educate consumers. Be sure to use common terms, not medical jargon, in educational advertising copy.

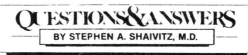

QUESTIONS&ANSWERS
BY STEPHEN A. SHAIVITZ, M.D.

Neurology Dept.,
Good Samaritan Hospital

Neurology Dept.,
St. Mary's Hospital

Adjunct Professor,
Florida Atlantic University

American Academy
of Neurology

American Association
for the Study of Headache

Palm Beach County
Medical Society

Stephen A. Shaivitz, M.D.

Board Certified
Neurology

(305) 478-1110

Headaches

"What are cluster headaches? Can they be treated?"

Cluster headaches consist of severe head and facial pain which last from 20 to 60 minutes, and occur several times each day.

Unlike migraines, which are accompanied by nausea, vomiting and sensitivity to light, cluster attacks cause the patient's face to appear flushed and sweaty. One eye will tear and the nose will run.

During the attack, the patient is agitated, often pacing for long periods. The victim is frequently awakened from sleep, and will hold his or her head, rocking and moaning from the excruciating pain.

These attacks occur frequently, in clusters, over a period of several days, weeks or months, before they end as suddenly as they began.

Cluster headaches are only rarely experienced by women. Though we do not know the cause(s), we do know that during the cycle of attacks the patient is extremely sensitive to alcohol. These headaches are treated by a variety of medications, usually with great success.

If you suspect a problem you should see a doctor. Also, if you would like more information on headaches or to receive Dr. Shaivitz's newsletter on "Headaches," please call us or write us for your free copy.

2161 Palm Beach Lakes Blvd., Suite 305, West Palm Beach, Florida 33409

FIGURE 15-6   Tucker's Law

ERNEST E. TUCKER was the city editor of Chicago's **American,** a major Chicago newspaper.

TUCKER'S LAW

1. Don't use no double negatives.

2. Make each pronoun agree with their antecedents.

3. Join clauses, like a conjunction should.

4. About them sentence fragments.

5. When dangling, watch your participles.

6. Verbs has got to agree with their antecedents.

7. Just between you and I, case is important.

8. Don't use commas, that aren't necessary.

9. Try to not ever split infinitives.

10. It is important to use your apostrophe's correctly.

11. Proofread your writing to see if any words out.

12. Correct speling is essential.

Good writing is a source of power, for writer and reader alike. Use it well.

BIBLIOGRAPHY

Ries A, Trout J: *Positioning: The Battle for Your Mind* 1981.

How to Write to Be Understood. *Communications Briefings* 1983; June.

Hospital Writers: Your Prose Is Sick, *Hospital Public Relations* 1983; July-August.

Misleading Health Care: A Preventive Approach. San Francisco, Calif., The California Association of Ophthalmologists, 1987.

Smith: When Testimonials Are Most Effective. *Strategic Health Care Marketing* 1985; April.

Clarke R, Kotler P: *Marketing for Healthcare Organizations.* Englewood Cliffs, NJ, Prentice Hall, Inc., 1987.

Does It Pay to Advertise? *Physician's Weekly* 1987; March 23.

Chapter 16

Yellow Pages and Other Directories

Ask some physicians if they engage in practice marketing, and they emphatically respond, "No way!" But ask them if they have a listing in the Yellow Pages of the telephone directory, and they'll tell you, "Of course!"

For many medical practices, the Yellow Pages constitutes the primary element of the marketing program. In fact, as you might suspect, for a good number of physicians, advertising in the Yellow Pages directory is the *only* promotional vehicle employed. But it's been our experience that this potentially powerful promotional tool is often not very well used, and may even be taken for granted by physicians unaware of the power of the Yellow Pages in consumer health care decision-making.

We discovered a classic example of this problem in the course of a consultation with a North Carolina obstetrician/gynecologist. In determining his sources of new patients, we asked what percentage were contributed directly or indirectly by the Yellow Pages. This physician had made a practice of carefully documenting how patients learned of his practice, and he confidently responded: "None. People in this area don't use the Yellow Pages to find a physician."

This ran counter to all of the studies we were aware of, particularly for a physician in his specialty. We asked him if we could take a look at his Yellow Pages listing. After about five minutes of searching, we finally found his ad. It was in the name of his professional corporation, which did not include his name. We concluded that anyone selecting this doctor's practice from his Yellow Pages ad would have to be attracted to the telephone number or the name of his corporation, neither of which held much promise, in our estimation.

YELLOW PAGES GROW IN POPULARITY

Studies show that 20 to 50 percent of the population use the Yellow Pages either as their primary source in selecting a physician, or to obtain additional information about a physician after they have the name. No matter what the reason, you need to be in the Yellow Pages as visibly as professional standards in your area permit.

In this chapter we are going to review some facts and suggest how you can use Yellow Pages advertising as an important link in your overall promotional mix. It's a link more and more physicians are discovering. Recently, Sheryl Bronkesh and Patricia Pritchard of Health Services Marketing, Ltd., in Scottsdale, and Steven D. Wood, PhD of Arizona State University reported on a comparison they did of physician advertising in the Yellow Pages in Phoenix, Ariz., and New Haven, Conn. in 1980, 1984 and 1988. In the 1980 Phoenix directory, only three physicians had in-column ads and none had display ads. By 1988, there were 165 in-column ads and 31 display ads by 25 specialties in the Phoenix directory.

In the more conservative New Haven community, there were no physician Yellow Pages ads in 1980. By 1984, there were eight in-column ads but still no display ads. Four years later, the 1988 New Haven directory had 75 physician in-column ads and 18 display ads by 26 different specialties. These numbers show that Yellow Pages advertising is rapidly being seen by physicians as the anchor to a cohesive practice promotion program.

More than one hundred years have passed since the first telephone directory, a single page in length, was issued in New Haven, Connecticut in 1878 (see Figure 16-1). In fact, this tradition even predated telephone numbers. Users of the directory simply told the operator the name of the individual or business they wished to call.

The 1878 directory was the forerunner of today's telephone directories and the beginning of a new era of communication and advertising. In the 1890's, publishers began the practice of using yellow paper to distinguish classified sections from alphabetical ones. The Yellow Pages were born.

Today, telephone directories are used by millions of consumers to find the products and services they want to buy. Almost every American business and household has a telephone and, of course, a Yellow Pages directory.

The Yellow Pages serves a function no other medium can match. It is a year-round medium that reaches consumers in actual need of medical services. And it is used. In a study commissioned by Southern New England Telephone (SNET), which publishes telephone directories, in November 1987, it was found that 53 percent of all Connecticut residents surveyed who had contacted a physician in the recent past had used the Yellow Pages in making that contact. Moreover, further studies have found that consumers rate the Yellow Pages just behind personal friends as the most valuable source of information in seeking a physician. They also view the Yellow Pages (along with trade journals) as the most appropriate vehicle for physician advertising. These statistics are significant, and merit analysis.

SOME FACTS YOU SHOULD KNOW

Let's take a closer look at what the Connecticut study found:

1. 53 percent of those people contacting a physician used the Yellow Pages in making that contact.

FIGURE 16-1 First Telephone Directory
This list of subscribers is historically considered to be America's original telephone directory.

LIST OF SUBSCRIBERS.

New Haven District Telephone Company.

OFFICE 219 CHAPEL STREET.

February 21, 1878.

Residences.	*Stores, Factories, &c.*
Rev. JOHN E. TODD.	O. A. DORMAN.
J. B. CARRINGTON.	STONE & CHIDSEY.
H. B. BIGELOW.	NEW HAVEN FLOUR CO. State St.
C. W. SCRANTON.	" " " " Cong. ave.
GEORGE W. COY.	" " " " Grand St.
G. L. FERRIS.	" " " Fair Haven.
H. P. FROST.	ENGLISH & MERSICK.
M. F. TYLER.	New Haven FOLDING CHAIR CO.
I. H. BROMLEY.	H. HOOKER & CO.
GEO. E. THOMPSON.	W. A. ENSIGN & SON.
WALTER LEWIS.	H. B. BIGELOW & CO.
	C. COWLES & CO.
Physicians.	C. S. MERSICK & CO.
Dr. E. L. R. THOMPSON.	SPENCER & MATTHEWS.
Dr. A. E. WINCHELL.	PAUL ROESSLER.
Dr. C. S. THOMSON, Fair Haven.	E. S. WHEELER & CO.
	ROLLING MILL CO.
Dentists.	APOTHECARIES HALL.
Dr. E. S. GAYLORD.	E. A. GESSNER.
Dr. R. F. BURWELL.	AMERICAN TEA CO.
Miscellaneous.	*Meat & Fish Markets.*
REGISTER PUBLISHING CO.	W. H. HITCHINGS, City Market.
POLICE OFFICE.	GEO. E. LUM, " "
POST OFFICE.	A. FOOTE & CO.
MERCANTILE CLUB.	STRONG, HART & CO.
QUINNIPIAC CLUB.	
F. V. McDONALD, Yale News.	*Hack and Boarding Stables.*
SMEDLEY BROS. & CO.	CRUTTENDEN & CARTER.
M. F. TYLER, Law Chambers.	BARKER & RANSOM.

Office open from 6 A. M. to 2 A. M.
After March 1st, this Office will be open all night.

- 14 percent used the Yellow Pages as their *primary* source in making their contacts, and
- 39 percent used the Yellow Pages as a *secondary* source; i.e., they already had the name of a physician or physicians in mind, but consulted the Yellow Pages for more information such as the telephone number, location, hours,
- services, etc.

2. 86 percent of the respondents agreed that physicians who advertise perform a useful service.

3. Use of the Yellow Pages to contact a physician tended to be higher among newer residents.

4. Yellow Pages usage among individuals with incomes above $40,000 per year did not differ from those with incomes below that figure.

5. 77 percent of the users were aware of the specialty guide, the section of the Yellow Pages within the physician category in which physicians of an individual specialty are grouped.
   - 86 percent of users with incomes over $40,000 were aware of the specialty guide.
   - 86 percent of users age 35–59 were aware of the specialty guide.
   - 80 percent of females were aware of the specialty guide.
   - 94 percent consider the specialty guide to be very useful.
   - 88 percent consider the specialty guide more useful than the main alphabetical heading.

The data from the Connecticut study is consistent with other studies. A nationwide survey of 1500 consumers conducted by National Research Corporation in 1986 found that 21 percent had used the Yellow Pages to select a physician, and another 11 percent would consider using the Yellow Pages to select one. This study also found that newer residents, younger persons, and women are more likely to use the Yellow Pages to find a physician. The only inconsistency between the two studies is that the NRC study found that consumers with incomes below $35,000 per year were almost twice as likely to use the Yellow Pages to select a physician as those with incomes more than $35,000. We don't know why this difference exists, but we suspect that variations between geographic regions must be taken into consideration.

Thumbs Up from Consumers. How do consumers view physicians advertising in the Yellow Pages? Very positively, according to a survey entitled "Consumer Attitudes Toward Advertising by Professionals."

In the study, Dinoo T. Vanier and Donald Sciglimpaglia, marketing professors at San Diego State University, asked consumers to rank the "most appropriate advertising media" for health care professionals. The winner: The Yellow Pages with an approval rating of over 80 percent. Moreover, consumers give favorable ratings to physicians who advertise, with the highest rating going to those who provide a great deal of information in their Yellow Pages ad, according to a 1987 study reported in the *Journal of Professional Services Marketing* by Cathy Cobb-Walgren and Halina Sleszynski.

In the previously cited study commissioned by SNET Publishing of Connecticut, it was found that 83 percent of the respondents tend to believe professional advertising in the Yellow Pages versus 59 percent who believe what is read in the newspaper.

SOME DISADVANTAGES

The Yellow Pages is a potent medium for promoting your medical services. It's the one media that helps you reach prospects at the best of all times—when they are in need of medical services.

But before we turn to suggestions for maximizing the effectiveness of your Yellow Pages advertising, it's important that you be aware of some of the disadvantages, problems and pitfalls of this media, so that you can avoid them if possible.

Your Competitors Are Listed With You. The competition factor within the Yellow Pages directory is intense. The ads of your colleagues/competitors appear on the same pages as your own. It is important to keep this in mind as you prepare your ad. An approach that may be very effective in a non-competitive environment may not work as well in the Yellow Pages. Your ad must be especially distinctive to stand out from this competitive clutter.

Your Ad Will Run for a Year. Since individual directories are published annually, you are married to your ad for a longer period than with other media. If your ad isn't doing the job, you can't pull it and try another approach. This places additional emphasis on the need to do it right the first time.

Design Limitations. Another drawback is the limitation of Yellow Pages ad design. With very few exceptions (the most notable being the use of red, and occasionally blue or green as a second color in some directories), you are limited to one color—black. Other limitations vary widely since each publisher makes its own regulations. They include restrictions on borders and illustrations, and sometimes even wording. This problem is further complicated by the fact that each state medical association and even the directory publishing company may address the use of Yellow Pages differently in its professional advertising code. Therefore, it is very important to determine at the outset what you can and cannot do or say in your ad.

The Sales Representatives. Although this is changing in some locales, another problem can be difficulty with the individual who sells Yellow Pages ad space. It is important to remember that these individuals are primarily order-takers. While many are extremely competent and have a solid advertising background, many others do not. Equally important, even if they have an advertising background, most have no knowledge whatever of the unique needs or ethical constraints facing a physician who wishes to use this promotional tool.

In addition, sales reps are usually assigned more clients than they can effectively handle, and this problem is aggravated as closing deadlines approach. Don't take anything for granted; double-check deadlines, insist on seeing a proof (a print-ready copy of the ad) and get everything in writing.

Ultimately, you are responsible for your ad, and it's too important a matter to leave to chance . . . or a harried sales rep. Mistakes happen in Yellow Pages advertising just as they do in other media. If the error is your fault, you have little recourse. If it's the fault of the publisher, you may have some recourse, but only if you can back up your case. Either way, you're still stuck with an imperfect ad for a year. So be sure to have written documentation of all that transpires between you and your rep from the moment you consider placing an ad. Check your proof carefully, because once you've signed off on it, you've signed away any right to demand changes or compensation. If a proof is not provided because of a deadline crunch, be sure you keep on file copies of the information you provided for your ad.

Measuring Effectiveness. A final Yellow Pages disadvantage, one that we will deal with in greater depth in Chapter 20, is the difficulty in measuring the effectiveness of Yellow Pages advertising. It's an accepted truth among advertisers that Yellow Pages ads are crucial, but it's difficult to prove a direct response from your Yellow Pages ad, unless it's your *only* form of promotion. People may turn to the Yellow Pages for your telephone number, location or other information after they've heard your radio spot, met a member of your staff at a social engagement, or seen a newspaper ad or article about your practice. If you have a multi-media campaign, how do you determine exactly which media caused the patient to call your office for an appointment? Dick Schleifer, the manager of professional ad sales for SNET Publishing, likens Yellow Pages advertising to the spy being sought by the FBI in a movie about World War II espionage. As the story goes, for days the agents staked out a house they thought was the head-quarters for a spy ring. In their report they stated that no one had entered or left the house during the period they had observed it. Yet each day, the mailman—who was in fact the spy—had visited the house. His visits had gone unreported, just as the effectiveness of your Yellow Pages ad may go unreported if you don't ask the right questions.

SELECTING THE RIGHT DIRECTORY

More and more types and sizes of Yellow Pages directories are being offered by a variety of publishers in cities large and small. All these choices create a dilemma for the physician. Which book do you list your practice in? All, some or only one?

The answer depends on your practice location(s), your target audience, the services you offer and the directories themselves. If you have a multi-location practice or one that draws from a broad service area, you'll prob-ably find it necessary to advertise in the metropolitan book (the big, hefty directory in major urban areas) as well as in one or more suburban books (depending on where you draw your patients from). One physician we know of was advertising in 11 different Yellow Pages directories. After doing a zip code analysis of his patient population, he found that he was drawing strongly from only three zip codes. He was able to eliminate his display ads in eight directories, using only a listing, and instead retained larger display ads in the areas from which he attracted patients.

If you're in a smaller area with only one main directory, you may still find yourself confronted with some of the new specialized directories. Look closely at the figures these publishing companies give you; ask questions about readership as well as circulation before making a decision to invest heavily in the optional books. You might even call one or two doctors who have advertised in these directories in your community or elsewhere, and find out if they felt their ad generated a reasonable response.

MAKING YELLOW PAGES ADVERTISING WORK FOR YOU

You have a wide variety of options in addition to display ads in the Yellow Pages. For example, there are space or *in-column* ads that appear in the listing column. These ads allow you to include various types of information, including a logo, to supplement the regular listing of name, address and telephone number. In most books, you can also purchase bold and semi-bold listings, alternate call listings (a second phone number and special calling instructions), anchor listings (including information to refer consumers to display ads), extra-line listings, and, of course, regular listings.

Size and Placement Considerations. In June, 1987, *The Physician's Advisory* reported that a three-line, type-only Yellow Pages ad was the most common size used by physicians, with 35 percent of physicians surveyed indicating they used that size. Another 23 percent used block ads over one inch.

In a study designed to determine the relative effectiveness of various sizes of Yellow Pages ads, Russell Marketing Research, Inc., asked some 200 Yellow Pages users to compare ads and decide which advertiser they would call first. Large ads outpulled medium-sized ads by almost two to one, and medium ads were considered more effective than small-sized ads by almost three to one.

Large ads are noticed in the Yellow Pages. A larger ad also allows you to provide more information about your practice and services, and the benefits you offer to potential patients. And that's what consumers are looking for when they turn to the Yellow Pages.

But let's face it. Not every medical practice can afford, or should have, a large display ad in the Yellow Pages. In some areas of the country, Yellow Pages display advertising for physicians is extremely low-key or not used at all. In these areas, an in-column ad or a low-key, small display ad may be a better way to make your statement without incurring peer disapproval. Also, display ads are usually grouped together at the beginning of the physician section, not in the specialty section. A consumer who goes directly to the specialty listing may miss your ad. So an in-column ad in the specialty section in addition to, or instead of, a display ad may be better for you.

But a small ad can also be effective. Cynthia S. Smith, author of "How To Get Big Results From a Small Advertising Budget," suggests that the key to selling a "solid and reliable" product or service in a "modest space" is absolute honesty. "No overstated claims, no lavish promises, no implausible statements," she advises. We would add that if budget or conservatism calls for a small Yellow Pages ad for your practice, don't attempt to cram it full of copy. Be judicious in the quantity of information you include, so that the type is large enough to be read. Use your logo, and work with a designer to make the ad effective.

The Right Place, the Right Time. As with so many aspects of life, being in the right place at the right time can make all the difference. In the Yellow Pages a desirable ad position is of critical importance. Position is determined by a combination of seniority and ad size. The larger ads are grouped together at the beginning of each section, progressing down to the smaller. Within each size category (half-page, quarter page, etc.) the order of placement is based strictly on seniority. The first year you advertise in any given category, your ad will be placed at the end of that category along with all other first-time advertisers. The first ad in each size category will belong to the advertiser who has held that size the longest.

The best advice that can be given under these rules is to vie for position. If you have a good position in your size category, weigh this factor carefully before you decide to increase (or decrease) the size of your ad. On the other hand, medical promotion is still a chaotic field, with many opportunities for climbing the seniority ladder. By anticipating what others are likely to do, by analyzing your directory carefully, by watching for opportunities, you should be able to improve your relative position.

Content: The Meat of the Matter. Graphics may grab the reader's attention, but content is the most important factor in successful Yellow Pages advertising. Given the importance of content, it is not surprising to see that such a high percentage of physicians are purchasing larger ads to get their message across. But the emphasis here should be on effective content, not length. Also, while content is critical, it should be devoted to consumer benefits rather than education. The person looking at your ad in the Yellow Pages is ready to use the type of services you offer. Your ad must convince them they should choose *you.*

See Figures 16-2 and 16-3 for examples of yellow pages listings and ads.

CREATING AN EFFECTIVE YELLOW PAGES AD

There is no standard formula for an effective Yellow Pages ad, one you can plug into for guaranteed success. Nevertheless, a careful study of the

FIGURE 16-2   Samples of Yellow Page Listings and Ads

Alternate Call Listing

JONES, RICHARD
Arthroscopic Surgery
2525 W Greenway ················· **993-0350**
5620 W Thunderbird Rd Glendale ············· **938-5800**
5251 W Campbell Av ···················· **247-9600**
Billing & Insurance ···················· **866-0758**
Rand David A 4232 E Cactus Rd ············· **996-0210**
JACOB, MARC
Arthroscopic Surgery
2525 W Greenway ················· **993-0350**
5620 W Thunderbird Rd Glendale ············· **938-5800**
5251 W Campbell Ave ···················· **247-9600**
Billing & Insurance ···················· **866-0758**

Anchor Listing — Reference Ad

Harris Keith H 550 W Thomas Rd ············· **264-0916**
HEMORRHOID CARE
C.A.R.E.—COLON & RECTAL EXPERTS
Painful Bleeding Hemorrhoids—Colon Diseases—See
Display Ad—Physicians & Surgeons M.D. (Medical)
14640 N Tatum Blvd ···················· **971-2610**

Johnson Gerald S, MD, PC
10575 N Tatum Blvd Prdse Vly ············· **991-7994**
Juarez Hilario
809 E Washington St ···················· **256-2044**
525 N 18 St ···················· **252-1510**

Extra Line Listing

SANDS, JON
Arthroscopic Surgery & Athletic Medicine
5040 N 15 Av ···················· **234-0303**
515 W Buckeye Rd ···················· **257-8201**
303 E Baseline Rd ···················· **268-5772**
SMITH, JON
Arthroscopic Surgery & Athletic Medicine
5040 N 15 Av ···················· **234-0303**
515 W Buckeye Rd ···················· **257-8201**
303 E Baseline Rd ···················· **268-5772**

Bold Listing

CATAWBA WOMEN'S CENTER PA
Richard V Surgnier MD
James William Wotring Jr MD
Joel B Miller MD
Scott T Chatham MD

In-column Display Ads — large and small

INDIANA CENTER FOR SURGERY AND REHABILITATION OF THE HAND & UPPER EXTREMITY

HAND SURGERY
ASSOCIATES
OF INDIANA, INC..

• JAMES W. STRICKLAND, M.D.
• JAMES B. STEICHEN, M.D.
• WILLIAM B. KLEINMAN, M.D.
• HILL HASTINGS II, M.D.
• RICHARD S. IDLER, M.D.
• THOMAS J. FISCHER, M.D.

Practice Limited to Surgery of the Hand
and Upper Extremities

TELEPHONE ANSWERS 24 HOURS

8501 Harcourt Rd Indpls In --- **317 875-9105**

GOLD, ALAN J MD
Rheumatology & Internal Medicine
1372 Peachtree St NE ···················· **892-2131**
If No Answer ···················· **898-0347**
HAAS, GEORGE R MD PC

ASTHMA & DISEASES OF ALLERGY
465 Winn Way Dec ···················· **294-4761**
2151 Fountain Dr Snivl ···················· **979-3796**

FIGURE 16-3 Examples of Effective Yellow Pages Ads

The headline "Complete Care. Complete Confidence."is brief but tells a great deal about the type of practice and services. It's much more effective than simply using the practice name. The "Health Care for Women" ad speaks directly to the target audience in the headline, illustration and copy.

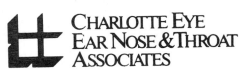

CHARLOTTE EYE EAR NOSE & THROAT ASSOCIATES

Complete Care.

Complete Confidence.

John E. Bourgeois, M.D.
Cornea & External Diseases
Cataract Surgery

David J. Browning, M.D., Ph.D.
Vitreoretinal Diseases & Surgery
Diabetic Eye Disease

Julian C. Culton, M.D.
General Ophthalmology
Cataract Surgery

Martin J. Kreshon, M.D.
General Ophthalmology
Cataract Surgery

Thomas K. Mundorf, M.D.
Glaucoma
Cataract Surgery

Timothy G. Saunders, M.D.
Pediatric Ophthalmology
Neuro-Ophthalmology

G. Cleveland Stowe, M.D.
General Ophthalmology
Cataract Surgery

John A. Young, M.D.
General Ophthalmology
Cataract Surgery

Accepts Assignment on All
Medicare Claims

1600 East Third St.—**372-3300**
Mercy Medical Park—**541-6677**

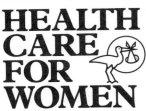

HEALTH CARE FOR WOMEN

DURING THE REPRODUCTIVE YEARS AND BEYOND

We are a caring team of professionals, using the most advanced methods and technology to serve the health and medical needs of today's busy woman - in a warm, cheerful atmosphere.

Kenneth Farhang, M.D., F.A.C.O.G., Diplomate,
American Board of OB-GYN
Emmajean McCreadie, R.N., C.N.P.
Female Certified Nurse Practitioner

■ Infertility counseling, treatment and microsurgery
■ Artificial insemination
■ Adolescent and adult gynecology
■ Gynecological surgery
■ Pregnancy prevention
■ Care of menopausal symptoms
■ Pregnancy care, gentle birth
■ Tying and untying tubes (band aid surgery)
■ Laser treatment
■ Premenstrual tension therapy (PMS)
■ Care of benign breast disease

Evening, Early A.M. and some Saturday appointments available.

Los Alamitos Medical Center East

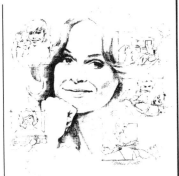

Alamitos Infertility & Gynecology Medical Group, Inc.
3801 Katella Ave., Suite 230, Los Alamitos 90720

213-598-9426
714-995-0333

information in this section, analysis of your competition, plus consultation with necessary professional resources should give you a feel for the direction your ad should take.

From the outset, it is important to determine your target audience and direct your advertising message specifically to these individuals. Copy and layout should work in tandem to attract the attention of this audience, with its specialized needs and values. Your ad should provide information, and create the overall image you want to achieve.

In general terms, prospective clients expect and respond to the following in a Yellow Pages ad:

Complete information
A prominent phone number
Your exact location, including information on how to find your office
Hours of operation
A listing of the services you offer
Years of experience
Professional titles
Insurance plans and credit cards accepted
An illustration that says something
Clarity of presentation
Proper balance between the size of the ad and the amount of information

Your years of experience take on special significance in light of a study showing that consumers perceive professionals who advertise as younger than their non-advertising colleagues. This study, commissioned by the Reuben H. Donnelly Company, a leading Yellow Pages publisher, also shows that professionals who advertise are perceived as slightly *more* competent, *more* client-oriented, and *less* expensive than the average professional.

Other factors you should consider including in your ad:

Special skills or equipment
Emergency service
Affordability/fee structure
Geographic areas served
Unique personal and practice features
Logo or insignia
Parking convenience
Professional association membership
Board certification
Slogan or advertising theme

And finally, we offer these suggestions for a dynamic, informative and uncluttered Yellow Pages ad:

1. Avoid generic, non-descriptive terms such as "General Practice."
2. Beware of phrases like "practice limited to . . ." This makes a specialty sound like a negative; rather, make it positive by using "specializing in . . ."
3. "Hours by appointment" is another phrase which is confusing at best, negative at worst. The implication is that without an appointment, the would-be patient can forget it.
4. A location map can be very effective since many Yellow Pages shoppers are looking for location.
5. Avoid the use of too many typefaces which can create a "cartoonish" effect inappropriate to professional advertising.
6. Avoid script typefaces. They can be very difficult to read. If used at all, script should be used only on a very limited basis for emphasis.
7. Depending on how it is used, boldface type can be a positive or a negative in your Yellow Pages ad. It can improve readability, especially in small ads, but if overused it can create a cluttered look.
8. As a rule, photos do not reproduce well because of the flimsy paper used in the Yellow Pages.
9. Avoid the temptation to add something new to your ad each year. The eventual result is clutter.
10. Effective use of white space can make an ad stand out on a page dominated by cluttered ads (see Figure 16-4).
11. Effective use of graphics or logo can attract "finger walkers" to your ad when it is grouped with ads dominated by straight copy.
12. The use of generic professional symbols such as the caduceus should be avoided since they usually have little meaning to the lay person, and they don't distinguish you from your competitors.
13. As a general rule, don't let the Yellow Pages art service create your ad for you. You're likely to end up with an ad that's a clone of 90 percent of the ads in your listing category. We strongly recommend using a professional designer for a distinctive ad that enhances your image. (Use the same designer for all your print pieces and ads, and you'll get a consistent look that builds professional identity for you.)
14. Consider an odd-sized ad—a strong vertical, for instance. It's one way to attract attention in a competitive situation. Horizontal ads, however, are easier to design. Or try an unusual border—one that curves at the top and bottom rather than following the angular edges of other ads. Set your ad apart through innovation.
15. It's better to spend your money on a larger single color ad than to invest it in red as a second color. If red is used, use it sparingly. A red border helps to unify other red elements in the ad.

As we've said, there's no secret formula for an effective ad. Study your market, your competition and your practice. Remember what research tells you about what consumers expect and respond to in a Yellow Pages ad. Heed the advice of experts in the field. Bring your graphic artist into the discussion from the beginning to get a creative point of view. Then determine the elements that will be included in your ad, ranking them in order of importance. That way, if you have to cut something out, you know where to begin. Now you're ready for copywriting.

FIGURE 16-4 A Final Checklist

As the elements of your ad fall into place, use this checklist to make sure you haven't forgotten anything.

1. Is your ad eye-catching (distinctive from other physician ads you expect to be in the next directory)?

2. Is the headline strong? Does it offer a benefit?

3. Is the ad easy to read (one or two compatible typefaces, no thin-stroke letters likely to fade in printing?) Is the print large enough for older eyes?

4. Does your ad have adequate white space used attractively and effectively?

5. Are the name and address correct and readable (either dominant or set apart from other copy elements)?

6. Does the ad include your logo (a graphic symbol) or your logotype (a distinctive typeface your practice name is consistently set in)?

7. Is the phone number correct? Is it highly visible?

8. Are special services mentioned (foreign language ability, professional specialties, etc.)?

9. Is your practice location pinpointed by reference to the closest intersection or nearby landmark or by inclusion of a map?

10. Do you have special office hours listed—Saturdays, evenings, etc.?

11. Does the ad complement and work well with your other advertising?

12. Can you back up all claims and offers for a full year?

13. Is your staff prepared to maximize the return on your Yellow Pages investment?

14. Is a system for monitoring your Yellow Pages ad in place?

YELLOW PAGES COPY: MAKE IT FACTUAL, GIVE IT PUNCH

Because consumers who use the Yellow Pages are looking for the facts, a good place to start with copywriting is to answer the basic five W's: who, what, where, when and why.

Who? Your name is probably less important than the nature of your practice. Avoid using your practice name as the headline of your ad unless it describes your practice (i.e., The Low Back Center) or unless you are already well-known in your community. In most cases, it's best to win your prospect's attention by reserving the headline to sell an important feature of your practice, and to place your name and telephone number further down in the ad in large or boldface type to make them stand out.

What? What service(s) do you offer? Is your specialty orthopedics, pediatrics, plastic surgery, or are you a family practitioner? It's important that your ad convey the type of practice you have and the care you offer. Some of the nation's largest Yellow Pages directories have introduced a "specialty guide" so consumers can easily locate the specific type of physician they need under the appropriate heading. Be sure that you describe your specialty in terms the average person understands. Otorhinolaryngology is impressive, yet few consumers know it's meaning. A better description would be "specialist in ear, nose, and throat problems." That is the information potential patients are looking for.

Where and When? Two more important elements of your Yellow Pages ad are the location of your practice and your hours of operation. The expanding availability of "locality" guides in Yellow Pages directories for large urban areas is making it easier for patients to find nearby physicians quickly and easily. Similar in layout to specialty guides, they allow physicians to be identified under the headings of the communities they serve. But you still must identify your exact location in your ad. This can be accomplished by mentioning nearby landmarks, intersections or highways. Another good idea is to run a small locator map in the bottom corner of your ad, if space permits. Don't forget to list your hours. Extended hours can be an important factor in the selection process.

Why? The question to answer here is why the patient should choose your practice over others competing for his or her attention in the directory. Remember, many Yellow Pages users are not looking for a certain physician by name, but one who can meet their specific needs. A striking and imaginative ad that calls attention to the features that make your practice unique can lead the prospective patient to select your practice. Answering the "why" question adequately may mean emphasizing any of the following special services that apply to your practice: 24-hour answering service, no appointment necessary, lab on premises, special consideration for children or senior citizens, house calls, bilingual abilities, etc. But don't be limited by this list. Include any other features or benefits that are unique to your practice and which may appeal to a specific group.

PUTTING IT ALL TOGETHER

At this point, you have a fairly definitive list (in order of importance) of the elements that will make up your Yellow Pages ad. The next step is to group similar components to create focal points that draw the reader's attention.

Group elements that relate to one another together. For example, information on location and your practice phone numbers might comprise one logical block. The services you offer might be another and the benefits yet another. And financial information (credit cards, insurance, payment plans) may also constitute a block of information.

Avoid being wordy. Use short phrases and statements. Prospective patients who use the Yellow Pages want to read the facts, not *Gone With the Wind*. Try to avoid the temptation to include every detail about your practice. Limit the information in your ad to those items of most importance to would-be patients. The ad must be graphically clean and pleasing in order to command attention. That means say what's necessary, and no more.

When you're finished, the copy should accomplish three objectives:

Attract the reader's attention
Be easy to read and follow
Prompt a response

When you're sure the copy effectively and succinctly answers the questions prospective patients may have, evaluate your ad from the standpoint of design. Does it visually leap out at you compared with the other advertisements likely to be in competition? Test it; set a copy of your ad layout on a typical page of your competitors' ads from the current directory and judge its impact.

IT'S NOT OVER TILL IT'S OVER

Your ad is done, the deadline met. Now you can relax and wait for the phone to ring with new patient appointments, right?

Wrong. Your work—and that of your staff—has just begun. Placement, size and content are important to the success of your Yellow Pages advertising efforts, but equally important is the total understanding and involvement of your staff.

It is absolutely necessary to keep your staff informed (or better yet, involved) concerning your advertising efforts if they are to successfully respond to inquiries generated by your advertising. Show them your ad. They should know what information is in it and any promises or offers that are made, such as a no-charge consultation visit. They should be able to tell callers, simply and clearly, how to get to your office. An informed staff can be your greatest resource. Advertising may be what prompts people to call your office, but it is the treatment they get once they do call that converts them from *potential* patients to *your* patients.

YELLOW PAGES CHANGES AND INNOVATIONS

The deregulation of AT&T, coupled with a new emphasis on marketing by Yellow Pages executives, has caused some interesting new developments in this once staid medium. Since January 1, 1983, a number of companies have entered the directory publishing field. Each has its own guidelines, requirements, and special services. Be sure to check with your local Yellow Pages office for the latest information regarding closing dates, and to be aware of any operating or procedural peculiarities unique to your region.

Other recent innovations, some experimental in nature, include the entrance by independent publishers into the business, with a wide range of neighborhood and specialty directories and generally lower space rates. As we stressed earlier, be cautious in using these directories, though. Just because it's put on the doorstep of everyone in town doesn't mean it's the directory referred to when it's time to look up a service or product. We don't advocate cancelling your Yellow Pages ad in "the big book" and substituting one of the lower-cost directories. It's a risk not worth taking, no matter what enticements or savings are offered.

A number of new directories are being introduced, including . . .

1. The Silver Pages, a directory for senior citizens introduced by Southwestern Bell.
2. Regional industrial directories and a nationwide professional engineering directory, both introduced by BellSouth.
3. Instant Yellow Pages Service, a computerized program that allows businesses to access information from every Yellow Pages directory in the country. This is primarily a sales and marketing tool.
4. Electronic Yellow Pages. A view data-tape system designed to bring computer access of the telephone directory into the phone customer's home.
5. Map Anchor Program (MAP). Added to a number of directories to help consumers pinpoint an advertiser's location, city maps set up on a grid are used in conjunction with three-digit identification codes included in ads and/or listings.
6. Two-volume directories. Available in many areas of the country, publishers issue two volumes, one for businesses and one for consumers.
7. Suburban editions. This practice is becoming increasingly common. Names and numbers still appear in the larger metro books, but you have the option of advertising only in your community, eliminating the "waste" audience and potentially lowering your Yellow Pages ad cost (or allowing you to go to a larger ad for the same cost as a smaller one in the metro book).
8. Talking Yellow Pages. A computerized information referral service, callers are given four listings in a given category and geographical area. This is an exciting, expanding trend, one that bears watching. Some physicians report excellent results in attracting patients with their promotion in the Talking Yellow Pages. If it's available in your area, it may be worth looking into.
9. Coupon sections. Results have been mixed to date, with some advertisers achieving phenomenal response and others minimal.
10. Red ink . . . and blue, and green. Referred to earlier, this option increases ad costs by 60 percent. The real value of ink colors other than black is in attracting attention. Southwestern Bell recommends that if you choose to go with red ink, you save it for really important, short attention-span elements such as a headline. Red will attract attention, but it won't hold it due to the poor legibility.
11. Asian Yellow Pages. A dual-language directory for Chinese- and Japanese-speaking people in the San Francisco Bay area.
12. 24-Hour Services Guide. A quick reference section listing businesses that have services 24 hours a day, it does not include display ads and is more expensive than regular directory listings.
13. Specialty directories. These books consolidate specialized information on given products and services such as health care.

These new programs are, for the most part, available only in selected areas. They do, however, attest to a new era of innovation introduced by deregulation. To determine whether specific programs are available in your area, contact your local directory representative.

AND FINALLY . . .

At the very least, consumers expect to find your name in the Yellow Pages along with your competitors. At best, they hope to find a substantial amount of information about your practice, and they expect to learn how they may benefit from calling you.

How you place this information—the format you choose, the quantity of information, the section(s) of the Yellow Pages in which you place your listing or ad, how your copy is written and the ad designed—all can have a tremendous influence on the results your listing or ad generates.

You can't afford to ignore the Yellow Pages, no matter what size or specialty your practice may be. It's a primary component of any marketing communication program. Spend some time planning your Yellow Pages insertion and training your staff to respond positively to patients who call as a result. It's time wisely invested.

BIBLIOGRAPHY

Bronkesh SJ, Pritchard PJT, Wood SD: *Yellow Pages Advertising by Physicians: A Preliminary Analysis*, the Western Regional Meeting of Decision Sciences Institute, April 1988.

Ad Factor/Millword Brown: Professional Yellow Pages Heading Study, conducted for Southern New England Telephone Co., January, 1988.

Jensen J, Miklovic N: Consumers Turn to Yellow Pages When Making Healthcare Choices. *Modern Healthcare* 1986; June 20: 40–42.

Cobb-Walgren C, Sleszynski H: Responses to Physician Advertising in the Yellow Pages. *Current Issues & Research in Advertising*, 1987: 129–152.

Chapter 17

The Print Media: Newspapers and Magazines

Newspapers and magazines have long been among the most accepted and acceptable media for physicians and other professionals engaging in advertising. For a long time, newspapers were the only medium (other than a simple Yellow Pages listing) that some state medical organizations allowed professionals to use to notify the public they had established their practice.

Today, the print media has a much broader application in the advertising efforts of medical professionals. Newspapers and magazines, shoppers and specialty journals, television guides and other publications are appropriate media for informing the public that you've established, expanded or relocated your practice. The print media also is good for educating and informing potential patients about new services you're offering, amenities in your practice that may appeal to them, events and educational seminars you're sponsoring, new technology that may help with a medical problem, and a host of other possibilities.

In this chapter, we'll help you see the pro's and con's of newspapers and magazines; we'll discuss how the print media can fit into your advertising strategies and objectives, and how you can target your advertising by selecting certain publications and sections of those publications that may appeal to your target audience. We'll offer guidelines for developing newspaper and magazine ads, and we'll help you determine the elements that belong in each. Even if you use an agency to prepare your ads or ad campaign, the information in this chapter will be valuable to you, since you'll be better able to judge its recommendations.

NEWSPAPERS

Newspapers are one of the best media for communicating with a local market, because they reach a mass audience in a defined geographical region. Even very small communities with no local television station usually have some sort of newspaper to keep residents abreast of local news—and such newspapers are generally very well read.

Some 70 percent of all adults in America read a newspaper every day. In an era when reading in general is being challenged by the electronic media, newspaper readers as a group tend to fall into the upscale end of the economic spectrum. That's good news especially for physicians whose services are elective, such as cosmetic surgery and some dermatology procedures.

Newspapers have remained strong in the face of competition from radio and television because they have learned to provide the in-depth coverage the electronic media can't offer. For instance, newspaper sections on science, food, business and living are creating many new print advertising options, according to *Advertising Age* magazine. Newspapers also have incorporated improvements such as color reproduction to improve their attractiveness to readers and advertisers alike. The goal for newspaper publishers now is to make strides toward attracting a greater share of the younger audience that currently favors alternative means of keeping up with current events.

MAGAZINES

With magazines, the major development of the past decade has been an increasing emphasis on reaching highly specialized audiences. Today, a magazine can be found for virtually every interest, age group, profession or business. There are magazines for lawyers and truck drivers, parents and grandparents, travelers, kids interested in science, health and fitness buffs, inventors and farmers. While their demise has been predicted for years, magazine circulation has actually increased 73 percent since 1950. Like radio, magazines have met the challenge of the electronic media by appealing to more specialized audiences.

Today, nine out of ten adults read an average or two magazines each week; the average reader spends 90 minutes per issue. Magazines appeal to an upscale audience; the typical magazine subscriber is 34.9 years old, married, and has a household income 24 percent above the national average.

FITTING PRINT INTO YOUR COMMUNICATION STRATEGY

The print media offer both advantages and disadvantages for physicians who are considering newspaper or magazines for their advertising program. Let's look at the pluses offered by newspapers first:

NEWSPAPERS
Advantages

1. **Consistent readership.** Newspapers are not subject to seasonal variations to the degree that TV and some other media are.
2. **Reach.** Newspapers usually outpull other media in a community.
3. **Image.** Newspapers do not have the credibility problems encountered by media

whose primary function is entertainment. People generally believe what they see in print, and they seek out newspaper ads, rather than regarding them as an intrusion.

4. Timeliness. Newspapers are current, with a short turnaround time on ad placement.
5. Flexibility. A variety of ad sizes and locations are available.
6. Permanency. Newspaper ads can be clipped and saved.
7. Targeted marketing. Many papers offer regional or suburban editions that allow smaller advertisers to target their message geographically.
8. Multiple readership. The average newspaper is read by at least two people.

Disadvantages

1. Lack of permanency. Yesterday's newspaper is yesterday's news. It is usually not retained to be read or re-read.
2. Wasted circulation. For most physicians and physician groups, large city dailies provide a waste of circulation, reaching readers far beyond the practice service area.
3. Ad competition. Newspapers can add pages to accommodate as many ads as they can sell. Your ad could face stiff competition.
4. Poor reproduction. Newspaper reproduction is poor compared to a slick medium like magazines. Photos can present a special problem.

MAGAZINES

These are some of the reasons you may want to consider magazines for your advertising media mix:

Advantages

1. Specialized audiences. If you want to reach women with a promotion on cosmetic surgery, you can choose a publication whose readers are overwhelmingly female and in the discretionary income bracket.
2. Quality reproduction. Magazines are usually printed on quality paper; ads reproduce well in both color and black and white. Photos are far more effective in magazine ads than in newspapers.
3. Long shelf life. Magazines are kept around longer and referred to more frquently than any other mass medium. One study showed that the average person picks up a monthly magazine four different times, a weekly magazine twice.
4. Image building. An ad in a high quality magazine lends prestige to the product or service.
5. Believability. Consumers find magazine advertising helpful, believable and an important part of overall magazine content.
6. Consistency. Seasonal audience variations, a common problem with television, are almost nonexistent with magazines.
7. Multiple readership. Magazines are seen by more than one reader.
8. High ad visibility. Page size and quality reproduction make magazine ads far less likely to be buried and overlooked.

Disadvantages

1. Long-range deadlines. Magazines are planned several months in advance, so your deadline may range anywhere from 21 to 60 days or more before the publication date. This long lead time makes it difficult to respond quickly to changes in market conditions with a new or revised ad.

2. Competition. Like newspapers, there is no limit on how many pages a magazine can have. While your ad may be more visible in a magazine, it can also face a lot of competing advertising. Some magazines can run more than 200 pages in length.

3. Wasted circulation. Even in a local magazine, unless you have several practice locations, your ad may reach many consumers who realistically can not be considered potential patients. You pay in the ad rates to reach those consumers nevertheless. Only specialists (and possibly some primary care physicians) with a geographically wide referral base should consider magazines. The cost is too high, the return likely to be too low, for most primary care doctors.

TARGETING YOUR MARKET WITH PRINT MEDIA

As a part of the total media plan, newspapers can get results for physician practices. Ob-gyn specialist Steven Kaali, MD, reported in the Feb. 16, 1987 issue of *Medical Economics* that a carefully thought out promotional plan for laparoscopic tubal ligation was extremely successful for his practice. It yielded 395 inquiries that resulted in 125 procedures, for a total income of $190,000. His expenses included $2,500 to develop ad copy, $47,436 for a six month ad campaign in 12 dailies and two monthlies, and $2,000 in miscellaneous costs. To assure a return on his investment, Dr. Kaali gave careful consideration to converting inquiring consumers to patients. Inquiries were generated with a coupon and a 24-hour telephone line, either of which permitted interested women to request a brochure on the procedure. A month after sending the brochure and a letter, people who had not responded got a second letter providing additional details.

The doctor wanted to ensure that new patients resulting from the ads stayed with the practice. When they returned a week later for suture removal, they received a personal thank-you letter from Dr. Kaali, along with three brochures describing other services of his practice. The women were also encouraged to have an annual check-up and pap smear. Dr. Kaali checked with his state medical society code to be certain his ad conformed to its code of ethics.

His ad campaign worked because he did his homework and spent enough time and dollars on the ad and media selected. He offered a call to action ("call for free brochure") that didn't require a commitment and therefore was more likely to generate a response, and concentrated on conversion and retention.

THE DAILY NEWSPAPER

The daily newspaper used to consist of one edition a day, with no variation in the contents or format when it was distributed to subscribers or street corner vendors who sold it to passers-by.

Gradually, as the capabilities and technology of newspaper printing presses broadened, several editions were added to each daily paper, incorporating the very latest news. Then, as communities became cities and cities became metropolitan cores surrounded by suburbs, regional and zoned editions were added. These "sub-editions" to the daily newspaper have been a boon to local advertisers.

Regional Editions. Many large suburban dailies publish regional editions with localized news and advertising. These regional editions allow you to reach consumers in specific geographical areas. In addition, many dailies publish suburban sections—supplements to the main newspaper— on specific days of the week. These special sections and editions are distributed to a limited geographic area and offer reduced rates compared with the regular full-circulation edition of the paper.

Special Sections. Occasionally, newspapers will publish special sections on topics such as physical fitness or health, real estate, travel or business. Such sections may offer special advertising opportunities; however, too often they are designed merely as a vehicle to sell advertising. If you are considering a one-time special edition or supplement, question the ad rep about the proportion of editorial copy to advertising, the types of articles to be included (are they primarily syndicated pieces, or will they be written by the newspaper's regular staff using local authorities), and who some of the other advertisers are. You want to be in good company with other professionals. At the same time, an excessive number of similar advertisers will overwhelm one another.

Special sections that are published on a regular basis on a specific topic may be very effective for professional advertisers. The *Washington Post* publishes a weekly magazine-format section on health, medicine and science focusing on current topics and concerns in those areas; it would be ideal for a physician advertiser.

Weeklies. Many small suburban or rural communities have a weekly or bi-weekly newspaper that is a prime source of local news (and even some friendly gossip) to residents of the community. These newspapers may be more effective promotional resources for doctors in the area than any other method (with the exception of word of mouth). Many of these small weekly newspapers are chatty, chock full of news, and the editor often is as friendly and accessible as the neighbor next door. Your ad in this paper should reflect the flavor of the community, the publication, and your practice.

One of the fastest growing segments of the newspaper industry is the suburban weekly. The term "weekly" is a misnomer, since some of these publications appear two or even three times a week. In considering the suburban press for your advertising campaign, keep the following in mind: 1) the quality of news coverage, which is as good an indication of readership as circulation figures; 2) the distinct targeting advantages of weekly publications, advantages not provided by the large dailies with which they often compete.

Specialty Papers. Specialty papers offer advertising possibilities in many communities, especially the larger ones. These newspapers may be geared to audiences such as senior citizens or children; ethnic groups such as Blacks or Hispanics; religious groups; fraternal organizations and labor organizations or professional fields such as law, communications or business.

MAGAZINES

There are so many magazine options that it is important to carefully evaluate those that are published for your geographic area. Only major metropolitan areas have their own city magazine, and not even all of them. For the most part, if you're in a smaller city or town, you probably won't need to reach the audiences of your nearby big city publication. While national magazines offer such data as rates, circulation and reader demographics, this information may be less readily available from local or regional publications.

Magazine sales representatives are a good source of information on a publication's reach, readership and audience demographics. Most can provide surveys and evaluations developed by research firms, as well as an editorial calendar that may indicate the best months for you to advertise based on the publication's article topics. Avoid lengthy sales pitches by requesting a media kit from magazines in which you're interested. Also, let magazine reps know what other magazines you're considering; they'll be happy to clue you in on weaknesses in the competition that you may not have considered. (Naturally, you must bear in mind the information source in reviewing a publication's strengths and weaknesses.)

Some Questions to Ask. Consider these questions when evaluating a magazine for potential advertising placement:

1. Will the publication reach the kind of people you want as patients (proper age range, sex, income, medical or health needs)?
2. Will your ad be seen by the magazine's readers, or is the size you can afford so small that it will be buried among other advertisers?
3. Are you investing your promotional dollars wisely, based on practical research, or are you simply seeking the prestige of having an ad in a certain slick publication?
4. Are you making a sensible business decision, or is your ad a good-will gesture? There's nothing wrong with expressing philanthropy by purchasing an ad in a charitable organization's publication or program, as long as you recognize the

gesture for what it is. Building good will in your community is important; just don't expect it to yield instant results.

RATES

Newspapers. Newspaper advertising offers the dual advantage of frequent exposure and regular contact with your potential patients. Ad rates are based on both size and type of ad. There are three basic types of ads available in newspapers, although probably only one is appropriate for physicians.

Display ads. Regular ads utilizing copy and art work such as photos, illustrations, logos, etc. Display ads appear throughout the newspaper and may be as small as one column by one inch or as large as a full page or even two full pages (see Figure 17-1).

Classified ads. Ads aimed at readers looking for specific products or services. Grouped together in a "classified" section, these listing ads may be worth considering in specialized newspapers (for example, a weekly business publication) if your budget is extremely limited.

Classified display ads. These ads appear in the classified section but usually include graphics, headlines, and other attention-getting devices (see Figure 17-2).

Advertising rates for display ads are usually quoted in column inches. A column inch is one inch high by one column wide. If you purchase an ad that is six inches high by three columns wide, you will be charged for 18 column inches. An advertising column in a newspaper may be a different width—usually narrower—than an "editorial" or copy column; check with your newspaper to be certain.

Some newspapers base their charges on line rates. Each line is 1/14 of an inch high by one column wide. If the line rate charged by your paper is $1 and your ad is 50 lines by two columns, your cost would be $100 for the ad.

As with other media, volume and quantity discounts are available from newspapers. The larger the space you purchase, the lower the cost per column inch or line. Frequency discounts are also available based on the size of your ad and the frequency. The rate for running an ad just once, called an "open" rate, is the highest.

Further complicating things, many newspapers charge different rates based on what you are advertising, or they may charge extra for a "preferred position" (requesting a specific location or page). ROP, or "run of the paper" ads can be placed anywhere at the newspaper's discretion. Despite the higher charge, preferred position ads allow you to target your audience and therefore should be considered. If, for example, you are aiming your message at men, the extra cost (if there is one) of being in the sports section rather than in the second news section may be worth it. Fortunately, not all newspapers charge extra for requesting a specific section.

FIGURE 17-1 Effective Display Ad
This is a very strong ad both graphically and in headline and copy. It conveys expertise, yet personal warmth. This is one of a series developed to promote individual physicians while at the same time creating an image for the Honolulu Medical Group.

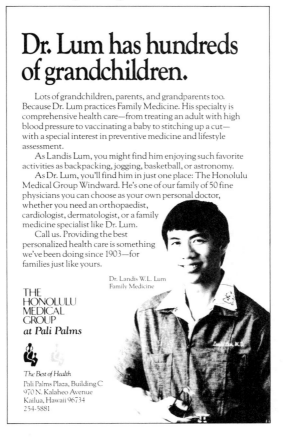

Classified ads are sold at a lower rate than display ads, and if your newspaper offers a professional classified section, you can appear regularly at a very attractive rate.

Consult your newspaper sales representative to determine how best to take advantage of the various discounts available.

MAGAZINES

The cost of advertising in magazines varies widely, depending on circulation, target audience and other factors. As a general rule, rates become lower as the geographic distribution of the magazine shrinks and as the special interest subject narrows in focus. This is because circulation usually decreases with each of these factors. (However, some very slick magazines

FIGURE 17-2   Sample Classified Display Ad
This ad is relatively inexpensive but by placing it in a weekly business newspaper, the ad targets the appropriate audience.

> # STOP SMOKING NOW!
> First deal with the addiction
> Martin Schwartzenfeld, M.D.
> 9876 E. Fairway
> Suite 456
> Anytown, U.S. 65432

with exclusive, upper income readership charge, and get, equally exclusive ad rates.)

While newspaper space is sold by the column inch, magazine space is sold by the page or fraction of a page. You can buy a full page, half page, one-third page, quarter page, even a sixth or twelfth page in many publications. You also have the option of vertical and horizontal ads, and you may encounter the following possibilities as well:

- Double truck: The center two facing pages in the magazine. Printing can spread over the whole two pages with no gap.
- Double spread: Also two facing pages, but not the center two. A double spread ad must be planned to jump the gap or "gutter" between the pages.
- Island: An ad surrounded by editorial copy. In theory, ads "bumping" copy achieve higher readership.

Most magazines use a sliding scale for ad rates, with the highest rate for a single insertion and progressively lower rates when a commitment is made to multiple insertions. To get the best rate, it's wise to plan ahead.

A word about regionals. Local consumer magazines are generally less expensive to advertise in than regional editions of national magazines. (A regional edition is one that contains—in addition to the national advertising and copy—editorial material and advertising that's focused specifically on the geographical region in which it is circulated.) Most regional editions are still too expensive for the solo practitioner, although for a larger group practice or multiple-location practices targeting a wide area, a regional edition may be cost-effective. Rates may start as low as $750 per full page based on a single insertion.

Magazines like *Time, Newsweek, Sports Illustrated* and *TV Guide* have regional editions. Regional edition rates are based on subscription circulation only. Newsstand copies will not contain your ad since they are not regionalized.

At least one firm, Media Networks, sells space in the regional issues of several magazines at a lower combined rate. To find out if your market is one of the 20 or so in which the firm operates, contact their home office in Stamford, Conn., or contact the advertising department of the magazine of your choice and request the name of a Media Network sales rep in your area.

MAKING YOUR AD SING

While the basic principles of creating an effective print ad are similar regardless of the medium, there are important differences to consider for newspaper advertising. Some of the factors to be aware of include:

1. The immediacy of the newspaper. People read newspapers for news, for current events, to learn what's going on around them. An effective ad plays on this characteristic. It should contain current, newsy-sounding information, if at all possible.
2. The limited amount of time people spend reading a newspaper. Most Americans read a newspaper every day, but few spend more than five minutes perusing ads. To make sure yours stands out, it must have both impact and appeal. It must be *obtrusive*, yet professional.

A good example of a print ad that's effective, attention-getting yet educational is the large ad run by a urology center in Dallas. The ad headline reads, "Blaming yourself is natural. Impotence is not." The ad then discusses this typical attitude of men who suffer from impotence, using a direct, easy-to-read approach. It goes on to refute the attitude, offering hope through the center's program. The photo of a concerned-looking older man with a woman's hands on his shoulders conveys the message of the copy. A pleasing graphic design complements the copy and ensures that the ad is seen and read (see Figure 17-3).

PRINT PUBLICATION AD BASICS

Now let's look at some of the basic components of any print advertisement.

The Headline. The headline is, quite simply, the most important component of the print ad. If it is effective, it attracts the reader's attention. If the headline fails, the advertisement fails. The headline must have impact. Promise or imply a benefit. Use "you" in the headline, not "we." Target your audience. Choose words that will appeal to your chosen readership. An example of a newspaper headline that meets all these guidelines is one used by a clinic in the south. The headline announces early detection and treatment of prostate cancer in big, bold type, and it introduces copy discussing a new test to detect early growths of the prostate. The copy also tells of a seminar being offered by the clinic. The headline talks directly

FIGURE 17-3   North Texas Urology Center Ad
Even sensitive topics can be dealt with in print if the copy, illustration, and design are carefully handled. Printed with permision of North Texas Urology Center and Universal Health Services, Inc.

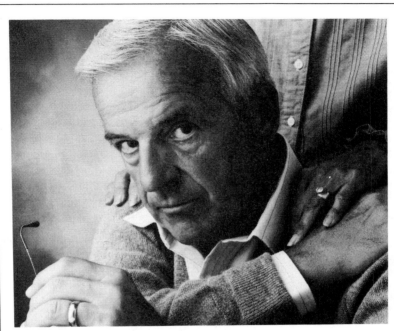

Many men don't want to talk about impotency. And still more do nothing about it. They accept it as a natural fact of aging, or as a consequence of other medical problems. Worse yet, they resign themselves to a life without sexual potency. The truth is, they don't have to.

Blaming yourself is natural. Impotence is not.

At the North Texas Urology Center, men are recovering from impotence through professional medical care.

If you are one of the over 10 million American men who suffer from this sensitive condition, contact the North Texas Urology Center. Our Board Certified urologists can help you lead a more fulfilling life.

Educational brochures on potency recovery and other urological disorders are available upon request.

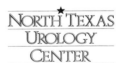

NORTH TEXAS
UROLOGY
CENTER

302 West Ninth Street
Suite BB
Dallas, TX 75208
214-942-2737

to the reader, offers a sense of immediacy, promises a benefit (early detection) and clearly defines its audience by including the words "prostate cancer." The ad got results, too; more than 65 people attended the seminar, and many calls and appointments followed in succeeding weeks.

You'll find more detail on headline writing in Chapter 15.

Body Copy. The body copy is the elaboration, the reinforcement for your headline. It makes good on what the headline promises. It provides the reasons and the facts. Use convincing arguments and get straight to the point. Be specific, friendly and believable. Make your copy long enough to do the job, but fast-paced, fact-filled. Then shorten it by rewriting until you are confident every word is essential. While you want the impact of your strongest arguments up front, end your copy with a bang, not a whisper.

With newspaper ads, copy should tend more toward the practical than magazine ad copy. People who read newspapers are usually in a hurry. They skim. If you have a lot of information, save it for the more leisurely pace of the magazine format, or come up with ways to entice your newspaper reader to want to learn more about the topic you've touched on. Use the words *you* and *your* in the body copy. Your practice is unique; your copy should reflect your uniqueness.

Graphic Elements. A successfully designed print ad means arranging all the graphic components—headline, copy, illustrations, photo, logo and border—to grab attention, create and hold interest, and impart the message. You'll have a far more attractive and effective ad if you hire a professional graphic designer to accomplish this. (See Chapter 22 for more information on working with a graphic artist.) Your choices for art work in both magazine and newspaper advertising include a photo, custom line art (illustration), clip art (purchased art work that's free of copyright restrictions), or no art work at all. Art adds visual impact to your ad, and helps carry your message graphically. But there's a major drawback to clip art, or to hiring an artist who is not very creative or original. That cute drawing of the old-time doctor with a stethoscope around his neck doesn't say anything new or unique about you and your practice. In fact, its stereotyped message may turn off potential patients.

With either magazine or newspaper, it's best to stick with simple art work, avoiding intricately detailed illustrations which may not reproduce well. Photos must be clear, sharp and of high contrast for both newspaper and magazine. Both types of publications require excellent photos—newspapers because there will be some loss of quality, and magazines because the superior photo reproduction will reveal every flaw in the photo. If you're using a photo of yourself in the ad, avoid the stuffy, posed studio portrait in business attire. Better to have a friendly yet professional photo, either with a patient or in a pose that has more of a candid feeling to it. (A professional photographer can take a photo that looks unposed even though it is.) Spend the money on professional camera work. It's worth it.

Whatever choice you make for illustrations, make sure your choice fits both the message and the image of your practice. You are a professional; your ad should convey your professionalism.

The Logo. Your practice logo is the one element in your advertising that doesn't change from ad to ad (except perhaps in size and position). Your logo is a reflection of your practice, creating your image in print. It also provides the element of repetition that makes your ads achieve cumulative impact. You must strive in all elements of your advertising to communicate the uniqueness of your practice, and the logo is one of your most potent weapons. Use it consistently.

PUTTING IT ALL TOGETHER

The actual production of a print ad—ordering type, designing the ad, then laying it out and pasting it up—is an involved process best left to a professional. However, it helps if you understand the steps in the process of creating a final ad. This knowledge can save you costly mistakes.

Newspapers usually offer you the services of their graphics department at little or no charge. Say "No, thank you." Newspapers offer a limited number of typefaces, and a less-than-creative graphics staff. The result: an ad that mingles listlessly with every other ad on the page. There is no excitement that makes your ad jump out. Pay an advertising agency or a graphic artist to achieve your goal: an ad that attracts attention by its visual presentation of the essential elements in a pleasing, yet noticeable, arrangement. You may have a great headline, an outstanding illustration, and award-winning copy, but if there's no creative design, these elements may not be noticed. Putting all the pieces together is as important a step as any in the process.

Here then, are the elements that go into producing an ad for print publications:

The Layout. The layout is a sketch of the final ad. It may vary from a rough sketch to a more finished "comp" (comprehensive, or a complete representative drawing of the ad). Either way, it's your opportunity to assess the ad design, type style, placement of headline, copy, and art work before it is actually pasted up.

When you're evaluating the rough layout, use these guidelines to judge it:

1. Avoid clutter. Don't fill the ad so full of details that nothing stands out. One element—usually the headline or illustration—should dominate and draw the eye into the rest of the ad.
2. Use white space. White space is the antidote to clutter. It adds a professional tone, and also sets your ad off from the rest of the page.
3. Select typefaces carefully. Choose for readability, simplicity, and clarity. Generally, this means a serif face for body copy, and a sans serif for headlines.
4. Make your illustration dominant. A large illustration or photo is preferable to several smaller ones, especially in newspapers, since reproduction can be a problem. Photos should have strong human interest qualities to lure the reader into the ad. The photo of the man in Figure 17-3 is a good example.
5. Be consistent in design. This will help you get more mileage from your ad-

vertising, since each ad will remind the reader of the next or previous one. (Consistency is another argument for hiring a designer to create your ads. You'll have difficulty getting a consistent look when every ad is put together by a different publication or individual.)

6. Avoid reverse type (light copy on a dark background) except for limited amounts of copy in large type. Especially in newspapers, a large quantity of reverse type is difficult to read, and probably won't be read.

7. Emphasize your logo. Your logo is critical to your image and to your ad's memorability, as well as creating a consistent look from one ad to another. So make the logo large enough to stand out. It should be at least as large as the largest type in the ad.

8. Position your headline for attention. Put it in a dominant position, and make it large and bold.

9. Consider color for magazine advertising. Color has been said to increase ad readership by 1500 percent. We don't recommend it for newspapers since so often there are problems resulting in blurred images.

10. Choose ad sizes carefully. Avoid square ads; they have little eye appeal. Save the cost of a full page ad by buying ad space a column narrower or a few inches shorter than full page. You'll still dominate the page, and you can use the money you save on production.

11. Provide a dominant element that takes up as much as two-thirds of your layout. Usually this will be the headline or illustration.

The Mechanical. Once you've approved the layout, or comp, a mechanical (paste-up) is prepared. The mechanical (also known as *camera-ready art work or art boards*) contains all of the elements of the ad in final form (type, illustrations, etc.). Careful proofreading is necessary at this stage. It's your last chance to catch typographical errors (but it's not the time for rewriting copy; major changes at this stage are costly). It's always wise to have several people proof your ad, including at least one not involved in your practice or the production of the ad.

A FINAL CHECKLIST

To a degree, the proof of an advertisement's effectiveness is in the results it achieves. Use this checklist to stack the odds for creating a winning ad in your favor:

1. Does the size meet the mechanical requirements of the newspaper or publication?

2. Does the ad attract attention? Is it eyecatching?

3. Are spelling and punctuation correct?

4. Is everything straight and even—copy, art, lines? Printing will only make these flaws more obvious.

5. Is the copy easy to read?

6. Is body copy set in at least 10-point type—or larger if your target market is primarily the elderly?

7. Are your practice name and telephone number prominent enough, and are spellings and addresses correct?

PRINT AS PART OF YOUR MEDIA MIX

You may decide that newspapers and magazines aren't an appropriate part of your advertising strategy. But more likely, if you are utilizing other media—radio, television, direct mail—you'll find print a vital part of a total campaign. Newspapers in particular support the message seen and heard on television and radio, and magazines lend strength and credibility to your image and services.

A good example of combining media for results is that of two board-certified general surgeons in New Jersey who formed "The Hernia Center." They chose hernia repair and began advertising to combat dwindling caseloads caused by intense competition from other physicians and HMOs. Ira Rutkow, MD, one of the surgeons, also has a PhD in marketing and economics, so he knew how to develop a media campaign and the ads themselves. The physicians researched their market before deciding to focus on hernia repair, selecting the procedure because of its common occurrence and because it was not as dependent on referrals from other physicians. They initially chose radio and newspaper as their advertising vehicles, devoting 20 percent of their annual gross income to their advertising budget. Their newspaper ad encouraged readers to call for a descriptive brochure; they also established a toll-free telephone line. Within a short period of time, the ads had generated enough business for the Hernia Center physicians to open a total of five offices. (They time-share space with other physicians.) See Figure 17-4 for the Hernia Center's newspaper ad.

Their media mix now encompasses radio, television, newspaper, magazines and billboards, and they're laying plans for construction of an outpatient facility for hernia repair. Their strategy, Dr. Rutkow says, is to "offer high quality care, treat patients nicely, empathize, get them better quickly, accept Medicare, and offer Saturday office hours and other conveniences."

AND FINALLY . . .

Physicians who choose advertising as one of their promotional strategies generally start with the print media, and for good reason. Newspapers and magazines provide very targeted audiences, both geographically and demographically. They allow a complicated or complex message to be disseminated. They also can be cost-effective if you've studied the media well, carefully researched your options, gotten accurate readership information from the media representative, and allocated a large enough budget to ensure a regular, frequent schedule.

FIGURE 17-4 The Hernia Center Ad
This ad is targeted to a specific group and, with the toll-free 800 number, offers a means of tracking response.

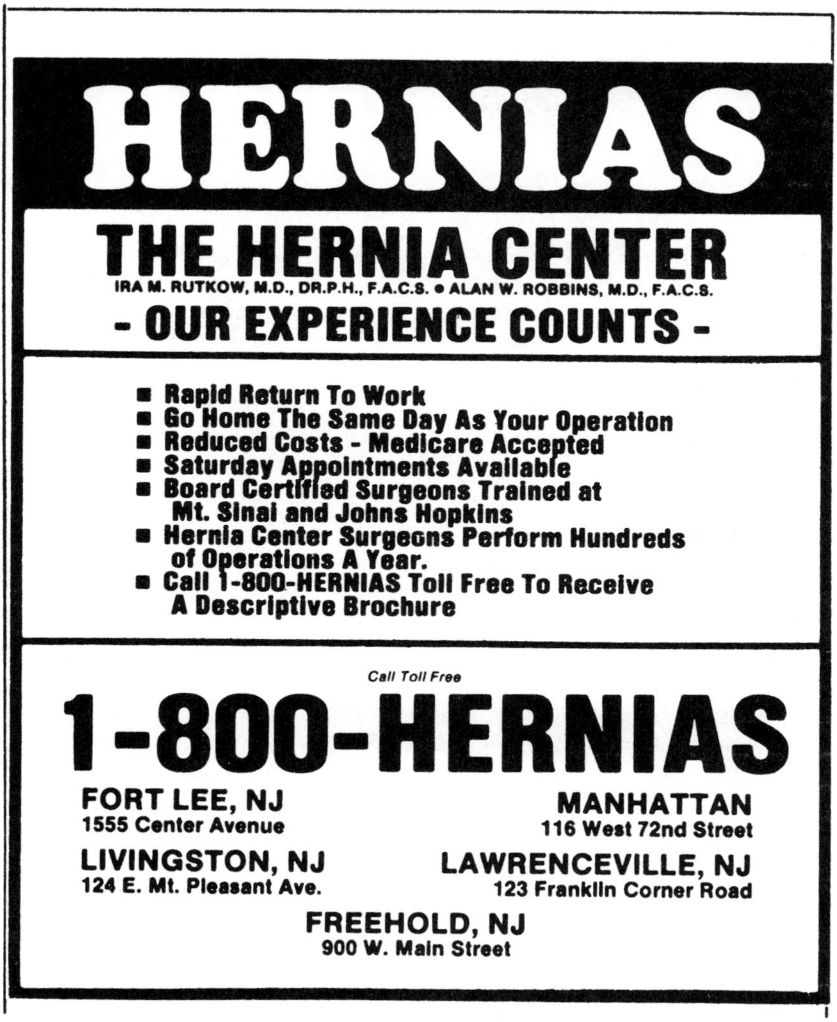

HERNIAS

THE HERNIA CENTER
IRA M. RUTKOW, M.D., DR.P.H., F.A.C.S. ● ALAN W. ROBBINS, M.D., F.A.C.S.
- OUR EXPERIENCE COUNTS -

- Rapid Return To Work
- Go Home The Same Day As Your Operation
- Reduced Costs - Medicare Accepted
- Saturday Appointments Available
- Board Certified Surgeons Trained at Mt. Sinai and Johns Hopkins
- Hernia Center Surgeons Perform Hundreds of Operations A Year.
- Call 1-800-HERNIAS Toll Free To Receive A Descriptive Brochure

Call Toll Free

1-800-HERNIAS

FORT LEE, NJ
1555 Center Avenue

MANHATTAN
116 West 72nd Street

LIVINGSTON, NJ
124 E. Mt. Pleasant Ave.

LAWRENCEVILLE, NJ
123 Franklin Corner Road

FREEHOLD, NJ
900 W. Main Street

Use the print media wisely, research it well, and readers may respond by becoming patients.

BIBLIOGRAPHY

Medical Economics 1987; February 16.
Does It Pay to Advertise? *Physicians Weekly* 1987; March 23.

Chapter 18

Advertising in the Electronic Media: Radio and Television

More and more medical practitioners are turning to the broadcast media—and getting results. Radio and television are no longer exclusively for big budget advertisers. Both radio and TV have become an excellent means of supplementing or even spearheading other promotional efforts for physicians in some specialties.

This growing trend is due largely to the recognition that our society depends on the electronic media for information and education, as well as entertainment. The time people spend reading today is a fraction of the hours they spend with radio and television. The mass audience attracted by both radio and TV means the per-person cost is relatively inexpensive.

Television and radio have much in common. Both are time-rather than space-oriented, selling advertising time in segments. Both utilize the public airwaves and must be licensed to do so by the Federal Communications Commission.

Advertisers new to the broadcast media will discover that it has unique needs. Unlike the print media, simplicity is a must in the advertising message. Broadcast messages are fleeting, and the audience is easily distracted. Furthermore, broadcast spots require a degree of showmanship not always appropriate with print advertising. Your message must attract attention; it must be intrusive in order to be seen or heard. Yet medical advertising in particular must remain professional; it can't be unsavory or abrasive.

Conversely, radio and TV are very different media. The TV advertiser has the visual element to help convey a message. But, through words and sound effects, the radio advertiser can create a visual image in the listener's mind. Therefore the production elements are very different. For this reason, TV and radio will be treated separately in this chapter.

THE RESURGENCE OF RADIO

Today there are more than 9,000 radio stations in the U.S. alone. There are more radios than people in the U.S., with an estimated 400 million sets in homes, cars and anywhere people can be found. On any given day, over 80 percent of all American adults listen to the radio for an average of more than three hours a day. In fact, during the morning hours, radio surpasses television audience size by a significant margin.

A Segmented Medium. For advertisers, radio is appealing because it permits selection of a narrowly defined audience. This means your message is targeted more effectively because each station's format appeals to a specific age and/or sociological group. The entire range of interests and tastes finds expression on radio.

Common radio formats include:

Adult contemporary
All news
Easy listening/beautiful music
Rhythm & blues
Classical/light classical
Country/western
Golden oldies
Middle of the road
Progressive rock
Jazz
Soft or "light" rock
Standard pop
Talk/discussion/interview
Top 40/contemporary rock
Christian/religious
Hispanic

The Advantages of Radio. The ability to target your message to a well-defined audience is considered one of radio's major advantages as an advertising medium. This allows you to reach those most likely to be the health care decision-makers. If you're a plastic surgeon wishing to inform people about innovations in cosmetic facial surgery, and you know the characteristics of your target market (e.g., women 30 to 65 who have discretionary income) you can select a radio format and time for your spot most likely to reach that audience.

Other advantages of radio as an advertising medium include:

1. Size. Radio is the biggest medium in terms of numbers. There are more radios than television sets or daily newspapers.
2. Reach. Radio is everywhere: indoors, outdoors, on the road, at work, at home and play.
3. All seasons. Radio audiences tend to remain consistent year-round.
4. Cost. Radio is an economical medium, providing the lowest cost per thousand audience members of all media.
5. Flexibility. Radio advertisers can change a message or advertising schedule on very short notice, eliminating the deadline delays common with newspapers, magazines, shoppers and direct mail.
6. Personal. Radio creates a one-on-one relationship that produces loyalty, believability and, most important, action.
7. High frequency. Repetition sells, especially with the broadcast media, and

radio's low cost and broad reach makes it a great medium for building frequency.

8. The motorist's medium. Radio reaches drivers and passengers. No other medium draws more than a passing glance from this important group.
9. Station loyalty. Radio listeners choose stations rather than programs; TV viewers do the opposite.
10. Inexpensive production. Radio spots can be produced at little or no expense.
11. Immediacy. Radio is a "fast-acting" medium, one that stimulates people to action right away.

The Disadvantages of Radio. Major drawbacks of radio advertising include:

1. Segmentation. How can an advantage be a disadvantage? With so many stations to choose from (some markets have as many as 25 or more), the market can become too fragmented and the choice of where to advertise confusing. You need to make sure you're paying a reasonable rate for the audience you want by scrutinizing rate cards and audience surveys. Even then you may discover that no single station attracts a majority of the market segment you want to reach.
2. Measurability. Sales reps will inundate you with surveys and statistics, but the truth is that it is difficult to accurately measure the radio audience. Unlike print, the broadcast media has no subscribers or newsstand sales that can be counted.
3. Attention. So many people listen to the radio while doing something else that gaining their full and undivided attention can be difficult.
4. Time and frequency. You must accomplish your message in a maximum of 150 words (for a 60 second spot) and you must repeat it often.
5. Limited availability. Unlike the print media, which can add pages to accommodate additional advertising, radio has a finite number of spots to sell. You may not be able to place your message exactly where and when you want it.

Types of Radio Spots. The most common lengths for radio commercials are 10, 30 and 60 seconds, although longer spots can usually be arranged with the individual station. Spots that are 30 or 60 seconds are the norm; the primary use for 10-second spots is name recognition and reinforcement of messages introduced in longer commercials.

The Radio Advertising Bureau identifies four major types of radio commercials:

1. Singing/Jingle. A time-proven approach, the singing commercial features an original composition or a recognizable tune. Without the visual element, music and other sound effects are very important for grabbing and holding listener attention.
2. Narrative. Usually a 60-second spot, the narrative commercial attempts to deliver a message by telling a story. It's a minidrama, usually involving more than one personality, and often depending on humor or the element of surprise.
3. Straight. The most common. A single personality delivers the message and

exhorts the audience to try the product or service. Music and humor are fairly common components of this genre.

4. Celebrity/Personality. A well-known celebrity or personality is tapped to deliver the message in hopes that the celebrity will bring credibility and appeal to the message. The caution in this approach is to make sure the personality does not outshine the message.

Many commercials make use of a combination of the above. Music, for example, can be effectively employed with all four, and a narrative approach may involve more than one celebrity or personality.

The Cost of Radio Advertising. The cost of radio advertising depends on several factors. The price you pay will be determined in part on the basis of how many listeners a station attracts, and on the demographics (age, income, sex, etc.) of that audience.

The length of the spot also is a cost factor. The general industry practice is to price 30-second spots at 80 percent of the rate of 60s, and 10s at 50 percent of the minute rate. In determining which length to purchase, however, message as well as price should influence your decision. Typically, 80 percent of radio spots are 60 seconds. In a 10-second spot, all you can do is identify yourself, announce what you are offering, and perhaps include a slogan. During a 60-second spot, and to a lesser degree a 30-second, you can also describe what you offer, explain the benefits of your service, support and reinforce your claims, and repeat your telephone number. Figure 18-1 describes some of the factors that may affect the cost of a radio ad campaign.

If radio is your only advertising medium, or even the principal one, 60-second spots are most effective. If your radio ads supplement other media, you may get good results from shorter spots. Many medical advertisers have found they can enhance the overall impact of their promotional efforts

FIGURE 18-1   Factors Affecting Radio Advertising Costs

Audience size

Audience demographics

Commercial length

Time slot

Time of year

Advance scheduling of spot

Number of spots run

Disc jockey appeal

Station broadcast power

by using radio to draw attention to their print ads. For instance, a radio spot can close with a live "tag" from the announcer saying, "See our ad in the "Lifestyle" section of today's *Journal*." With a live tag, the recorded spot is ten seconds shorter (i.e., 50 seconds on a 60-second spot) in order to allow for the tag.

The time slots in which your ads run will also affect the price you pay. Radio attracts the largest number of listeners when they are captive—in the car on the way to and from work. This is called "drive time" and commands the highest rates. These are typical time classification categories:

AM Drive Time	5–10 am, Mon–Sat
Daytime	10 am–3 pm, Mon–Fri
PM Drive Time	3–7 pm, Mon–Fri
Evening	7 pm–12 midnight, Mon–Sun
Overnight	12 midnight–5 am, Mon–Sun
Weekend Drive Time	10 am–7 pm, Sat–Sun
Sunday AM	6–10 am, Sun

You pay less for advertising time when radio listeners are fewer in numbers. This does not mean these times are ineffective. Not everyone lives on the same schedule, and it may be that your particular target group comprises a large portion of listeners during the off-hour programming. Radio is a companion for many night shift workers, for example. In general, however, radio is considered a daytime medium; the night belongs to television.

Other factors that may affect what you pay include the selling power of a station's on-air personalities, and the power of the broadcast signal. And even on the same station, the price of a spot in a given time period varies.

Since radio can't increase the number of hours in a day to accommodate advertisers, many stations have developed "grid" systems to get the most for the time they have to sell (and to encourage advertisers to buy the less popular time slots). Grid systems are basically sliding scale rates based on supply and demand.

When demand for spots is low and supply is plentiful, stations ask a lower rate. As the available number of spots decreases, however, the station will start asking progressively more for each spot. Each time classification may be selling at a different grid level. For example, there may be a big demand for spots during morning Drive Time, but a lot of spots available during daytime. The morning Drive Time spots would sell at a higher grid rate than would the Daytime spots.

By using such a system, the station can keep a balanced number of commercials throughout the day, while securing the highest rates the market will bear. Typically, it's the last-minute advertiser who pays top rates. The advertiser who plans well in advance can usually buy spots at the lowest grid, saving money and still acquiring desirable time slots.

Meet with your station sales rep and discuss both cost and availability of spots. Be sure to obtain as much information as possible, including the demographics and size of the station's audience (see Figure 18-2).

Most radio stations offer a number of package plans for budget-conscious advertisers, a category most physicians will fall into. A common package approach is the "total audience plan" that provides a combination of spots designed to reach all the station's listeners in a given time period. Stations will often throw in free spots, usually in the evening or overnight time categories, to encourage you to buy a package plan. Weigh the cost of the package, however, against the cost of targeting the audience you want, to determine the better value.

Using Radio Effectively. Radio's flexibility offers medical advertisers a variety of options for maximum utilization. And the more stations in your market, the wider the range of promotional opportunities available to you.

Station loyalty of listeners is an important factor in selection, as is the following of its individual radio personalities. Unlike TV, radio stations tend to attract loyal listeners. Many people leave their radio on one station all the time.

One approach that has proven helpful to many small radio advertisers is to use one station for a given time period, say 12 weeks. Then you can switch to another for 12 weeks, and then another (as long as the audience demographics for these stations fit your target audience). This way you will not only find out which station performs best for you, but you'll also gain better total market penetration.

Once you've selected a station or stations, your next decision is how

FIGURE 18-2 Time Buying Tips for Radio from the Radio Advertising Bureau

1. Don't choose a station just because it's your favorite station. You'll hear your own commercials, but you may not be reaching your target audience.

2. Pay attention to audience surveys and demographics.

3. Listen to a variety of stations in your market. Your subjective opinion adds a human element when you review the surveys. Does the station have the proper image to promote your practice? A rock station may have the highest audience figures in town, but the raunchy morning disc jockey who reads your live spots may do you more harm than good.

4. Plan ahead in order to get the best times and rates.

5. Get it in writing. Finalize your buys with a contract and written instructions regarding which ads are to run in which spots.

6. Track your spots on the air, and request "make goods" if they don't air as scheduled, or if a live announcer shortchanges you or goofs up while reading it.

your message will be delivered. You may use spot announcements, or sponsor your own program or a station feature.

A spot is a commercial of 60 seconds or less. It has the advantage of flexibility. The number of spots can be varied according to the desired impact and budget, and they can also be concentrated during specific time periods. You can promote different services, yet retain "image" continuity through a consistent message. You can also spread them among a variety of stations as was suggested earlier.

The number of spots you run will depend on your budget, but generally, more is better. Repetition is a broadcast necessity.

One approach is to maintain a fairly consistent schedule throughout the year, with increases at times when seasonal demands or practice needs dictate. Another approach is to advertise heavily for a period, then stop for a period. Such intermittent ad periods are called "flights," or "surge" advertising, and they allow you to concentrate your spots for maximum impact.

In addition to spot advertising, a physician can also use radio to promote his or her practice by sponsoring regular station features such as newscasts, weather and traffic reports, sports reviews or health programs. By doing so, you achieve identification and recognition, and possibly community prestige for being associated with a popular and respected feature.

Program sponsorship is a very soft-sell kind of advertising, more image than sales-oriented, making it a "safe" way for a physician to enter the advertising arena (as long as your ad content is subtle and appropriate). It won't result in immediate response or action (i.e., calls to your practice) but it will help people remember your name or practice. If sponsorship advertising is combined with more aggressive forms of promotion, it can be highly effective.

Time Is Fleeting. Whether you choose spots or sponsorship, remember that your message must air frequently if it is to be effective. You can't count on potential patients hearing your message unless you give them repeated opportunities to do so. It is this quality of radio that makes it seem so expensive to the small-budget advertiser. But again, it can be used effectively to supplement other forms of promotion, especially print and Yellow Pages advertising.

Radio is particularly good for this because it is intrusive. Prospective patients may not be thinking about health care and therefore will ignore your print ads. A well-done radio spot is more likely to intrude on their thoughts and make them think about their health or that of their family for at least a few seconds. Repeated advertising efforts build upon this.

Creating a Spot. Radio has been called theatre of the mind. It creates images through the use of sound, the way a print ad employs creative copy and expressive pictures to trigger a favorable response.

What parent would not respond to the sound of the crash of furniture followed by the piercing shriek of a small child and the wailing cry, "Mommy!" Such is the power of words. When coupled with other sound effects, music and the soothing voice of Dr. Jones caring for little Jennifer's minor emergency, the message is clear.

Too many advertisers, unfortunately, simply read their print ad copy on the air or play the audio of their television ad on radio. Though all your ads should have a recurring theme, each should be specifically created for the medium in which it is used. Radio advertising should be written to take advantage of the unique characteristics of radio.

The first step is to decide where you will have your spot produced—at a radio station or an independent production studio. The local station may be cheaper, but production studios have more sound effects and greater capabilities. (You don't have to have the spot recorded at the station where it is to run. Any radio station offers production services.)

First, find out what studio effects are available. If you choose to rely on station production facilities, your sales representative can be an invaluable source in formulating and producing your spot. Don't overestimate your rep, however. He or she is first a salesperson, although years of exposure to the business undoubtedly make him/her knowledgeable. The sales rep can put you in touch with production people and on-air personalities who can assist in the creative development of your ad. Some stations will produce your commercials at a reasonable cost (and in some cases, at no charge). You will pay a "talent" fee if you use a station personality as the voice on your commercial.

Radio copy begins with a concept. As with print, all elements of the ad should create a single impression of you and your practice. The impression must be consistent with your practice image and positioning; it must also be consistent with your other media promotions.

As with print, you must zero in on your target audience and let them know within the first few seconds that your message is directed to them. A nebulous, misdirected ad will defeat what you have accomplished through careful media selection.

Radio: The Personal Medium. Radio is a personal medium, so direct your message to a single listener. Make every listener feel you are talking *only* to him or her.

The majority of radio listening occurs in automobiles. Drivers make excellent listeners. Research continues to prove that drivers are more attentive to radio messages than the average listener at home, so this is who your message should be directed to.

But even with the advantage of a captive audience, you are still competing for the listener's attention. Always remember that you are dealing with *listeners* on radio. Just as a print ad must be visually appealing, a radio ad must be audibly appealing. Words may send your message across the air waves, but it will not be retained without sound cues for the listener.

Sound effects and music also give color and body to your ad, the same way a photo adds an extra dimension to a print ad. Don't fill every second with noise, though. Audio "white space" is just as important as white space in print. (In fact, a pause should be considered one of the building blocks of a radio ad.)

Still, audio ornamentation does make a difference. The simple addition of appropriate sound effects or theme music can add immeasurably to the appeal and effectiveness of a strictly verbal ad. It is not necessary to have a jingle written specifically for you. Instead, you can create identity by having the same background music in every ad.

Choosing a Voice. The selection of an announcer is also very important to your message. A distinctive voice can become as identifiable with your practice as a few bars of an instrumental theme. Your choice of an announcer will probably depend a great deal on who is available at the station with which you're working. You may wish to use their on-air personalities for a pre-recorded spot, which offers the advantage of consistent quality. Many local radio personalities have a strong hold on their audiences, and if he or she believes in you, and sounds like it, you'll get a very credible spot.

Or, you can provide a script for the announcer or disc jockey to read live. Enthusiasm adds a dimension to live commercials and capitalizes on the announcer's own style and popularity. Having your spot read live also adds spontaneity, giving your message a greater sense of immediacy and timeliness.

Vocal quality is another important consideration. Would your target audience be more responsive to a commanding male voice, or would a sympathetic female voice have more appeal?

Be Wary of Humor. A word of caution on the use of humor in your radio spot. Humorous commercials wear out much faster than straight pitches, and therefore must be changed more frequently. Also humor in medical promotion must be handled with great delicacy and care, for an individual or family's health, after all, is a serious matter. Our advice is to leave use of humor to professional advertising agencies pitching cars or soap.

Writing the Radio Script. The first step in producing a radio ad is developing the script, with dialogue, sound effects, music and other non-narrative elements indicated.

Radio copy must be simple. In a 30-second spot, you have only 65 words to get your message across to the listener. To accomplish this goal, it's best to present one basic idea several different ways. A good formula for writing broadcast ads is the old adage, "Tell them what you are going to tell them; tell them; then tell them what you told them." You are doing well if listeners understand and remember one point, so don't try to include all of the features of your practice in one ad. If you include a telephone number, it should be repeated at least three times. Better still, refer listeners to the telephone directory; that way they don't have to remember your number.

The image to be conveyed in all of your advertising is that of a trained, caring professional, not a fast-talking patent medicine salesman.

Radio is personal. Make it work for you by writing conversationally. Don't be afraid to use incomplete sentences and phrases in radio copy. They make sense to the ears, and that's what you're writing to. Remember, people don't talk in complete sentences, let alone the complex, grammatically correct sentences that are appropriate in written language.

The Imagination Medium. Use your imagination to make the ad interesting. Radio is an imagination medium, and innovative ads have the power to capture listeners and, better yet, motivate them to action. People respond to radio requests for action. They call a station to banter with a disc jockey or to request a song. If they can do that, they can call you immediately, too—if you give them a reason to. Incite listeners to action. It's a good way to measure the effectiveness of an ad or a particular station.

Timing Counts. Radio is both timely and timed. Air time is planned in seconds, so your message must be timed to run the exact length of contracted time or slightly less (see Figure 18-3). If you are purchasing 30-second spots, it's a good idea to create a 28-second spot. If you run long, your ad could be cut short on the air. If your message is too complex to tell in 30 seconds or less, then buy 60-second spots. The last thing you want is to have your ad read faster than it should be to squeeze it all in. If your message is educational, a longer spot may be needed. Like the editorial ad in print, educational radio spots have the appearance of a public service spot rather than advertising—a plus to physicians concerned about peer reaction.

Even when repeated, telephone numbers and addresses are difficult to remember. Listeners will seldom write down a number or address, so don't expect them to. If you use a telephone number in your radio spot, consider a simplified phone number or an acronym phone number that spells out a word or phrase according to the letters on the phone dial. For addresses, simply mention the nearest intersection or the medical building where your practice is located.

Whatever approach you choose, listen to your ad before it runs. Better still, play the entire ad within a taped sample of the station's regular

FIGURE 18-3 Sample 30-Second Spot

Sound Effect: A-CHOO!

Announcer: If you're constantly sneezing and congested and your eyes are always watering, you may have allergies. You need professional diagnosis and treatment by physicians who specialize in allergies. Call the Cove Creek Allergy Center, 555-5555, for a comprehensive evaluation, and stop sniffing and sneezing. Call today. The Cove Creek Allergy Center, 555-5555.

Sound Effect: A-CHOO!

---

programming so you can get the full effect of what the audience will hear. That will give you the best insight into the appropriateness and impact of your message.

Radio Copy Guidelines. The Radio Advertising Bureau suggests that in writing ad copy you should:

1. Write conversationally. Person to person, not writer to reader.
2. Talk benefits such as health, fitness, good looks, immediate care, comfort about family health.
3. Be direct and to the point. Use short sentences. Don't back into a thought; say it.
4. Repeat key elements, such as the practice name, as early and often as you can.
5. Use positive action words like *now, today, forever.* Take advantage of the urgency and immediacy of radio.
6. Write for the listener.
7. Put the listener in the picture. Radio is theatre of the mind. Make sure the audience is involved.
8. Use simple descriptive words that form pictures, give dimension and color.

Radio is well-suited to medical promotion. It is believable, targeted and can be cost-effective even for small advertising budgets if it is carefully planned, and incorporated as a part of an overall promotional campaign.

TELEVISION, THE POWER MEDIUM

Television is the fastest growing advertising medium. Since the first commercial station began operation in New York City in 1941, the number of U.S. stations has grown to more than 700 (excluding cable). And the number of households owning television sets has risen from nine percent in 1950 to more than 98 percent today.

A major reason for television's advertising success is the fact that it is a demonstration medium. It combines sight, sound, color, drama and action, and it reaches people where they live—at home. Television is the next best thing to hiring someone to personally visit the homes of your potential patients.

But is television truly a viable medium for medical practice promotion? Isn't it for the big guys . . . the HMOs backed by national advertising budgets and extensive expertise?

While it's true that TV's primary application in the medical profession is by practices with multiple locations and large group practices, its very potency and reach make it difficult to dismiss without careful investigation. A study conducted by R. H. Bruskin Associates for the Television Bureau of Advertising revealed that adults spend more time with TV then with all other media combined. The average adult spent over four hours a day watching television in 1985, compared with less than three hours a day devoted to newspapers, magazines and radio combined.

Use of the medium by professionals is growing rapidly. In fact, TV advertising by the medical, dental and ocular professions reached $125.6 million in 1985, an increase of $36 million over the previous year, according to the Television Bureau of Advertising. Just during the first half of 1987, TV advertising expenditures for the medical and dental profession increased 20 percent.

For the right physician in the right specialty, a good television ad campaign can make a big difference. A solo plastic surgeon in Milwaukee reported that he doubled his practice volume in two years by running a series of 10 TV spots. His annual ad budget was $150,000, an expenditure that's not unreasonable for television advertising. It overwhelmed his practice with new patients. The specialist generated a four-to-one return on his ad dollar. For a specialty like plastic surgery, television is an obvious choice. It's a visual medium, one that can depict the benefits of cosmetic procedures.

Of special interest to advertisers with limited budgets is the fact that recent increases in TV viewership have occurred outside of the prime viewing hours. Increases in viewing are occurring in morning, afternoon, late night and weekend periods.

This means that, depending on the audience you are trying to reach, television can be an especially good buy during these non-prime-time viewing segments, when advertising time is less expensive. Stay-at-home mothers, for example, make up the majority of afternoon TV viewers, while senior citizens comprise a large portion of early morning television viewers. The young mothers would be the perfect target for a large pediatric or family practice group, whereas older audiences would appeal to an ophthalmologist, an internal medicine specialist or orthopedic surgeon.

TV: The Pluses and Minuses. Before we examine the basics of TV advertising, let's look at some of the medium's major advantages and disadvantages. On the plus side, television advertising offers:

1. Impact. The combination of audio and video is a potent one; no other media can match it.
2. Mass coverage. Some 98 percent of all U.S. homes have at least one TV set, and no other medium can even approach that level of saturation. TV is the great equalizer. You don't even have to be able to read and write to "get the picture."
3. Repetition. With television, you can repeat your message as often as you like. Familiarity breeds business.
4. Flexibility. TV offers sight, sound, color, action. It can set a mood, demonstrate, make an announcement.
5. Prestige. TV is perceived by the public as the "big time." Unless your spot is poorly conceived, your image will likely improve by your presence on television.
6. Targeted marketing. You can direct your message to the audience you wish to reach by carefully choosing programs and time slots.
7. Credibility. Viewers consider TV an up-to-date, authoritative medium.

8. Scheduling immediacy. You can get in the TV station's schedule right away if you have a spot produced.
9. Intrusiveness. TV is the most intrusive of all the media, combining sight, sound and emotional appeal.

Television does have drawbacks, of course, not the least of which is cost. Others include:

1. Commercial clutter. Not only are 30-second spots increasing, now advertisers are using more and more 10-second spots on TV. Shorter messages add to the confusion of TV advertising.
2. Fleeting messages. TV commercials come and go quickly, leaving no second chance to reach a viewer who uses a commercial break to leave the room, or who simply "zaps" a videotaped TV spot.
3. Cost. The cost per thousand viewers may be low, but many solo or one-location physician practices have no need for the mass TV audience, and can be priced out of the market. Production costs also can be sizable.
4. Wasted audience. Your message will go to people who are not really potential patients. You pay to reach them anyway.
5. Reaction time lag. Viewers seldom react the first time they see a message. You must reach them again and again to generate a response.
6. Long lead time. TV commercials take a long time to produce, making it more difficult to respond to immediate practice needs or patient demands.

TV Advertising Timing. As with radio, there are a variety of commercial lengths available. While 30-second spots are the overwhelming favorite on TV, 10-, 15- and 60-second spots are also fairly common. The spots shorter than 30 seconds, however, are generally used by advertisers who have already established a TV identity and are reinforcing an established theme or message.

Ten- and 15-second spots also can be used to create a TV image for practices that have no public image. By utilizing frequent, simple messages at fixed time periods, these short spots can be very effective.

How Rates Are Determined. TV advertising rates can be misleading. A sales representative may quote a tiny "CPM" rate (cost per thousand viewers), and you may be impressed. But remember that much of the mass audience under discussion may be "waste" audience for you—viewers not within your service area—so the CPM is meaningless for you. Of course, if you have numerous locations convenient to most people, or if you offer specialized services that people are willing to drive a long distance for, television's mass audience may be desirable. TV is a viable option for any physician or group practice with sufficient budget to utilize it effectively.

Like radio, TV is sold in grids of progressive rates. A grid rate is based on the popularity of the adjacent programming. Other rate-affecting factors include the type of spot: a choice of fixed spots, (you choose the program); pre-emptible (you risk being bumped by an advertiser willing to pay the higher fixed rate); or run-of-station spots (the station decides when it will run).

Package plans are also available. They are appealing to small advertisers because they offer a number of spots at a lower cost.

Like radio, TV is segmented into time periods. Standard TV time periods (Eastern Standard Time) are Early Morning (sign-on to 10 am), Daytime (10 am to 4:30 pm), Early Fringe (4:30 to 6 pm), Early News (6 to 7:30 pm), Prime Access (7:30 to 8 pm), Prime Time (8 to 11 pm), Late News (11 to 11:30 pm), and Late Fringe (11:30 pm to sign-off).

Individual programs within a time period attract different audiences. Your media sales rep (or advertising agency if you're using one) can determine which times are best for your ads, based on the audience you're trying to reach.

Some TV Research Findings. Here are some trends in television that any potential advertiser should be aware of:

1. Seasonal variations. November through March are traditionally high viewing months, July and August tend to be lower.
2. Viewer variations. The higher the income and education level, the less time spent watching TV. However, individuals with higher income and educational levels are heavier cable users. The penetration of cable is causing more fragmentation of network and independent viewing audiences.
3. Household characteristics. The larger the household, the more time spent watching television. Households with children watch more TV, as do women and older adults.

The Role of the Station Representative. If you'll be developing your TV ad campaign yourself or with a staff member, you should meet with as many station representatives as possible. Be prepared to answer questions about your objectives, your target audience and your budget. Ask about getting *geographic audience estimates*. This custom research can determine where viewership is actually coming from in a given locale. The sales rep will provide you with viewer information and, later, a written proposal. The price you pay for TV advertising time will depend on supply and demand. The greater the demand for a time, the higher the price. Scheduling in advance will enable you to negotiate better prices. Great buys are available during the summer and after Christmas. It's also possible to negotiate a lower package cost if you're willing to make a major commitment to one station.

Producing a TV Commercial. Because broadcast messages are fleeting, it's vital that yours be effective and repetitive. You have a limited amount of time to communicate your message, so every word, every image, is critical.

Where do you start if, like most physicians, you have no experience with TV advertising beyond what you see on your own set?

If you were to analyze the commercials you see, you would find that the most effective ones use a single selling point rather than a barrage. They attempt to create a single, consistent image.

Your objective is to plant an image of your practice in the viewer's mind. Then, when it's time to call a doctor, your practice is likely to be recalled.

Writing the TV Ad. To create an effective TV spot, start with an idea of interest to the viewer, back it up with a benefit, then present the idea in the most interesting and original way possible. Every effective commercial has a unique selling proposition based on an analysis of your practice, your target audience, marketplace and competition. How does your practice differ from others? That's your unique selling proposition.

As in other forms of advertising, simple is better on television. Too many visual images in too short a time burden the viewer and dilute the impact of your message. Your commercial should have a "key visual" that the rest of the spot builds up to. This visual will be the picture remembered by the viewer.

Because health care is a personal service, it's best to personalize your appeal with actors who have a low-key, friendly, but professional presentation.

TV Advertising Basics. Here are pointers to remember for creating an effective TV advertisement.

1. Know your audience. If you are to *reach* your target audience, they must identify with your message.
2. Simplify. A 60-second spot contains about 150 words, so every word counts. Be conversational, avoiding technical terms, and keep it brief. Never use a long word when a short word will do the same job.
3. Listen to your words. Read copy aloud, listening for awkward or unclear spots.
4. Be sincere. Television must be believable. Consider the needs, desires and fears of your viewing audience, then address them in a positive manner.
5. Be consistent. Continuity among all of your ads, and within various TV spots, is one element of repetition that can increase recall.
6. Grab viewer attention with a provocative statement or visual, a sound effect or jingle.
7. Call for action. Close your spot as strongly as you open it.
8. Identify yourself. Repeat your practice name several times during the course of the spot.

The Storyboard. The storyboard is a series of sketches that provide a rough blueprint of the sequence of events, the action in a commercial. More than likely, you'll require the assistance of a professional television production firm if your commercial is complex enough to require a storyboard—that is, if it consists of more than a single individual speaking to the camera without much action.

Kinds of Commercials. The most common commercial formats include:

1. Straight announcement. This involves a person looking at the camera and delivering the message. It can be dramatic and have impact with the right technique or personality (e.g., a close-up of the person speaking, shot against a dark or plain background). If shot routinely or poorly, the straight announcement comes off as the "talking head" commercial and is a waste of your TV ad budget.

2. Demonstration. This is an especially effective vehicle for television. People are interested in what you can do for them or how you do it; the best way is to show it. For example, if a key feature of your practice is a 10-minute maximum wait policy, you can demonstrate a physician reception room crammed with people, reading thick books, knitting, looking at their watches—then next door, your reception area, where patients are alert, being called in for appointments, watching educational programs, and smiling. The point is demonstrated instantly, effectively. Or you can demonstrate a procedure or technique (avoid surgery demonstrations; most people won't respond positively).

3. Testimonial. A sophisticated variation of the straight announcement, in which a patient is used to discuss the practice. If you use testimonials, it's important not to permit patients to discuss your professional or medical skills.

4. Dramatization. A brief story or scene is used to get the message across.

5. Dialogue. Two or more people talking tends to involve the audience more than a straight announcement.

6. Animation. Not for a sophisticated audience, and an expensive approach, but it can be good for presenting difficult or distasteful ideas.

No matter which technique your television spot uses, you must come across as warm, believable. The relationship you develop with your patients is based on trust. Warmth fosters trust, and that will attract patients faster than any fancy gimmick or high-tech approach.

While these techniques and approaches may seem a little elaborate for the advertising you are planning now, they give you an idea of what is available to you and what direction you may choose to go in the future.

Film or Videotape? There are two ways to produce a television commercial—film and videotape. Most locally produced spots are videotape; most national spots are film. Film is much higher quality; it's also more expensive. It's possible to spend $100,000 or more for a single filmed spot, and many major advertisers spend far more than that. But you don't have to spend mega-bucks; a good quality film production can be created using professional talent for $5,000 to $10,000.

At the more reasonable end of the cost range, it's also possible to produce an effective videotaped commercial for about $1,000, depending on the complexity of the spot and the talent used.

You can call on an advertising agency or a quality production company in your area. But if your budget is limited, you may wish to consider using a local television station to produce your ad. Most local stations have complete production facilities and offer this service as a loss leader to get your spot on the air. If this is the way you choose, work with your station representative. He or she can help you find talent, arrange the production schedule and more. Since producing a television spot is a complicated task, we recommend you leave it to professionals who do it daily.

A few physicians have a camera presence, a charisma; they make a memorable appearance in a television spot. Most do not. If you're not sure (and we think it's best to err on the side of doubt), your production studio can "screen test" you.

A Final Checklist. As your commercial proceeds from concept to completion, many decisions have to be made. Here are some practical guidelines that will help you steer a course toward a TV spot that attracts phone calls and patients:

- Make sure the promise or benefit your commercial gives is unique to your practice.
- The value of repetition can't be overstated. Your message and your name must be firmly implanted in the viewer's mind.
- Don't let attempts at creativity get in the way of your message. Balance the creative concept with the message content.
- Choose the right person to deliver your message. Unless you're a persuasive communicator with "stage presence," leave the job to a professional . . . and choose the professional carefully.
- Television is a visual medium. What the viewer sees should have as much or more impact as what he hears.
- Music can add immeasurably to a commercial's impact.
- Be patient. TV advertising depends on momentum, multiple impressions and mental imprinting. If you choose to advertise on TV, make a commitment to it. Results don't happen overnight.
- Tracking is especially important with TV advertising, in part because of the heavy expenditure it requires. You'll want to have your office staff record on what station patients heard about your practice, and what time the calls come in, so you'll know which spots are doing you the most good. (People tend to act at the time they hear your message; you want to know what those times are whenever possible.)

Don't Forget Cable. In addition to commercial television, cable TV is becoming more of a force with TV viewers. Cable television offers the usual advertising options of local and network TV such as 10-, 30- or 60-second spots.

Because cable TV stations are far more targeted than commercial stations, cable may be valuable for medical practices with a service or message of narrow scope, or appealing to a very defined audience. Cable also offers the opportunity to develop an advertising message of greater length—20, 30 or even 60 minutes—for conveying complicated information. Be certain if you choose this route that the station has the audience figures, during the time slot you'll be running it, to make developing a program of this sort worthwhile.

A new concept that has recently developed is a multi-media approach using a combination of direct mail and one- or two-minute cable TV commercials or 30-minute cable "commercial" programs. In some areas, cable subscriber lists are used for the mailing; otherwise, a mass mailing to target markets is done. The half-hour info-commercial and direct mail campaign has yielded tremendous results for advertisers who have tried it. Health care advertisers' experiences have not been reported yet. However, the concept seems to have great potential, particularly for specialties like obstetrics-gynecology, plastic surgery, dermatology and sports medicine. The significantly higher discretionary income and educational level of cable subscribers, combined with extremely low cable media costs, make it worth considering.

Television: It May Be for You. Television can work for physicians, whether solo or group practice. You must have the budget to develop a professional spot, for an amateur or second-rate one shrieks "Cheap!"— and that's an impression you don't want to leave with patients. And you must have the budget and the commitment to advertise with enough weekly spots and over a long enough period to assess results.

AND FINALLY . . .

Television and radio may not be the answer for all medical practices, but in an era of increasing competition, consumer sophistication, and dependence on the electronic media for education, news and entertainment, radio and TV certainly warrant consideration as a media strategy to complement your print advertising.

BIBLIOGRAPHY

Let the Airwaves Take Your Practice Message to the Public. *Physicians Marketing* 1987; April.

Boom in Health Care TV Ads *Modern Healthcare* 1987; October 23: 16.

Gray: The Selling of Medicine 1986. *Medical Economics* 1986; January 20.

MDs Say Patients Get Health Information From TV. *AMA News* 1987; November 6.

Tele-Mail—A New Revolution in Direct Marketing. *Direct Response* 1987; June.

Chapter 19

Direct Mail: The Personal Approach

Direct mail is a broad term that refers to virtually any type of promotional piece that's mailed to a carefully selected list of recipients. It usually works best in harmony with other communication tools to help reach desired practice objectives.

An increasingly popular promotional strategy, direct mail expenditures rank third behind newspapers and television. Direct mail permits a personal, targeted appeal to individuals with like characteristics and habits. It's effective, too. A survey by the U.S Postal Service indicates that 78 percent of all advertising and promotion material sent through the mail is opened and read.

For physicians, direct mail is appealing because it offers the opportunity to communicate personally with patients and potential patients. An assortment of approaches, from newsletters to practice brochures to a notice about a special flu shot clinic or health education class, make direct mail adaptable to almost any situation.

Direct mail is an effective method for physicians to test practice promotion concepts. For example, a conservative physician in Phoenix mailed a 4″ × 5″ card on high quality stock announcing the opening of his practice in obstetrics and gynecology. The card was very similar to the announcements once routinely placed in the daily newspaper by local medical societies for physicians. Recognizing that a simple announcement probably would not attract a large number of new patients, this physician also listed his areas of specialization and services on the card, such as pregnancy care, infertility evaluations, colposcopy, menopausal disorder and family planning. He distributed it via a service (called *marriage mail or co-op mail*) which bundled his mailing in with a number of other advertisers in order to reach a large number of homes at relatively low cost. (Actually, as tasteful as his practice-opening announcement was, we suspect he would have gotten more impact had he spent the extra money to mail it in its own envelope, perhaps with a personal letter outlining his practice philosophy, his training and additional details about his services.)

SOME DIRECT MAIL OPTIONS

These are some of the options available to physicians interested in direct mail marketing:

Personal Letter. Inexpensive and effective if done well, the personal letter has multiple applications. It can be duplicated, professionally printed or computer-generated.

Postcards. The postcard is an effective tool for brief announcements and messages, and like the letter, it's also inexpensive to produce and to mail. It can be simple or highly stylized, subtle or more to-the-point.

Brochures. The brochure is usually a high-quality printed piece providing practice information. It generally is most effective when mailed in an envelope with a cover letter. It has applications beyond direct mail.

Mailgram and Simulated Mailgram. A variation of the personal letter, this piece conveys immediacy and adds impact to the message it contains. Western Union offers a variety of electronic mail options that may at times be appropriate for your practice communication strategies. You'll find a sample mailgram letter in Figure 19-1.

Newsletters. More and more practices are finding the newsletter an effective way to stay in touch with current patients and attract new ones. Unlike other forms of direct mail, the newsletter is published on a regular basis, and is an information piece which can double as an action-oriented communication. It also has a personal, friendly feeling if done properly.

Coupons. Often used in conjunction with a personal letter or other direct mail piece, the coupon provides the consumer with a concrete call to action, usually with a limited time frame. Coupons carry the danger, however, of appearing to promote "discount" medical care, which connotes lower-quality medical care. Be very careful in using coupons.

Invitations and Notices. An invitation through the mail to a special event, a health fair, a class or other practice-sponsored event is a very personal way of keeping in touch with patients and others.

Direct mail includes anything that can be mailed. You are limited only by your imagination and your budget. Doctors have successfully employed posters, calendars, folders, magnets and other specialty items and a variety of other print materials as direct mail vehicles.

A MULTI-PURPOSE MEDIUM

Because it's a specialized, yet broad medium, direct mail is flexible enough to achieve a variety of communication goals. Perhaps these ideas will get you thinking about how you could use direct mail in your practice:

- Announcing a new location, associate or service
- Regaining "lost" patients
- Welcoming new or potential patients
- Thanking patients for their patronage and/or referrals

FIGURE 19-1   Sample Mailgram Letter

A mailgram letter from Western Union has a look of urgency and importance. It can be a good way to invite patients to a class or health fair, or to inform them about a new service or treatment.

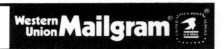

```
        WESTERN UNION PRIORITY MAIL      Western Mailgram
        1651 OLD MEADOW ROAD             Union
        MCLEAN, VA 22102

        9811700000111  900521    DTSK


                                                     ***BUSINESS REPLY***
►       L. B. JONES
        32 SOUTH MAIN ST.
        MAPLEWOOD PA 15219


        YOU HAVE IN YOUR HANDS ONE OF TODAY'S MOST EFFECTIVE VEHICLES FOR
───     BUSINESS COMMUNICATION, A WESTERN UNION MAILGRAM.  WITH A MAILGRAM    ───
        MESSAGE, YOU CAN REACH VIRTUALLY ANYONE, ANYWHERE, OVERNIGHT.

        WHEN YOU ABSOLUTELY HAVE TO REACH EITHER JUST A FEW OR A FEW HUNDRED
        PEOPLE BY THE NEXT DAY, NO OTHER SERVICE CAN DO IT AS EFFECTIVELY
        AND AS ECONOMICALLY.

        MAILGRAM ALSO OFFERS YOU THE FLEXIBILITY OF THE FOLLOWING FEATURES:

             *  POSTAGE PAID BUSINESS REPLY ENVELOPE.
             *  CERTIFIED MAIL, RETURN RECEIPT REQUESTED IF YOU REQUIRE
                PROOF OF DELIVERY.
             *  OFFICIAL LEGAL DOCUMENT, RECOGNIZED BY FEDERAL REGULATIONS.
             *  TEXT INSERTS TO PERSONALIZE THE MESSAGE FOR EACH RECIPIENT.
             *  MESSAGES OF UP TO 7 FULL PAGES OF TEXT.

        SATISFIED MAILGRAM CUSTOMERS ARE USING MAILGRAM TO:  ANNOUNCE NEW
        PRODUCTS, RAISE FUNDS FROM MEMBERS, GENERATE SALES LEADS, ISSUE
        PRESS RELEASES, CONTACT DEALERS AND DISTRIBUTORS, COLLECT ON
        DELINQUENT ACCOUNTS AND OTHER IMPORTANT CORRESPONDENCE.

        FOR ADDITIONAL INFORMATION ON WESTERN UNION MAILGRAM MESSAGES, CALL
───     1-800-336-3797; IN VA 1-703-449-8877.                                ───

                                MICHAEL MURPHY
                                VICE PRESIDENT MARKETING


        ***REFOLD ENTIRE LETTER SO THAT RETURN ADDRESS AND PERMIT NO.SHOW***
        ****THROUGH WINDOW OF BUSINESS REPLY ENVELOPE. NO POSTAGE NEEDED.***

                        FIRST CLASS PERMIT NO.   2197 MCLEAN      VA
                        -----------POSTAGE WILL BE PAID BY ADDRESSEE----------

        RETURN TO:              WESTERN UNION PRIORITY MAIL SVCS.
                                TELEMARKETING DEPT.
                                P.O. BOX 1037
                                MCLEAN, VA  22101


        TO REPLY BY MAILGRAM MESSAGE, SEE REVERSE SIDE FOR WESTERN UNION'S TOLL - FREE PHONE NUMBERS
```

5241 (R 7/82)

- Publicizing special events such as an open house
- Creating and reinforcing an image for your practice
- Providing news and information about medicine and your practice
- Stimulating calls for appointments during slack periods in your schedule
- Creating interest in seasonal programs or services
- Announcing specialized programs or clinics to a targeted audience
- Retaining current patients by maintaining contact

THE PLUSES AND MINUSES OF DIRECT MAIL

Compared with other media, direct mail is:

The Ultimate Personal Medium. No other form of communication, other than personal, face-to-face communication, comes close to the personal touch conveyed by a mailing specifically addressed to an individual or household. Direct mail is a unique form of one-to-one communication.

A Detail Medium. Unlike other media, there are no time or space limitations on direct mail pieces. Rather than having only sixty seconds or a quarter page to get your message across, you can develop your points as fully as necessary. If you want to explain a complex or detailed procedure, such as removal of spider veins or the importance of knowing cholesterol levels, direct mail allows you to do so.

Selective, Targeted Marketing. With direct mail, you can reach precisely the audience you want. If you're an internist who wants to reach business people with your executive health/fitness exam, you can purchase a mailing list of executives, for instance, and narrow the list still further, to executives over 40 with incomes of $50,000 plus.

Flexible Format. What you can do with direct mail is limited only by your imagination and budget. From postcard to poster, from specialty item to coupon, the possibilities are limitless. And pieces can be combined for maximum impact and effect.

Attention Getting. Direct mail captures your audience's attention better because it does not compete with other media (except other direct mail), and because the recipients choose to read it when it is convenient for them.

Timely. You mail when you want, when it's more appropriate for your practice needs. No need to worry about waiting for the next issue or missing a deadline.

Like every promotional strategy, direct mail also has its *disadvantages*. The major limitations include:

Cost. With production and mailing costs considered, direct mail can be an expensive promotional medium. This is somewhat tempered, however, by the selectivity factor. If your promotion reaches precisely the right audience and stimulates a response from them, then direct mail is very cost-effective. And compared with television or newspaper ad costs in most metropolitan areas, direct mail is far less costly.

Poor Image. The term "junk mail" has probably done more to create an image problem for direct mail than any other single factor. Nevertheless, direct mail is read by its recipients. A high quality, targeted piece will not be lumped by the recipient into the "junk mail" category.

Mailing List Quality. The effectiveness of your direct mail will be determined in part by the quality of the mailing list you use. And mailing lists are a mixed bag—some very good, some not so good.

Competitive Clutter. While your promotion has the competitive advantage of being self-contained, it also competes with other direct mail arriving in the same day's mail.

Organizational Restrictions. Direct mail can be limited somewhat by your state or local medical society. Some have regarded direct mail as an inappropriate medium for professional promotion. Most of these restrictions have been successfully challenged. Nevertheless, we suggest that you check your own state codes or local medical association guidelines before you proceed. It's also wise to consider collegial reaction to any promotional effort, and its potential impact on your practice and patient referrals.

MEASURING SUCCESS

With direct mail, more than any other medium, you are in control. You can take as much or as little space as you need to make your point and sell your services. You don't have to fit into any editorial environment or compete with other advertisers on the page. If you reach the proper audience, and if you grab their attention (the two key challenges to successful direct mail promotion) you can achieve success.

How do you measure success in direct mail marketing? In narrow terms. A response of one to three percent of the audience is generally considered acceptable by direct mail professionals; five percent is considered phenomenal. Of course, the "universe" or total audience from which such figures are derived is usually at least 10,000 or more. A one percent response for a mailing of 10,000 would be 100, and if only 20 percent of those became patients, your promotional effort would probably be judged very effective.

FIRST DETERMINE YOUR OBJECTIVES

Like any promotional effort, a successful direct mail campaign begins by knowing why you're doing it. What do you hope to accomplish with your mailing? Do you want to attract new patients? What kind? For what services? From what age group, sex, income or geographical area are you seeking patients?

To set objectives for your direct mail effort, first evaluate these elements of your practice:

■ Features—the services and amenities that attract patients and that set you apart from other similar practices

- Benefits—how do the features of your practice benefit potential patients?
- Strengths—what are the strong points of your practice? Location? Staff courtesy and expertise? Your specialized training? Unique practice environment or decor?
- Weaknesses—what are the weak areas of your practice, and how can you correct them or convert them to strengths? (You can't ignore them!)
- Patient characteristics—what are the common characteristics of your patients? Knowing them will help you target your direct mail effort.

Next, decide who you want to reach, and why. List the characteristics of your target audience, and determine what features of your practice will be perceived as benefits to this audience. According to Ed Burnett, a leading direct mail consultant, your best mailing list is one that mirrors your current customer profile (unless you're establishing a completely new service in your practice, with a different target market). This means that you must have a demographic profile of your current patients. (If you've done a patient survey, you should have a good picture of your patients.)

State your goal in measurable terms, e.g. "to attract 50 new patients for the Diabetes Clinic," or "to generate 75 requests for information about infertility options." Having a measurable goal is the only way to determine whether your direct mail effort achieved the results you sought.

KNOW YOUR AUDIENCE—AND YOURSELF

No matter what your goal, you must tell potential patients what's in it for them—why they should call your office for an appointment, why they should select you as their physician. Direct mail is a very personal medium. It doesn't convince with an approach directed to everyone. It persuades with an approach that reaches one person individually—your reader.

But how do you achieve this personal feeling in a direct mail piece to someone you don't know personally? You must know as much about yourself, your practice and your intended recipient as possible. You must be able to tell your audience what's really special about you. And you must know something about your audience so you'll know what appeals to them. You must have some way of making them feel you really do know their concerns and needs.

One way to find out about your potential patient is through your mailing list. Somewhere in each list, if it has been selected appropriately, you will find a characteristic or common factor that you can use to give your message a personal touch. If, for example, your list came from the membership roster of a local parent-teacher association, you could begin a direct mail letter like this: "Since I have school-age children of my own, I know the problems you face in trying to keep your children healthy when they seem to prefer TV and junk food to exercise and vegetables."

Understanding yourself means discovering what makes you (and your practice) unique. You must discover, isolate and dramatize the reasons a person should see you rather than another doctor.

To test whether you've found your uniqueness and emphasized it in your direct mail piece, go through the copy after it's written. Wherever your practice name is, cross it out and insert a competitor's practice name. If the copy decribes your competitor as well as it does you, start rewriting.

No two physicians conduct themselves or their practice in exactly the same manner. Nor does every physician enjoy working with the same type of patients. There are as many variations among practices as there are medical specialties.

Couple your uniqueness with a personal appeal and you have a very potent form of communication. One way to personalize your appeal is by stressing benefits instead of features. By focusing on benefits, you take the point of view of the reader, your potential patient. Instead of saying, "I strive to provide good medical care," say "You will feel healthier and more fit."

The average person is bombarded by more than 1,000 media impressions per day. Radio, billboards, signs and other stimuli compete for our attention. In an effort to cope with this information explosion, we activate a built-in selector. It sorts and instantly accepts or rejects the constant barrage of information, based on this simple principle: "Is there something in it for me?" Be sure your potential patients know exactly what's in it for them individually when you address them via direct mail.

Since some of the primary formats used in direct mail—newsletters, brochures, educational material—are the subject of discussion in other chapters of this book, we'll focus in this chapter on the letter that often accompanies another printed piece.

THE DIRECT MAIL LETTER

The direct mail letter is a flexible medium in terms of the messages it can convey, and printing and graphic considerations are generally far less complex than for brochures and other forms of direct mail. For example, letters are best typed, not typeset. Typesetting hinders the personal communication appeal of a letter, and adds to the cost as well. A letter should not look or sound too polished or slick; the content must be informal, personal yet persuasive. The direct mail letter should look like and read like a personal letter. Writing a direct mail letter is probably one of the most difficult of all copywriting tasks. To be assured of a successful letter, it is best to hire a specialist in direct mail marketing.

THE AIDA FORMULA

If you choose to create your direct mail piece yourself, you must acquaint yourself with some guidelines for direct mail. If you hire a consultant, these rules will help you evaluate the job.

A good letter follows the time-honored "AIDA" formula: Grab Attention, Heighten Interest, Create Desire and Call for Action. Take a good look at the next sales letter you receive in the mail; you'll find that the ones that make you act (or consider acting) follow the AIDA pattern.

Attention. To create attention, open with your strongest appeal or benefit. Your opening paragraph is vital; if it intrigues the reader, he or she will read on. If not, your letter and the rest of your mailer may be tossed. The attention-grabbing benefit will depend on your specialty, your practice, and your objective with the letter. There are a variety of approaches. A question builds curiosity and reader involvement (but it must be thought-provoking to be effective). A dramatic narrative opening tells a story and speaks to the reader in a very personal way. Whichever approach you use, remember that you must immediately answer the reader's question: "What's in it for me?" Fail that at the outset, and you'll lose your reader and waste your promotion dollar.

Because these approaches are more subtle than simply stating your strongest benefit, you may wish to use a headline with them above the salutation. Strong headlines can coexist with the personal salutation and writing style of a letter.

Interest. The next step is to sustain interest. Don't give all the details of your offer right away. If you do, there is no reason for the reader to go on reading. Rather, intersperse them through the body of the letter. Entice the reader to continue reading.

Desire. Once you've caught the reader's attention and captured interest, you must stimulate desire. This does not imply that you are creating desire where none exists; no marketing person can accomplish that. But by creating awareness of your service, you create awareness of the individual's need for it. This translates to desire. For example, if your direct mail letter is addressed to those business executives we mentioned awhile back, you may explain in your letter the risks of improper diet, lack of exercise, the effect of undiagnosed stress on the heart, and the need for everyone to know his blood pressure, cholesterol level, and cardiac risk factors. Throughout the letter, you're describing the services available through your group practice's executive fitness/diagnostic center. You strike a chord of identification in the executive who's reading the letter as he sits at his desk wolfing down a lunch of corned beef and swiss cheese and potato chips before heading into a high-pressure board meeting. He decides to call your program for an appointment and learn what his level of fitness is, and what he can do to increase it. Our executive has been aware for some time that he should do a better job of health maintenance. Your letter serves as the stimulus to action.

While personal and friendly, a direct mail letter should be bold. Direct mail writing is forceful. In medical marketing it must also be the ethical, bearing in mind the prohibitions against self-aggrandizing statements, exaggerations and other forms of hope that are not only distasteful and unprofessional, but may be contrary to Federal Trade Commission advertising guidelines or those of your local or national medical organization.

Action. By now, you've gotten the reader's attention and created interest and desire. The next step is to ask for action. Always close your letter by telling the reader exactly what to do, and how and when to do it. It's easy to put off a decision, so give an incentive for acting now. Establish a time frame for your offer. For the overstressed executive, your letter might simply close with the encouragement: "Call 234-5678 today for your personal Executive Fitness Profile appointment. We have a time slot to fit your busy schedule." A postscript can urge, "You're probably sitting by the telephone as you read this letter. Why not pick up the phone and call 234-5678? We can schedule your appointment *immediately*."

Another more subtle approach is suggested by Trey Ryder, national direct mail consultant. In the September 1985 issue of *Direct Marketing* newsletter, he suggests that in order to get a potential patient to call your office, you should set up a no-pressure situation that allows a commitment-free call. For instance, offer free information, a brochure, a newsletter or helpful hints. Ryder says if the information helps, the individual becomes a serious prospect for your services. This approach is a good way to attract people who otherwise would not call. An effective, trained receptionist can also translate calls for information into appointments, without being high-pressure.

The Mandatory P.S. The P.S. is your parting shot; every letter should have one. It's one of the best-read parts of a letter. Tests show that 95 percent of the time it will increase response. Use the P.S., as in the "executive fitness" example earlier, to touch again on a point previously made within the body of the letter.

SAY WHAT YOU HAVE TO SAY

Don't be afraid of a long letter, but don't write just to make your letter long. As a rule, letters to people you know and who know you (such as your current patients) can be shorter than those sent to people who are unlikely to know of your practice.

Letter Talk. The language of a direct mail letter should be as similar as possible to spoken language (without obvious grammatical errors, of course). Use short words, short sentences, short paragraphs. Make your letter as warm and friendly and easy to read as you can. Be specific, using facts with impact. Know your audience and what they'll respond to. Don't waste time getting to the point. You've got five seconds to convince readers to keep reading your letter. Grab them immediately.

Mix short sentences with an occasional longer one for rhythm. Use "you" liberally to involve the reader in your message. Then insure a smooth flow to your letter by using the transition phrases listed later in this chapter.

Testimonials add credibility to what you're saying, but make sure that patient testimonials don't attest to your medical or professional skills.

(You'll find more on testimonials in Chapter 17.) Also, testimonials must be by actual patients; if a composite is used, you must identify it as such.

Command your reader's attention. Inform him. Build conviction and belief in your practice and your health care services. When appropriate, ask a question that gets the reader to agree with you. Show that your thoughts and beliefs parallel his or her's. Write to one person, not the 5,000 people on your mailing list. That one person is the only one who matters.

Avoid trite phrases, exaggerated claims and farfetched statements.

Figures 19-2 and 19-3 offer some of the "hot" words and transition phrases that are helpful in direct mail copy. Use them for reference and ideas, but don't overuse them. Remember that your copy must reflect you and your practice. Make your letter sound like *you* talking.

FIGURE 19-2   Direct Mail "Hot" Words

These "hot" words trigger a reaction when used in direct mail copy:							
All	Change	Easy	Fun	Help	Love	Now	
Awesome	Crazy	Emerge	Gap	Home	Money	Peace	
Awful	Crucial	End	Give	Least	More	Proven	
Beauty	Death	Final	Greed	Less	Most	Quiet	
Begin	Destroy	Free	Growth	Life	New	Result	
Birth	Die	Frontier	Health	Live	None	Right	
Safe	Self	Survive	Value	Vision	Want	War	
Wrong	You	Your					

FIGURE 19-3   Direct Mail Transition Phrases

Give your message a smooth flow with these connector phrases:

But that's not all
And now you can see why . . .
Even more important than that . . .
But there is one more thing
Here's all you have to do,
Better yet,
So that's why . . .
When you first . . .
Here's the next step . . .
Within the next few days . . .
But here's a way to be sure . . .
And in addition . . .
You may wonder why . . .
You see
But please remember that . . .
As you may already know . . .

SOME VISUAL TIPS

Regardless of the length of your letter, it should be visually appealing. Use short paragraphs, no longer than seven lines, and indent them. Use bullets to set off important points.

Underscore and CAPITALIZE for emphasis, but don't overdo it—you have a professional image to maintain. **Occasional boldface type** (like this) helps to emphasize important thoughts. Any thought that demands major emphasis may be indented and surrounded by extra spacing above and below. (Just like this paragraph.)

Use page turners—sentences split at the bottom of the page so you have to turn to the next page to finish reading them. And finally, consider printing your letter in two colors, which usually outpulls a single color. If you print the letter on colored stock (pastels like ivory, cream, pale peach), it's best to use black ink. But don't be afraid to use a warm second color for emphasis. Boldfaced words, underlining, subheads and the signature might be in a second color.

THE ENVELOPE

The envelope is equally as important as what's inside. The envelope can persuade the reader that the contents may be of interest, or the envelope may lead him/her to toss the whole piece unopened. Envelope size, shape, color, the method of addressing, wording (or lack of it) on the outside, type of postage—all these lend impact to your printed piece.

The Teaser Copy. Many direct mail experts recommend using the envelope to promote the contents of a direct mail piece. Copy on the outside of an envelope to encourage the recipient to look inside is called a "teaser." For example: "Inside: 10 Health Care Tips to Help You Stay Well This Winter." Or "What You Should Know about the Disease Nobody Talks About."

There are two schools of thought on the subject. The first is that teasers tip off the prospect that your piece is advertising mail, allowing it to be tossed unopened. The second says that chances are you're going to tip the prospect off anyway. If you use a label, the recipient knows it's not a letter from Grandma.

For this reason, many consultants recommend teaser copy. However, we believe physicians especially must exercise judgment. For some direct mail pieces, teaser copy is appropriate and helpful (for instance, a newsletter might have a teaser that refers to one of the articles inside.) For others, the teaser copy may make your printed piece appear less professional.

Teaser copy establishes a context for the information inside. There are two kinds of teasers: the first arouses curiosity with an intriguing statement; the second touts a specific benefit or offer.

Teasers do not have to be located on the address side of the envelope. Studies have shown that teasers on the back of an envelope also achieve high readership.

Other Considerations. When you are selecting an envelope in which to enclose your letter, card, invitation, brochure or newsletter, keep these suggestions in mind:

- Ivory, cream or gray are considered better envelope colors than white.
- An envelope with a window almost always improves response. (It looks like an invoice, so it usually gets opened.)
- A stamp, rather than metered postage, looks more personal.
- If you're mailing a series of closely-spaced promotions or informational pieces to the same list, be sure to change your envelope with each mailing.
- Odd sizes or shapes for envelopes are attention-getters, but also expensive. Check first with the post office to be certain the size you're considering is not considered oversized or nonstandard. If it is, there will be a postage surcharge (and it may possibly weigh more than one ounce, in which case you'll pay extra postage as well).
- Depending upon what you're mailing, consider hand-addressing to your mailing list. Studies show a 60 percent improvement in the response rate for direct mail that's hand-addressed rather than typed or computer-generated.

DIRECT MAIL PACKAGING

Packaging can play a role in the success or failure of a direct mail endeavor. While many mailings consist of a single piece, usually a letter or card, others include up to five or six enclosures.

Those who advocate multiple enclosures find it too easy for the recipient to toss one piece if their interest is not sufficiently aroused. However, if the envelope is stuffed with a number of pieces, the individual will probably take the time to glance, at least briefly, at several or possibly all of them. If you include four pieces in your mailing, you have not one, but four opportunities to catch the interest of your reader. An example of a multiple enclosure direct mailing by a physician is one that would include:

- Letter from the physician
- Practice brocure
- A magnet or sticker with emergency telephone numbers and the physician's practice number
- A business reply card (BRC) to be filled out by the reader and returned in order to receive additional information, become a newsletter subscriber, etc.

Alternately, one of the enclosures could be a short handwritten note from the physician with a line or two inviting the reader to visit the office and meet him and his staff. If the original note is written clearly in black ink, it will reproduce well and have a personal feeling to it.

If you decide on multiple enclosures, be sure to include your name, address and telephone number on each piece. Then if the recipient throws away part of your mailing, the pieces he returns will have sufficient information to act upon.

A sample direct mail piece with multiple enclosures, done by a group practice, is shown in Figure 19-4.

THE COUPON IN DIRECT MAIL

A survey by A. C. Nielsen showed that two-thirds of all households use coupons as part of their regular shopping habits, with housewives age 31 to 45 the highest users.

The coupon provides a handy tool for monitoring the results of a direct mailing. But in the medical profession as indicated earlier, coupons must be used with great caution.

Coupons have been effectively used to promote consumer awareness of sports physicals, first office visits, screenings, minor emergency care and a host of other medical services. If you incorporate a coupon into your direct mail promotion, it's important to include an expiration date. It is this element that makes coupons immediate traffic builders—and also that allows you to judge the success of the coupon promotion.

Coupons can help increase response to your direct mail piece. Use of a toll-free 800 number can improve your rate of response. More and more doctors, particularly those in metropolitan areas, are finding that toll-free numbers attract patients from outlying towns.

CO-OP OR "MARRIAGE" MAIL

Co-op direct mail efforts, also referred to as "marriage mail," couple print pieces from several advertisers in one envelope. You reduce postage, printing and mailing list costs with this method, but you should first determine who the other advertisers will be. You don't want to include your professional practice in with exterminating firms and carpet cleaners. With co-op mail, it is important that all advertisers have similar target audiences. If you're considering co-op direct mail, try to find a firm that brings together professionals in one mailing—attorneys, dentists, etc. And be sure your fellow mailers have good reputations.

In co-op ventures involving only professionals, each professional often is responsible for printing his own individual piece based on a few guidelines. The cost of printing a cover letter and envelopes is shared. The cover letter briefly explains that the mailing is done as a benefit for families who require professional services.

DIRECT MAIL AND THE LAW

Direct mail is a form of advertising. It requires that you follow the same guidelines and limitations that you must for any other medium. To assure that a direct mail advertising campaign is not false, misleading or deceptive and thereby not susceptible to scrutiny by a government regulatory agency or professional association, follow these guidelines in preparing direct mail promotions:

1. Do not misrepresent or distort any fact in any manner.
2. Do not attempt to qualify or modify a totally false or untrue statement.
3. Avoid ambiguous statements that may be susceptible to multiple interpretations since the ambiguity will be construed against the advertiser.
4. Insure that all claims are verifiable, or don't make them.
5. Don't fail to disclose material facts whereby the effect would be to deceive a substantial segment of the advertising audience.
6. Don't use statements which may be deceptive even though they are not literally or technically construed to constitute misrepresentation.
7. Insure that services can and will be performed according to the terms, conditions and price (if listed) as set forth in promotional material.
8. Make only claims or representations that can be performed.

THE ALL-IMPORTANT MAILING LIST

The strongest reason for using direct mail is that you can select your audience. Therefore it's important to use the best mailing list possible. Here's how to find that list:

Compile Your Own List. This can be a time-consuming process, but such lists often outpull all others. Start with your patients and former patients; add everyone you and your staff have contact with. Pass around a sign-up sheet at speaking engagements and public events sponsored by your practice. Use directories (obtainable at libraries) that contain names listed by street address. Your Chamber of Commerce, banks and other sources can provide the names of new residents and homeowners, although they'll probably charge for this list. Or consider exchanging lists with fellow professionals in non-related specialties.

Once you have developed a list, keeping it current is of paramount importance. As many as 25 percent of the names on a typical list can change in some way in a single year.

It is also helpful to code your list, or to group entries into several categories for different purposes. You may wish to sort names by geographic location, age, sex, employment, interests or income.

Mailing House Lists. Mailing houses are perhaps the most expedient way to obtain a mailing list. These companies compile a variety of lists based on a number of factors including geography, income, length of time in the area, employment, automobile ownership, household size . . . almost any characteristic you could wish.

When renting a list from a mailhouse, consider how well the list is

FIGURE 19-4   A Multiple-Item Direct Mail Piece
This group practice invitation contained several printed items that would appeal to patients and encourage retention of pieces and recall of practice name.

Dear Scottsdale Resident:

On behalf of The Scottsdale Clinic we would like to welcome you to Scottsdale.

The Scottsdale Clinic is a multi-specialty medical group serving Scottsdale and the surrounding area. That means we can handle your medical needs from a simple immunization to sophisticated diagnostic technology. Our doctors and their specialties are listed on the back of your Health Check.

To help you stay healthy and to help us catch any warning signs of illness, we are sending you our Health Check, a guide to medical services and their frequencies according to age and sex. Take a minute to look over the chart to make sure you are up to date.

We have also enclosed a special invitation for you to come tour our new facility. We are looking forward to meeting you.

Warm regards,

The Medical Staff of The Scottsdale Clinic

THE SCOTTSDALE CLINIC

*Cordially Invites You
to its new facility at
9220 E. Mountain View Road
For Your Personal Tour and
Introduction to our Fine Family of Physicians*

Call: 860-1200

The Scottsdale Clinic Health Check

By providing the minimum recommended medical services and frequencies according to age and sex, The Scottsdale Clinic can reduce risks for death from: ✓ heart disease, ✓ cancer, ✓ diabetes, ✓ and other disease through early detection. For information contact The Scottsdale Clinic 602/860-1200.

MEN AND WOMEN					
Test	16-20	20-40	40-50	50-60	Over 60
Blood Pressure	yearly	yearly	year y	yearly	yearly
Comprehensive History/Physical		every 5 yrs.	every 5 yrs.	every 3 yrs.	every 2 yrs.
Blood Cholesterol	one time	every 5 yrs.	every 3 yrs.	every 3 yrs.	
Rectal Exam			yearly	yearly	yearly
Stool for Occult Blood			yearly	yearly	yearly
Proctosigmoidoscopy				every 3-5 yrs.*	every 3-5 yrs.*
Tetanus/ Diphtheria		every 10 yrs.	every 10 yrs	every 10 yrs	every 10 yrs
Influenza Immunization					every year
Pneumococcal Pneumonia vaccine					one time only
Chest X-Ray	Not generally indicated*				
EKG	Not generally indicated*				

WOMEN					
Test	16-20	20-40	40-50	50-60	Over 60
MD BREAST EXAM	Self Exam each month	yearly	yearly	yearly	yearly
Pelvic Exam	*	every 3 yrs.*	every year*	every year*	every year*
Pap Smear	*	every 3 yrs. *	every 3 yrs.*	every 3 yrs.*	every 3 yrs.*
Rubella/ German Measles	one time only				
Mammography		**	*	every 1-2 yrs.*	every 1-2 yrs.*

** At age 35 discuss with your Scottsdale Clinic Physician the possibility of a base-line mammogram.
* Discuss this with your Scottsdale Clinic Physician since the frequency will depend on your personal situation.
* After two normal exams one year apart.

YOUR HEALTH CHECK

The Scottsdale Clinic
9220 E. Mountain View Road   *January*   19 *88*
Scottsdale, Arizona 85258
602/860-1200

Pay to the Order of *SCOTTSDALE RESIDENTS* | 1 ,HEALTH CHECK |
_____ *ONE HEALTH CHECK*

First Bank of
Good Health

For *A healthy body* _____ *The Scottsdale Clinic*

MEDICAL STAFF

INTERNAL MEDICINE - David Franey, M.D.; Kent Lyon, M.D.; Beverly Tozer, M.D.; Helen Trop, M.D.
ARTHRITIS / RHEUMATOLOGY - Thomas Disney, M.D.; Emilio Rodriguez, M.D.
CARDIOLOGY - Berkley Benneson, M.D.; Frederick Simonie, M.D.
CARDIOVASCULAR / THORACIC SURGERY - Richard Mushorn, M.D.
COLON/RECTAL SURGERY - Edmund Leff, M.D.
DERMATOLOGY - Glenn Yarbrough, M.D.
EAR, NOSE and THROAT - Joel Cohen, M.D.; Jack Weiss, M.D.
DIABETES /ENDOCRINOLOGY - Kent Lyon, M.D.
GASTROENTEROLOGY - Robert Leon, M.D.; Franklin Lewkowitz, M.D.
GENERAL SURGERY - John Giedraitis, M.D.; William J. Hyde, M.D.; William Marsh, M.D.
GYNECOLOGY - Ingrid Haas, M.D.; John Malfetano, M.D.; Bruce Miller, M.D.; Bea Garcia Stamps, M.D.
HYPERTENSION / NEPHROLOGY - David Cherrill, M.D.
NEUROLOGY - Eric Erlbaum, M.D.; Jeffrey Steier, M.D.
PSYCHIATRY - Thomas Bittker, M.D.; David Boyer, M.D.; Robert Posner, M.D.
FAMILY COUNSELING - James Bell, M.C.; Judith Slepian, M.C., N.C.C.
PULMONARY - Bradley Gordon, M.D.; Richard Levinson, M.D.; Ian D. Miller M.D.
RADIOLOGY - Jack Crowe, M.D.; Sam Hessel, M.D; Jonathan Levy, M.D.
UROLOGY- Donald Boatwright, M.D.

maintained (kept current), whether it can be arranged by zip code, how the names are furnished (mailing labels, computer tape or direct addressing of your material), whether recent names can be furnished on a continuing basis, what guarantees you have on deliverability, and finally, the cost. Lists usually range anywhere from $15 to $100 per thousand names.

List Brokers. List brokers are specialists whose primary function it is to find a direct mail market for a product or service and to arrange a transaction between list users and list owners. The knowledge and experience of a broker costs nothing, since he is paid by the list owner. You pay the list owner for use of the list.

With a list broker, you simply outline your specific requirements; they do the research and legwork. You should contact a broker while you're in the planning stages, not when you're ready to mail. The broker performs a vital function in locating lists for the mailer. This individual constantly seeks new lists for your consideration, verifies the information provided by the list owner, reports on the past performance of a list, and helps assure the smooth completion of your mailing.

To locate a list broker or mailing house, look in the classified section of your telephone directory under Mailing Lists or Addressing and Lettershop Services. Figure 19-5 contains a list of sources for direct mail lists and brokers.

CRITERIA FOR SELECTING A LIST

No matter who you purchase your list from, you should ask these questions to assure the best possible selection of names for the money you'll spend:

1. Is it a stock list or can it be customized for my mailing?
2. Where did the list come from? Who originally developed it?
3. Can I insert names (such as friends, relatives, staff members, etc.) to confirm that the item was packaged and mailed according to instructions and in a timely fashion?

FIGURE 19-5 How to Find a Mailing House or Broker

You can contact the following sources for lists of services and brokers:
- Direct Mail Advertising Association, Inc., 230 Park Ave., New York, NY 10017
- Directory of Mailing List Houses, B. Klein & Co., 27 East 22nd St., New York, NY 10010
- National Council of Mailing List Brokers, 55 W. 42nd St., New York, NY 10036
- National Mailing List Houses, Small Business Bibliography No.29: U.S. Small Business Administration, Washington, D.C. 20416
- Standard Rate & Data Service, Direct Mail List Rates and Data, 5201 Old Orchard Rd., Skokie, IL 60076

4. Is this same list available for future mailings?
5. What format are names provided in? (The most common formats for labels are 4-across ungummed Cheshire labels for machine affixing, or 4-across pressure-sensitive labels that must be removed and affixed by hand. Cheshire is usually preferred by mailing houses; it's also cheaper. You should ask the mailing house you're using what format they prefer if you're getting the labels from another source.
6. Are there guaranteed delivery dates and refunds for undeliverable names?
7. When was this list last updated and cleaned of duplicates? List compilers generally update lists every three months, as the new phone books appear.
8. What is the minimum number of names required for an order?

MANAGING THE MAILING

Your direct mail compaign begins with a phone call to the post office to check on permits that may be required, positioning standards for teaser copy or postal mailing imprint (called the *indicia*), size specifications on self-mailers and current postal rates.

The more work you put into sorting your mailing the better rate you will get. Third-class mail, which must be sorted and bundled prior to delivering it to the post office, is substantially cheaper than first class. Tests show that it usually pulls as well as first class, but remember—third class is much slower, so allow plenty of time if you're mailing timed material.

Some other tips and options to consider:

1. It takes only 200 pieces to qualify for bulk rate.
2. You can apply for a permit for a postage indicia which is then printed on your self-mailer or envelope. However, remember that pre-printed postage doesn't have the personal look of a postage stamp.
3. Zip codes are required for direct mail.
4. For faster delivery, pre-sort your mail by zip code, whether it's required or not.
5. Be sure postage is accurate. Check your postage meter when weighing a sample piece.
6. Mail first class material Monday morning in order to have a Tuesday delivery when mail is lightest.

TESTING DIRECT MAIL

For relatively little cost, valid tests may be constructed to determine which of a number of variables draws best. Only one variable at a time is tested in order to insulate cause and effect.

To test, there must be certain constants. For example, if two different copy appeals are to be tested, both must be mailed the same day, in the same type of envelope, to names from one list.

It's also necessary to select a representative yet random group of names from a mailing list. Generally it is best to use the smallest sampling possible for results that can be projected to the total list. That way, when you know what works best you can send it to the rest of your list.

When you analyze returns to determine viability of a mailing, look at the long-term factor. If a mailing yields a patient for a $38 first-visit, that person is probably worth a great deal more to you than the $38 you charge. There's a long-term profitability associated with every patient you get and hopefully keep in your practice.

The required response to a mailing depends on the cost of the mailing, the cost of the service you're offering and the overall value of the individual responding.

Of course, everything hinges on your being able to monitor results. Your staff should be made aware of the mailing, especially if people are being asked to call for an appointment or information. If you use coupons or other response devices, it will be easier to check results. In any case, it's important to monitor response to a mailing so that you can repeat a winning formula. Resist the temptation to change for the sake of change. As long as the returns justify it, go with what works.

DIRECT MAIL GUIDELINES AND CHECKLIST

Here's a synopsis of direct mail pointers:

Color. Two-color letters and brochures usually out-pull one-color, but color is totally ineffective unless used with discretion.

Envelopes. Number 9 and 10 envelopes are usually most effective in mailing to business, while consumer mailings work best in larger formats. Variety in type, size and color of envelopes usually pays in a series of mailings to the same group.

Letters. Form letters with paragraphs indented will out-pull those that are not. Two-page letters on separate sheets will out-pull a letter run on both sides of one sheet. A separate letter and circular will generally do better than a combined letter and circular. Underscoring pertinent points aids readership and increases response. A special offer with a time limit usually increases return. A testimonial in a letter increases its pull.

Illustrated enclosures. A brochure dealing with a specific offer contained in a letter will usually be more effective than a brochure of an institutional nature. A brochure, unlike a letter, should be typeset.

Addressing. Label addressing frequently produces the most economical response but hand-addressing may be effective in some cases, depending on the audience and the product being mailed. An invitation gets a better response if it is hand-addressed.

Timing. A direct mail letter that produces a satisfactory number of responses on the first mailing can usually be repeated 30 to 60 days later to the same list and produce an additional satisfactory response.

AND FINALLY . . .

Direct mail is a very specialized field. Unless you have a great deal of time and knowledge of direct mail—or a staff member who does—you may be wise to use a firm specializing in direct mail. Chapter 22 explains how to use outside resources; refer to it. Direct mail specialists help with everything from developing mailing lists to getting postal permits. They'll advise you on your direct mail piece, or even develop it for you, from concept through completion. They'll test your mailing to be sure it generates an acceptable response, and often they'll guarantee list accuracy and even results. If you're developing a simple direct mail piece—a newsletter, a brochure and cover letter, you may only need a marketing, advertising or public relations firm for assistance rather than a direct mail specialist. Either way, it's wise to recognize when you need help, and seek it early, even if only for preliminary advice.

BIBLIOGRAPHY

Huey: *The Direct Marketing Executive's Workbook.* Torrance, Calif., 1987.

Barasch: *Marketing Problem Solver.* Fullerton, Calif., Cochrane Chase & Co., 1973.

Marketing Memos, *Direct Response,* 1987; 2; June.

Health Care Marketer/Target Market 1986; 1; Nov 10.

Hodgson: *The Greatest Direct Mail Sales Letters of All Time.* Chicago, IL, The Dartnell Corp., 1986.

Chapter 20

Monitoring Advertising and Public Relations Effectiveness

There are no tried and true precepts that will guarantee the success of your practice promotion program. If there were, advertising agencies would be unnecessary and media costs would be much lower.

However, you can influence the ultimate success of your endeavors in two critical ways:

1. By adapting basic public relations and advertising concepts to the unique attributes of your practice and to the characteristics of your present and potential clientele—your target market(s).

2. By monitoring and revising your overall program to capitalize on what works for you and for your practice.

The second of these factors is the subject of this chapter. Throughout this book, we discuss various practice promotion strategies and their benefits and negative features. We explain how to conceive, develop and implement each of these strategies, whether you're doing it on your own or with the assistance of professionals.

No matter what methods you choose to incorporate in your marketing program, each will take time and/or money. To make the best of your investment, it is crucial that you monitor every effort, whether it is public speaking, holding an educational seminar for the public or physician office staffs, placing stories with the media, mailing a newsletter or brochure, or advertising in the *Daily Bugle*, KTOK radio and WSEE-TV.

A tracking strategy will tell you much about the media you use and the patients your efforts attract. In this chapter, we'll delve into the reasons why monitoring should be a requisite element of every public relations or advertising effort, how to establish a tracking system, and how and why to make adjustments to your tracking system as well as your promotional/advertising program as you go along.

TRACKING IS A MUST

Even if your marketing program generates a significant number of telephone calls and new patients, if you don't know which ads and media or which public relations strategies are accomplishing your goals, that exciting, expensive creative concept and big promotion budget will have limited long-term value.

Moreover, it's possible that a public appearance or an advertising campaign will stimulate a flurry of phone calls or mail. But stacks of telephone messages and a mailbox full of filled-out-coupons don't necessarily translate to a heavily scheduled appointment book. The wrong media, poorly worded copy, a radio or TV ad aired during the wrong time of day can result in responses from people who can't afford your medical services, or who don't actually want or need medical care or treatment but may have responded for some other reason. Tracking your promotional efforts—particularly your advertising—will help you narrow your media selection and ad message(s) to those that produce qualified responses (i.e, patients who will remain with your practice on a continuing basis).

MONITORING PUBLIC RELATIONS EFFORTS

Before we go further into a discussion of how to monitor your advertising, we want to emphasize the importance of tracking public relations efforts as well. While it is not a clear-cut, simple task, evaluation of public relations strategies is essential to your overall marketing effort. You'll want to know if holding educational classes for patients and the public is worth the time, effort and money poured into it. You'll want to know if spending time scheduling and doing a radio interview is worth the calls that may result. You'll want to know if your annual holiday reception for doctors results in increased referrals during the following year or referrals from physicians who previously had not sent you patients.

At the same time, it is a given that some of your public relations effort will go toward image- and awareness-building and developing community good will, rather than immediate growth in new patients or patient services. Therefore, while we strongly urge tracking mechanisms for every promotional strategy, we can't say that you will know immediately, for instance, that an open house was a worthwhile venture. (We would speculate, however, that if 600 people attend your open house, and your goal was 300, you can assume that it was a successful event. And you can even track beyond attendance figures, by having people sign a guest book, fill out a door prize coupon, or sign up for free health information or your newsletter mailing list. Then you can follow up on those names and eventually determine how many become patients.)

There is no "publicity tracking guide" or "special event response evaluation form" that will meet every need. However, on an individual basis, there are tactics you can incorporate into various public relations approaches, such as media publicity, special events, public speaking or distributing educational material. Here are some ideas that may work for you.

HOW TO MEASURE RESPONSE TO PUBLIC RELATIONS EFFORTS
Media Publicity (TV/Radio, Newspaper or Magazine)

■ Offer an informational brochure or handout on the interview topic (for example: "Achoo! 7 Signs of Allergy Problems") to viewers/listeners/readers who write or call. Sometimes the station or newspaper will permit the audience to request the brochure or information directly from it.

Special Events (Open House, Health Fair, etc.).

■ Have a guest book for people to sign when they arrive.
■ Have a door prize drawing for which entrants must sign up.
■ Have a sign-up sheet for more information about a special procedure, treatment, health tips, etc.
■ Have your appointment book at the event and schedule office visits for participants who would like to be seen by a physician regarding a specific problem or procedure.
■ Register people there for educational classes/seminars/programs on health related topics.

Community Speaking Engagements.

■ Have a sign-up sheet available for individuals who wish to be on the mailing list for your practice newsletter (a copy of which you've provided every audience member).
■ Have cards available for individuals to fill out with their name/address as well as health or medical subjects they would like to see discussed in further speaking engagements, or as topics for educational programs.

ADVERTISING EVALUATION: IT NEVER STOPS
Your initial media mix is developed on the basis of the best information available to you at that time. You determine a realistic budget, select your target market, and evaluate the media available to you. But once your ads run, you must continually evaluate the results. You should know as precisely as you can exactly which ads in which media have attracted calls, appointments, requests for information, registrations, etc. When you track results in this manner, your next ad series or campaign will be based on the added knowledge of what worked and what didn't. Futhermore, you should know how many new patients resulted from the calls and requests for information. A comprehensive tracking system will help you with this.

Too often, this is where a practice promotion program breaks down. A harried physician, having already invested more time in developing a campaign than was originally intended, sees his ad in print or on the air. Satisfied that the promotional campaign is completed, he then returns to the practice of medicine.

However, once the ad appears, the effort must continue. If a tracking mechanism has been developed and implemented, the office staff need only complete the steps of the process with each new patient. A weekly or monthly evaluation determines if changes or modifications are needed in the promotional efforts.

The effectiveness of your promotional campaign can improve with each new series of ads, with each additional TV news interview or community talk, as awareness broadens and the cumulative effect of past advertisements intensifies. But if you don't monitor results, you are destined to make the same mistakes over and over. This is a senseless waste of your time and your staff's as well as a squandering of your promotion dollars.

The Traffic Sheet. Evaluating advertising effectiveness is one of the most difficult aspects of a practice promotion program, and is therefore frequently neglected. The physician who runs just one ad in a single medium hasn't much difficulty knowing if the ad worked, but as soon as the single ad becomes an advertising program, with different ads in a variety of media, evaluation becomes complicated.

The key to successful monitoring is the traffic sheet. The effectiveness of this process depends on accurate recording of information on traffic sheets completed each day by front desk personnel. By tabulating the results each month, you can deternine what medium is generating the most responses and what ad or service is generating the most interest.

On the traffic sheet is listed the date, the name of the caller, whether the call resulted in an appointment, and how the caller learned of your practice. Gaining this last bit of data is accomplished by using separate columns for each publication or station where your ads are currrently running. You should also have a column for any public relations efforts you may have been involved in—a talk show appearance, a newspaper article on your practice, etc. As your media mix and PR strategies change, columns are added or subtracted.

Traffic sheets can be as simple or as complex as necessary to fit your media mix. The important thing is to have your staff keep accurate daily records so that at the end of each month you will know how many calls were triggered by each medium.

Figure 20-1 shows a sample traffic sheet.

At the end of each month or quarter, your traffic sheets can be totaled and converted to percentages. This makes analyzing your advertising effort much easier. The monthly or quarterly summary is called a **recap sheet** (Figure 20-2). For each week, list the number of calls received from each ad source [the daily newspaper, radio station(s), TV, Yellow Pages, etc.], transferring the information from your traffic sheets.

Based on these numbers, you then figure the percentage of total calls for each medium. In the far right column, place the total number of calls for each week (100 percent of the calls received due to your advertising program.)

The bottom two rows on the recap sheet pull all the information together

Promoting Your Medical Practice

FIGURE 20-1 Sample Traffic Sheet

TRAFFIC SHEET

DEC 1987
MONTH

DATE	YELLOW PAGES	LOCAL NEWS	MALVERN Comm. Tms.	MAIL-LEADER	SENIOR VOICE	DIRECT MAIL	REFERRALS	RADIO
12/3/87	/				/	/		
12/4			/				/	
12/7	/						/	
12/8			///					
12/9	///		////		///	//		
12/10	/		/				////	
12/13				/				
12/14	/		/			/		
12/15						/	//	
12/20			//				/	
12/21	//		///			///		
12/22	/						/	
12/27	/							
12/28			/		//			
12/29					////			
	11	—	17	1	10	8	12	—

and make it possible to analyze the effectiveness of each medium during a given month based on expenditures for each. In the "monthly totals" column, place the total number of responses for each medium or ad source and the resulting percentage. In the "expenditures" column, list the total amount of money spent on each medium for the month and the percentage of your total monthly budget that figure represents. Now you can compare the percentage of responses from each medium to the percentage of your budget committed to that medium.

Multiple Ads in a Single Medium. If you place more than one ad in a single medium, it is wise to adjust both your traffic sheet and your monthly recap sheet to reflect the responses generated by each. If, for example, you are running two radio spots simultaneously on the same station—one promoting a spider vein program, the other advertising an acne clinic—simply make separate response categories for each.

For ease of tabulation, some physicians have found it helpful to key their ads. One way to do this is to indicate in the ad a specific name to ask for when calling for information or an appointment. By using a different name for each ad, your staff will automatically know which ad generated each call. (The names, by the way, don't have to be actual staff members. You can still designate one person to handle all the calls, as long as everyone knows who to turn the call over to when the caller asks for "Mary," "Lisa," "Robin," or any other names you've specified in your advertising).

The alternative is simply to include a question for new patients on the registration form asking how they learned about your practice. This method is not as reliable, however, since a patient might say "the Yellow Pages" when in reality she learned about you through a newspaper ad, but then looked you up in the directory just before calling the office. Since the Yellow Pages was the last place she looked, that's the source she may recall.

Two other methods that can help you keep responses straight are coupons which vary (at least slightly) from one ad to another, or asking patients to bring the ad with them for a special gift, a free screening, etc. And of course there is the possibility of having a well-known radio or television personality instruct listeners to "Tell Dr. Evans that Tom Tate sent you," or to mention that "you heard it on KTOK radio."

Additional Determinations. The traffic sheet and monthly recap sheet suggested here are both fairly simple. As your expertise and your advertising progresses, you can add categories to increase the sophistication of your monitoring program. For example, you may wish eventually to determine the *total dollars* generated by each new patient brought in by a specific ad, or even the *gross profit* per patient. By so doing, you may discover that although one medium produces more respondents than another, this difference is offset by a higher dollar volume or profit per patient with another medium. You may learn, for instance, that ads in the weekly "shopper" generate plenty of consultation visit patients, but that they never return to the practice or schedule the procedure or treatment discussed. On the other hand, a 30-second spot on the local classical music station may result in far fewer consultation visits, but more of them may become actual continuing patients.

FIGURE 20-2 Sample Recap Sheet

MONTHLY RECAP SHEET

MONTH

WEEK OF	YELLOW PAGES	MALVERN Comm. TIMES	MAIL-MEMBER	SENIOR VOICE	TOTALS
12/3/87	# of calls _11_ % _23_	# of calls _17_ % _44_	# _1_ % _19_	# _10_ % _26_	# _39_ % _100_
12/10/87	# of calls ___ % ___	# of calls ___ % ___	# ___ % ___	# ___ % ___	# ___ % _100_
	# ___ % ___	# ___ % ___	# ___ % ___	# ___ % ___	# ___ % _100_
	# ___ % ___	# ___ % ___	# ___ % ___	# ___ % ___	# ___ % _100_
	# ___ % ___	# ___ % ___	# ___ % ___	# ___ % ___	# ___ % _100_
MONTH TOTALS	# ___ % ___	# ___ % ___	# ___ % ___	# ___ % ___	# ___ % _100_
EXPENDITURES	$ ___ % ___	$ ___ % ___	$ ___ % ___	$ ___ % ___	$ ___ % _100_

MIX YOUR MEDIA MIX

The data you gain from the traffic sheet and recap sheet will allow you to adjust your media mix accordingly. If, for example, your newspaper ad is pulling a higher response percentage than the money you've invested in that medium, and the opposite is true of your magazine ad, you probably should redirect your advertising dollars away from magazines and more heavily into newspapers. (This is assuming that the ad copy and design are similar for each medium, or that each ad is different but appropriate to the audience of the publication.)

As you compare results, keep in mind the benefits of a good media mix. Unless one medium is overwhelmingly more effective than all others, it's wise to retain a diversified mix. Placing all your promotional eggs in the same media basket can nullify the positive complementary effect gained from a multi-media advertising program.

You'll find your ability to interpret the results of your recap sheet improving each month. After all, you have an inside knowledge of your practice that nobody else has, and as your advertising instinct improves, you will develop a feel for the media mix adjustments that will benefit your practice the most.

Productivity Index. Eventually you may wish to develop a productivity index to help you adjust your media mix according to the number of new patients you would like to atttract. If, for example, you spend $1,000 on your Yellow Pages ad over a period of three months, and the ad brings in 25 new patients with average charges of $82 each, you are spending $1 on Yellow Pages for each $2 generated (25 patients × $82 = $2,050). Dividing $2,050 by $1,000 gives you a productivity index of 2.05.

If your radio spot generates 20 new patients at a cost of $1,200 during the same period, the productivity index is $1.36. You gain $1.36 in revenue for each $1 spent on radio advertising, assuming the average radio respondent also requires $82 worth of health care.

As you can see, your Yellow Pages ad is more productive. But you can carry this process a step further. If you want to attract 100 new patients to your practice during a given period, you can determine how much you need to spend on a certain medium to generate the additional patients and, more important, which medium would be most cost-effective. Theoretically, an additional expenditure of $4,000 on Yellow Pages for one quarter could generate 100 new patients. To generate the same number of patients via radio would cost an additional $6,000. This process is not as precise as it sounds, however. You'll recall that there is some cross-fertilization among the various media, as well as some misinterpretation by patients as to how they learned of your practice.

Other Tracking Techniques. Other less involved monitoring techniques may also be helpful in tracking ad results. As mentioned earlier, it's a good idea to ask each person who calls your office, "How did you hear about our practice?" Then record the response on a tally sheet that lists all the various options, i.e., Physician Referral, Family/Friend, Yellow Pages, Newspaper Ad, Radio, Magazine, TV, Hospital Physician Referral Program, Newspaper Article, etc. The name of the referring physician, family member or friend should be written down and, if you advertise on several radio stations or more than one newspaper, the caller should be asked which station or which newspaper.

Additionally, the new patient information sheet should ask "How did you hear about our practice?" with the same check-off responses as were asked on the telephone. You should then compare the results of the patient's telephone response and the written form, because they will not always be the same. These results should also be tallied monthly.

A patient survey is another way to gain information about the sources from which you attract patients. With a patient survey, responses are not immediate, they are reflective. Survey questionnaires can ask patients how they learned of your practice as much as a year or two after the first visit. So while you will get a general picture of what brings your patients in, it is certainly not as specific or reliable as the advertising monitoring method discussed.

Advertising, like most promotional strategies available to physicians, is somewhat unscientific despite the many dollars spent each year evaluating audience reach, share, and target markets. While we encourage you to maintain a traffic sheet and other monitoring techniques, you should be aware that advertising can produce delayed and even long-term response, in addition to the calls and appointments generated at the time your ad or ad campaign runs.

To a certain extent, every promotional method you use helps to raise public awareness of your practice and services. And even advertising for a specific service or program creates general awareness of your practice among consumers, including those who have no use for the service you're advertising. Yet months later, recollection of an ad may stimulate an individual to call you (and they may or may not cite it as the factor that prompted the call). Advertising, along with other promotional strategies, then, should be seen as an investment with benefits that can accrue over an extended period of time.

THE QUALITY FACTOR

One variable to consider in all of this is the quality of the ads you are running in each medium. If your newspaper ad is superior to your radio spot, the ad quality—rather than the media used—may account for its effectiveness—and the type of patients it generates. And be sure your ads in all media adhere to the guidelines outlined in this book.

AND FINALLY . . .

Monitoring advertising effectiveness can be as simple or as complicated as you want to make it. The important thing is to start keeping records immediately when your campaign commences. Begin with the basic forms, improving their complexity and the sophistication of the information you seek as you progress.

Remember, too, that public relations efforts work hand in hand with paid advertising. One complements and enhances the other. To a certain extent you must trust your instinct. As you accumulate experience, it will become a valued ally in tracking and adjusting your media mix and your overall promotional campaign.

Promotion Budget and Strategy

Chapter 21

Setting Promotional Priorities and Budgets

Not long ago we visited with an allergist at his practice in a medium-sized Alabama community. He had read an article we had written on marketing and asked us to assist him. After a short while it was evident that this physician had a good understanding of marketing theory and principles. We asked him, "How can we be of assistance?" His reply was not uncommon: "I know there are a lot of promotional opportunities available to me, but I don't know which ones to use and how much I should spend."

The answers to those questions, like other aspects of marketing, don't come without a little work. In this chapter we are going to take you through the steps we have found to be important to maximize the return on your promotional investment. We will examine a number of common marketing goals and various promotional strategies to meet those goals. We'll inventory the options available to you in carrying out those strategies, go through a prioritizing process, and examine the budgeting process.

WHAT'S YOUR DESTINATION?

STRATEGIC PLANNING

It is often said, "If you don't know where you're going, no road will get you there." This certainly applies to setting your promotional priorities.

Before you launch a promotional campaign you must know what you want to achieve. This may sound obvious, but we constantly encounter physicians who want to advertise their services, or who want a practice brochure, and we find ourselves advising them against doing so. The reason? They don't have a strategic plan. They don't know what they want to accomplish, let alone how to achieve it.

Strategic planning involves deciding where you want to be at some point in the future—usually one to three years—and how you intend to get there. To develop a strategic plan you must look objectively at your situation and establish goals. Only then do you lay out the road map (in the form of specific strategies and tactics) that will take you there.

A typical strategic planning process goes something like this:

Examining your practice situations. This step is essential if you are to set realistic and attainable goals for yourself. As we pointed out early in this book, you must look at your practice environment, both internally and externally:

Internally

- What are your products and services? Do your patients request or need services that you could provide, but do not? Are your patients and referral sources satisfied with your services, the way they are treated by staff, and by you?
- What are your weaknesses? Do you have limited resources (e.g., you know that your patients would benefit from additional on-site diagnostic testing, but you are unable to buy the needed equipment at this time)? Do you have few or no established specialized skills (e.g., you are a general internist and your community is well supplied with generalists)? Poor location (e.g., your office is located five miles from the new medical office building where the majority of your referral sources have rented space)?
- What image is projected by your office setting? What is your schedule of hours? How do you handle after-hour calls? Is your practice location convenient to the majority of your patients?
- What do your patients think about your fees? Do they understand what they are being charged for? Do they understand what they are not being charged for? Do they understand the ways you help them with their health problems at low or no cost?
- What are you spending now on promotion? Do you have a system of tracking the results on your promotion efforts so that you can measure your return on investment?

Externally

- What are your external strengths? Do you have good-sized patient and referral bases?
- Who are your competitors? Where are they located? What amenities or services do they offer that you also do—and that you don't?
- What are your opportunities? Is your practice area growing and prospering? Are there prime locations available for expansion? Are your patients or other groups interested in services or programs that will enable you to expand your services and/or location?
- What threats do you face? Are your target patient groups moving to another area? Are health maintenance organizations expanding rapidly in your community? Are your patients using "nontraditional" health care providers for services that you could be providing?

These and other questions must be answered. Get objective answers wherever you can: ask your patients and the physicians who refer patients to you what they think of your practice and how it compares with your competition.

SETTING MARKETING GOALS

Once you have honestly and objectively answered the questions above, you are ready for the next step in strategic-planning: setting realistic and achievable goals. Within any medical practice the physician(s) (and the staff) should be working toward separate sets of goals that at the same time—personal, professional and practice goals. Strategic planning demands that you enumerate and examine these goals so that you can identify areas of commonality and disparity. With this information, and data gathered in examining the practice environment, you can then formulate group, or strategic practice goals.

The goals you set must be **SMART;** that is, they must be

SPECIFIC
MEASURABLE
ATTAINABLE
RELEVANT
TRACKABLE.

Let's look at how you achieve SMART goals.

Specific. Your goals should be as specific as possible. You should clearly state what the goal is, to whom it is directed, within what time frame it is to be achieved, and what criteria will be used to measure their achievement. For example, one of your goals may be "Within six months to increase by six the number of physicians who regularly refer patients to me." To measure this goal, you can use the simple tracking question on your new patient information form: "Who referred you to this practice?" or "Name of referring physician."

Measurable. Your goals should, when appropriate, include specific numbers (100 additional patients or procedures), percentages (25 percent more market share), time frames (within six months, by the end of the year), or areas (within a 10-mile radius of this office).

Attainable. It does you no good to have specific goals if they are neither realistic nor attainable. You may wish to capture 50 percent of the marketplace, but how realistic is such a goal? Can it be done?

Relevant. Does the goal relate to your overall mission? Does it help you achieve your ultimate desires for you or your practice?

Trackable. Are your goals stated in a way that allows them to be tracked over a period of time? Tracking is critical in order to determine if your plans are working and if you are reaching your goals. Tracking is also necessary in order to know when to modify strategies you've implemented. Once consensus has been reached on strategic practice goals, decisions on the allocation of personnel and financial resources become less cumbersome, and usually more productive. In working with a large multi-specialty group in the midwest we found that the group had never committed itself to a formal strategic plan. Every decision made by the group was a board matter, or as one member of the group quipped, "a bored matter."

The problem they faced was that they had no sense of direction, and therefore every opportunity or threat that confronted them had to be evaluated in isolation, rather than in terms of the group's long-range plan. This posed an insurmountable barrier to achieving the group's full potential. Their case is unfortunately not unique.

Since the readers of a book like this presumably already understand the importance of strategic planning, we can dispense with more of the dos and don'ts on this topic and turn our attention to the most common marketing goals and their implications in planning promotions. (If you don't have a comprehensive understanding of strategic planning, we recommend reviewing our earlier physician marketing text, *Marketing Strategies for Physicians: A Guide to Practice Growth.*)

COMMON MEDICAL MARKETING GOALS

Patient retention. Let's say you are a general surgeon doing in excess of 500 surgical cases a year. From this bit of information there are several assumptions we can safely make:

1. Your practice is well-established.
2. Your have a fairly large base of referral physicians.
3. You gain a substantial number of new patients from former patients who have recommended you highly.
4. You are very well-liked by your hospital's administrator.

In summary, you have what every new general surgeon wants: market share. But no physician or practice retains market share without retaining patients. A practice in which new patients must be continually generated in order to replace departing patients is a practice in severe trouble.

Like many other health care marketing professionals, we believe that the greatest challenge facing physicians today and in the years to come is retention. Physicians spend many years and substantial amounts of money to achieve large bases of patients and referral sources. Specific strategies must be developed to help ensure that this valuable investment of time and money is not wasted, and that such investments don't produce smaller returns than they could.

In the case of the general surgeon, retention goals might include maintaining specific ranges of referrals per referral physician per quarter. This is a measurable goal that when tracked will provide the surgeon with an "early warning system" to detect a drop in referral patterns by one or more physicians.

Attracting new patients. What about the physician with a practice that is not as busy as it could be? We encounter this situation most frequently when a physician is just establishing a practice, but we also find many mature practices faced with the need to attract new patients. Obviously, even the busiest physician needs new patients simply because he or she loses patients each year for reasons beyond his or her control. Word of mouth works well for a physician in this situation, but what about the practice that has just added a new associate who is not working at capacity, or the physician who finds that the number of competing physicians (and alternative care providers) is increasing at a rate faster than the population supporting them?

We know there are any number of reasons why a medical practice must continually and aggressively seek to expand the number of new patients to the practice. Fortunately, there are also an equal number of strategies available to ethically attract new patients. The decision may be made to expand the practice service area by establishing an additional location, or specific groups of patients can be targeted based on age, sex, risk factors, health care needs or occupation.

Each of these strategies requires a slightly different approach to promotion. Again, the key to selecting the right channel is knowing what you want to achieve.

Establishing a niche for yourself. Before you say that this is simply too much "marketingese," consider a situation we encountered a few years ago. We had been retained by a 25-member multi-specialty practice in a rural community to evaluate the market potential of establishing a primary care practice in an adjacent county. Our analysis showed the feasibility was excellent, and we were asked to develop a marketing plan for the new practice. Following a meeting with the physicians in which we presented the marketing plan, one of the young internists asked us if we had any ideas on how he could increase his patient base at the main facility.

In a discussion that followed, we learned that this physician was reasonably busy, but he was not happy with his practice because he was not treating the kinds of problems he was most interested in—namely, cardiac patients. Further probing revealed that he was especially interested in the rehabilitation of cardiac patients. At that time the nearest cardiac rehabilitation unit was approximately 40 miles away. We encouraged him to think through and do some research on what would be required to establish a cardiac rehabilitation program in the community, both in terms of equipment and personnel, as well as additional training that would be required on his part. He did his homework well and a year later the group opened a cardiac rehabilitation program with the internist as its director. This is an example of how one physician established a niche for himself and not only increased his satisfaction from practice, but also benefited his patients and his group.

INCREASING YOUR PROFITABILITY BY CHANGING YOUR PATIENT MIX

In helping physicians develop their marketing plans we always ask them to complete a Physician Self-Assessment Questionnaire. It is not uncommon for a physician to respond as follows:

1. I want to *decrease* my practice *hours.*
2. I want to *decrease* my patient *load.*
3. I want to *increase* my practice *income.*

Inconsistent? Not necessarily, providing the physician is willing to make the investment required to change the mix of patients served. By "mix" we mean the composition of your patient base, defined in specific terms such as medical problem, age, place of residence, method of payment, economic status, and so on.

When a physician is starting out in practice, he or she is usually willing to provide a wide range of services simply because some business is usually preferable to no business. Over time, as the physician's patient and referral base grows, it often seems that the increased hours devoted to the practice do not translate into commensurate increase in income.

When we encounter a situation like this, our first step is to undertake an analysis of the types and frequency of services provided. As we all know, not every service carries the same profitability. For example, let's look at two patients treated by a gynecologist. One patient is self-referred, the other is referred to the practice by a physician:

Self-referred patient. During the first year this woman has a routine examination with basic laboratory work, and one acute problem that requires additional laboratory work. The economics of this example might be as follows:

Services	Fees	Variable Costs
Examinations (2)	$ 75.00	$20.00
Laboratory	40.00	25.00
Totals	$115.00	$45.00

*Marginal Contribution: $70.00

*Marginal contribution is the difference between the fee for providing a service and the variable or marginal cost of providing that service. That is, it is the additional revenue or income generated by a given service that is available for compensation or to cover overhead. Variable, or marginal costs, are the non-fixed costs associated with providing your services. For example, costs of supplies used in diagnosing specific patients in the lab or examining room would fall into the category or variable of marginal costs.

Physician-referred patient. In this second example, the woman was referred by a physician who suspected a problem that was subsequently confirmed, resulting in a needed surgery:

Services	Fees	Variable Costs
Surgery	$375.00	$10.00
Pre & Post Op	Incld.	20.00
Laboratory	30.00	15.00
Totals	$405.00	$45.00

Marginal Contribution: $360.00

This example clearly demonstrates that in this case, strategies directed at physicians to increase referrals can have tremendous impact on the bottom line, and that just being "busy" isn't necessarily an end in itself.

In Summary. Each physician must develop his or her individul marketing goals. Well-established practices may be quite satisfied with a goal of retaining their present patient base, whereas another equally well-established practice may want to build its patient base or change the "mix" of patients. Regardless of the specific goal, the important thing is to know *why* you have set the goals you have, and to have goals that guide your decision-making and allow you to approach promotional efforts with clear objectives in mind.

DEVELOPING YOUR PROMOTIONAL PRIORITIES

In the broadest terms there are two types of promotional objectives: those that are product-oriented and those that are image-oriented. Both are effective in achieving specific desired outcomes:

Objective	Desired Outcome
Product-Oriented	■ To achieve awareness of the uniqueness of a product or service (attraction)
	■ To maintain a patient or referral base (retention)
Image-Oriented	■ To develop and maintain the image of your profession
	■ To develop and maintain a favorable image of your medical practice

Product-Oriented Vs. Image-Oriented. Traditionally, physicians have been image-oriented in their promotion. Ethical standards, qualifications, and other profession-oriented messages have been communicated to the public by national and local associations. Today, armed with new technology and training, physicians who were not traditionally thought of by the public as providers of particular products or services are able to change that perception through the effective use of promotion. This enables them to provide services to their patients that heretofore were referred to specialists. National specialty organizations like the American Academy of Family Practice, the American Academy of Dermatology, the American Academy of Pediatrics and the American College of Surgeons, among others, have reacted by launching national campaigns to inform the public of the advantages of receiving care from their members. That's appropriate on the specialty or academy level, but what about for the individual specialist?

In 1985 we were retained by a specialty group to help them increase and retain their patient base. In assessing their promotional expenditures we found that a substantial portion of their investment was going into an advertising cooperative that was dedicated to promoting their board-certified specialty. In addition, each member of the group was paying into the national academy for a similar advertising campaign. While we supported their belief that the promotion of the specialty was important, we explained to them that they had to increase the funding of their *product-oriented promotion* if they were to achieve their marketing goals. They followed the advice and achieved their goal while continuing to support the image of their profession, both through contribution and patient education.

Why is product orientation necessary? Product orientation is consumer orientation, and medicine has become consumer-oriented. The American public is less inclined to purchase medical care on the physician's terms only. Convenience is on everyone's mind. People want to know about your convenient schedule of hours and the range of services available from you under one roof. In addition to convenience, people want to know that your practice is especially prepared to help them with their special problems. In most cases, consumers are looking for products or services to help them with problems; they are not necessarily seeking a particular medical specialty. For example, consumers look for psoriasis care (product), not dermatology (specialty).

Women's health, elder care, sports medicine, nutrition counseling, and the myriad of other programs gaining acceptance are consumer-oriented. They offer what the consumer wants. Image promotion usually does not help a consumer find the help he or she is seeking.

We don't want to give you the impression that we think image-oriented promotions are inappropriate. On the contrary. The image of the medical profession has been tarnished over the past decade, and you need to subtly address that fact in your communication efforts. For example, misleading stories sometimes appear in the press that physicians are benefiting inappropriately at the expense of their patients. It is important that the public also be made aware of what your practice is doing to help needy patients and to keep costs to a minimum. It's necessary that your patient and potential patients know that you are concerned about their needs and that you support the community that supports you—that you give to it in a variety of ways, not necessarily medical. Community involvement efforts subtly convey this message.

Priorities Change. As circumstances change, your priorities change. As a practice matures, the need to constantly promote its products and services to the public may diminish, but patient retention becomes more important. However, if competition increases, or if expansion is undertaken, the need to engage in public promotion can quickly rise in priority.

If your promotional investment is to be effective, you must be prepared to modify your promotional plan as circumstances change.

BUDGETING YOUR PROMOTIONAL INVESTMENT

Once you have thoroughly analyzed your practice situation and settled on a set of realistic goals, you're ready to move into the fast lane of promotion and marketing communicaton. Fasten your seatbelt, it's a different world!

Throughout this book we have described the multitude of options for ethical practice promotion. At the same time, we've suggested how to avoid some of the pitfalls that could be expensive both financially and professionally. As you are reviewing all these options, you must determine potential costs of those you are seriously considering. In earlier chapters on advertising, we discussed the importance of knowing how many people and what specific demographic groups the various media reach. You must narrow your choices to those that reach your target audiences. Finally, which of all the available options will fit your budget?

Establishing a budget for your promotion and communications efforts is your next step. It's a process many physicians back away from, because it requires closely evaluating both the chosen strategies and projected practice revenues. Let's look at how you go about it.

How Much Should You Spend? The first question some physicians ask when we begin to discuss finances and costs is "How much should I spend on promotion?"

And our answer is: No more than you have to, but as much as it takes to achieve your goals. This may sound easy, but it's not, for it usually takes more to achieve a practice's goal than the physician(s) anticipate.

For example, we recently were working with a group of 26 physicians who had joined forces and formed a single multi-specialty practice. Our work included overseeing the practice's grand opening which was to be a public event. The goal of the event was to draw as many people to the facility as possible so that word would quickly spread about the comprehensive services available under one roof to the area's residents.

The investments made in planning and carrying out a large-scale event of this nature are not insignificant, particularly on the heels of a major construction project. Things to be planned (and paid for) include food and drink, invitations, advertising and publicity, giveaways for the public and VIP gifts, flowers, photographer, rental tables and chairs and other odds and ends. There may be overtime pay for staff. Each event carries its own list of expenses—and if the event is to be judged a success, it's best to economize carefully. Cut back on the number of flower arrangements, if necessary, but don't cut out the advertising to promote the event to the public.

When we presented the multi-faceted promotional plan to the administrator—one that included several special events for different audiences, plus extensive publicity for the public open house—he initially balked at the cost, and wanted to reduce the program to save money. We convinced him that the worst thing he could do would be to carefully plan a relatively expensive event no one knew about. We went forward with the promotional program that we had proposed. The series of events were attended by more than three thousand people, and the practice took off at a rate no one had dared hope for.

Calculating Communication Budgets. In performing a marketing audit of a medical practice, we always look at the total marketing communication investment as a percentage of the gross receipts. If this percentage is below two percent, we often find that the practice is beginning to stagnate. There is no magic percentage, but it's safe to say that a practice in a normal market must invest three to five percent of the gross receipts in various internal and external communication efforts to maintain a solidly growing patient base. In a highly competitive market this percentage may easily reach five to 10 percent.

We find that an investment of up to 15 percent (or even higher in certain cases) of projected gross revenues is required for promotion in introducing a new product or service (see Figure 21-1).

Clearly this percentage varies due to a number of factors:

■ growth goals of the practice
■ competitive environment
■ specialty
■ product or service being promoted
■ geographic area in which practice is located.

So, while we'd like to give you a set percentage of gross receipts that you should invest in marketing communications, we cannot. However, there are some rules that will help you maximize the return on your promotional dollar.

1. Set objectives. Like any other investment, your investment in promotion should earn you a return. What's acceptable? The first year you establish a promotional plan, your investment should be structured so you break even after expenses (but still follow the minimum percentage figures outlined previously). Usually you measure potential return in terms of the average annual revenue generated by a new patient multiplied by the number of new patients projected. You can determine this amount by analyzing a sample of new patients in your practice. If you find that on the average a new patient represents $500 in revenue during the first year, you can divide the proposed promotional budget by this average

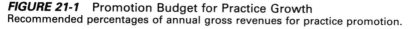

FIGURE 21-1 Promotion Budget for Practice Growth
Recommended percentages of annual gross revenues for practice promotion.

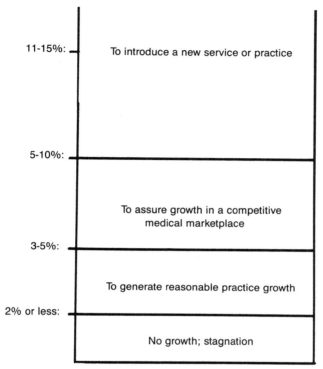

to determine how many new patients you need to generate from the campaign to cover the costs involved. If the number seems reasonable, the campaign is worth pursuing; if not, you will have to evaluate the promotional plan to determine if the potential for success is great enough to justify the risk involved.

Specifically, if you know that a particular promotional activity will require twenty new patients to cover the cost of the ad program, what are the consequences if it only produces half that number? If you find that it is a hardship to pay for the activity, can you afford the risk of not being successful? We can't answer that question for you.

2. Plan an annual budget and adjust quarterly. Because promotion requires repetition, you must plan your budget over an extended period of time, usually a year. While it's recommended that you plan your budget and activities for the year, it is usually not advisable in a medical practice to commit to one or more strategies for the whole year at once. This is because you will be continually evaluating the effectiveness of your promotions.

3. Get some professional assistance. If you're going to be successful in promoting your practice, you must project a professional image to the public. A poorly prepared ad, an amateurish-looking brochure or an ill-conceived public event can have damaging effects. Some up-front dollars spent on professional design and copy can make the difference between success and failure.

4. Track your results. If you don't establish a system to track the results of your

promotions you will never know if your investment was worthwhile. Everyone likes to hear their ad on the radio or see it in the newspaper, but that doesn't pay the bills; new patients do. Not every ad or promotion you try will be successful, regardless of how well you do your homework. That doesn't mean that you shouldn't promote your practice. It just means that you should know what works, so you can continue it, and what doesn't, so you can invest your dollars more wisely.

Composition of a Typical Promotional Budget. Let's now look at a specific case that produced the results desired. The practice was a two-physician family practice group with modest lab and x-ray. While the practice was very busy, the volume was not quite high enough to support a third physician who would be joining the group in twelve months.

The service area was rapidly growing, the local economy was strong, and the physician supply was lagging behind the demand. During the previous year the practice had attracted approximately 500 new patients, which brought the active patient base up to roughly 4,000. Two marketing goals were given priority over the next twelve months:

1. To maintain good communication with the existing patient base.
2. To attract 750 new patients to the practice, an increase of 50 percent over the previous year.

A survey of the patients had revealed that they would be very receptive to a patient newsletter and that they wanted more patient education than the practice had been providing. Market research revealed that there were approximately 40 new families moving into the practice area each month. Out of our strategic planning session, the following promotion budget was developed:

Reprint Patient Brochure (1,000 × $.75)	$ 750.00
Patient Newsletter (5000 × $.60 × 4)	*12,000.00
Health Education Brochures (3000 × $1.00)	*3,000.00
Direct Mail (500 New Residences @ $.75)	**375.00
Newcomer Information Program (500 × $2.50)	1.250.00
Specialty Items (5000 × $.30)	1,500.00
Yellow Pages Ads ($250.00 per Month)	*3,000.00
Newspaper Ad Campaigns ($1,500.00 × 4)	*6,000.00
Special Events ($500.00 × 2)	1,000.00
Total	$ 28,875.00

*This figure includes design costs for ads, publications, etc.
**Includes postage at bulk mail rates.

The extensive marketing communications campaign was a success. More than 800 new patients were attracted to the practice, and existing patients noticed the increased communication and interest in their health, and increased their referrals. The promotional costs and all the other marketing costs were more than covered by the increase in new patients over the prior year. It was established that each new patient brought the practice approximately $35 in revenue over expenses related to the promotional campaign during the first year.

You Must Consider Your "Indirect Sales." The above calculation of return on the promotional investment is conservative in that it fails to take into consideration what we call "indirect sales." In a medical practice, one of the greatest sources of new patients is satisfied existing patients. It is not uncommon for a physician to receive 40 percent of his or her new patients in this manner. Looking at this statistic from a marketing perspective, we can say that each new patient attracted through your communication activities actually represents 1.4 patients. Therefore, in calculating the return on an investment, it is quite appropriate to take this "indirect sale" into consideration.

Another example of an indirect sale is the fact that a patient usually remains with a physician for more than one year; this is of course particularly true in primary care, but the concept also applies to specialty fields. You should know what the "lifecycle" of the average patient is in your practice. Armed with this information, you will be able to make better decisions on whether or not you should make a particular promotional investment.

AND FINALLY . . .

We've gone through a process that can permit you to set your promotional priorities and budget effectively. We hope our message is clear: that marketing communication efforts and their attendant costs require a great deal of planning and a reasonable budget. But doing so will help you to maximize the return on your promotional investment.

Chapter 22

Working with Outside Resources

Even the most ardent do-it-yourselfer can be stymied when it comes to some aspects of marketing and promotion. This is particularly true in the medical field. As a physician, your training is in identifying and treating human medical problems. Creating a promotional plan, writing ad copy, developing a newsletter or calling a reporter to suggest a feature story quite likely are not within your realm of experience or expertise.

However, as we have pointed out in this book, it is possible to carry out much of your promotional plan yourself, competently and professionally, with the assistance of your staff. If you follow the suggestions and formats we've provided in the preceding chapters, you should see tangible results.

On the other hand, if you opt to hire a marketing, public relations or advertising consultant or firm rather than doing it yourself, it's vital that you know the ground rules. As practice marketing consultants ourselves, we've worked with a large number of physicians over the years. And what we have found is that all too often physicians come to a marketing or communications consultant with one or more of the following misconceptions:

- Unrealistic expectations of what a consultant can or should accomplish for them.
- An expectation that the responsibility is all on the part of the consultant.
- Unrealistic expectations of what a marketing or communications professional's time and/or services should cost.
- Expectation of results without research. (The "I just want a brochure" syndrome.)

Your consultant—whether writer, artist or full service firm—will require approval from you at every step of every project. (This approval process protects you as well as them, and assures that the product you get meets your needs and wishes.) You therefore must have at least a basic familiarity with their working methods, techniques and terminology, and their expectations of you. You also should know what you can and should expect of them.

In most cases you'll find it necessary (and more productive) to blend doing-it-yourself with hiring outside resources. If you're an ob-gyn with a series of pregnancy-parenthood preparedness classes and you want an explanatory brochure, you may choose to write the copy yourself (or have a staff member do it). Yet in order to achieve a polished, professional look that enhances your image, you should hire a graphic artist to handle the design and typesetting. Or you may use an advertising agency for your print and radio ads, but want to handle other efforts yourself. You'll require a printer for brochures, newsletters and other printed pieces, and working with a printer can be frustrating and tedious if you don't understand the terminology and options available. (In fact, it's such a complex topic, we've devoted a section of the Appendix to working with printers.)

No matter how many or how few consultants you use, a sophisticated, well-coordinated communication program cannot be developed and administered in a hit-and-miss fashion. Competition has increased, the consumer is becoming increasingly sophisticated, and your alternatives have become more complex. You must be able to deal knowledgeably with the resources available to you in order to assure a top-quality promotional campaign that's also cost-efficient.

THE CHOICES AVAILABLE TO YOU

In the final analysis, the decision regarding use of professional resources should be based on your needs and budget. But first, let's take a look at the function of each of these resources, one or more of which you may require as you develop your marketing and communication campaign. Notice that none of the resources listed covers every base—marketing, research, advertising, public relations, etc. Be wary of any individual or firm who claims they can do it all without calling on outside resources themselves. Remember, even physicians rely on specialists. So should communication professionals (see Figure 22-1).

MARKETING CONSULTING FIRM

A marketing firm looks at your practice from the viewpoint of the consumer, determining his/her wants or needs relative to your practice/services. A marketing firm researches all the elements of your practice—location/accessibility; pricing/fee structure; services; how you communicate with your patients and referral sources; your competitors; your patients and potential patients. Working with you, the marketing firm then determines your positioning and target audience(s), formulates practice objectives and the strategies and tactics for meeting these objectives. A marketing firm may also implement recommended strategies, such as writing and producing a brochure, developing a newsletter, creating an ad campaign, etc. Marketing firms may have in-house resources such as writers and artists or hire them as needed.

FIGURE 22-1 Services Provided by Communications Consultants

- Strategic marketing planning and implementation
- Public relations counseling
- Market research and analysis
- Patient surveys and demographic analysis
- Referral source and community surveys
- Focus groups
- Product/service/practice positioning
- Special event planning, publicity and execution
- Logo and identity development
- Referral source communication programs
- Media preparedness training
- Ongoing media relations
- Targeted publicity for special events or services
- Speechwriting and scheduling
- Community relations program planning
- Employee "customer awareness" training
- Employee communication programs
- Practice brochures, special services brochures
- Patient education brochures
- Newsletter development and implementation
- Video and audiocassette programs
- Copywriting
- Graphics/design
- Advertising planning and implementation
- Advertising placement (media buying)
- Printing coordination
- Direct mail planning and implementation
- Ad specialty planning/coordination

ADVERTISING AGENCY

An advertising agency is an organization of business and creative people dedicated to making advertising succeed. An ad agency studies your service(s), its strengths and weaknesses, and how it compares to the competition. Then it analyzes the market for your product or service, determines the best media to reach that market, and formulates and executes a creative campaign that will accomplish a pre-determined objective. Finally an ad agency conducts (or should conduct) ongoing market research to determine the effectiveness of your advertising campaign.

PUBLIC RELATIONS FIRM

The goal of a public relations firm is to increase or improve your image and visibility in the public eye. The functions of a PR firm include analyzing your current and desired image with all of your "publics" (referring physicians, patients, health care professionals and organizations, the community, etc.), and determining strategies for creating or enhancing your desired image with these groups. These strategies may include making contact with the local media and providing them with information and new developments regarding your practice; increasing your community involvement and visibility; and arranging speaking engagements and appearances on local radio and television programs. A public relations firm or consultant should develop a coordinated public relations plan based on your goals, needs and target audiences.

FREELANCE OR INDEPENDENT WRITER, ARTIST

By definition, a freelancer is a self-employed person offering professional services, usually without long-term contractual commitments to any one employer. Writers and graphic artists often work as freelancers, but it is possible to hire the services of almost any professional on a freelance basis. A freelancer will coordinate his/her efforts with other consultants you may be using or will bring other freelancers to you and work in tandem.

MARKETING/PUBLIC RELATIONS DEPARTMENT OF YOUR HOSPITAL

More and more hospital PR and marketing departments are providing marketing and promotion assistance to their medical staff. Some provide this service free—although generally it's less personalized—while others charge for individualized assistance. Check with your hospital's office to determine the extent of service they offer physicians (if any).

MARKETING/PUBLIC RELATIONS STAFF OF YOUR MEDICAL SOCIETY

Some medical associations and specialty groups offer services to their members, including practice management, promotion, public relations and other services of a similar nature. Many of the national organizations provide extensive assistance to members. For example, the American Academy of Family Practice has a kit called "Honing the Competitive Edge" with sample press releases, speeches, marketing articles, Yellow Pages guidelines, etc. Other specialty societies have similar programs. Check with yours to see what may be available.

Bear in mind that help from your hospital or medical association, whether free or not, is not likely to be as comprehensive or personalized as it will be from a consultant you've hired. You should weigh these considerations when selecting professional help.

DETERMINING YOUR NEEDS

The problem of determining which combination of alternatives is best for your practice is complicated by the fact that there are large agencies, small agencies and individual consultants. Some offer marketing, public relations and advertising services, some only one of these services or a combination. As a general rule, a smaller agency will usually provide better service to smaller clients. (Be aware that client size is measured in billings, not number of employees, number of practice locations or practice size.) In fact, many one-man agencies survive and thrive by offering highly personalized service to a limited number of small clients. With larger agencies, there is a tendency to assign less experienced staff to smaller clients, saving the seasoned professionals for the big-money accounts.

For the physician who has some marketing expertise and who enjoys a more direct involvement in piecing together the components of a promotional campaign, freelancers may be a good choice. They can also be cost-effective if your particular need is limited to the freelancer's area of expertise. If, for example, you have a staff member who is a good writer and can create your brochure copy, you may need only a graphic artist to develop the design.

THE CALL FOR SPECIALIZATION

More and more these days, a number of advertising, public relations and marketing firms are calling themselves health care specialists. While we advocate selecting a firm that has a background and documented experience in health care, we would advise that you question closely any firms or individuals you're considering who call themselves health care or medical specialists. Find out precisely what their experience is; look at samples of their work in health care; ask them specific questions about practice promotion, and listen to their answers. Talk to their present or previous health care clients (and if they have none, yet call themselves specialists, show them the door).

THE SELECTION PROCESS

Finding the right individual or firm for your practice is an important but time-consuming process. With the help of these guidelines, however, the process can be greatly simplified (see Figure 22-2).

First, it's wise to work with an agency that specializes in health care or physicians, if possible. Otherwise, you must educate your consulting firm not only in your practice philosophy and services, but also in the intricacies of the health care field. If there are no individuals or firms in your community that specialize in health care or physicians, be very selective. Physician marketing and promotion and the ethical considerations involved are too complex and sensitive to turn over to a firm or individual totally unfamiliar with it.

There are several ways to find a good agency or individual:

1. Consult with your colleagues in non-competing specialties, particularly those who have promotion programs of their own, to see whom they use or recommend.

FIGURE 22-2   Considerations for Choosing a Consultant or Firm

---

- Do you feel comfortable with the people you're meeting with—and will they be your account reps? A client-consultant relationship is, after all, a personal relationship as well. You must like and respect the people you'll be dealing with.
- How long have clients been with them?
- What has been achieved for their clients?
- What is the extent of experience with your specialty or with physicians in general?
- How much emphasis is placed on research? Don't expect a marketing, advertising or public relations firm to jump in and start producing brochures, newsletters, ads or other communication efforts without learning about your practice, your patients and potential patients, competitors and service area demographics. If they do, you should question their commitment, capability, and understanding of health care.
- Will they talk about fees and charges up front? How heavily are outside services marked up, if at all?
- Have lavish promises or exorbitant claims been made? Just as no physician will guarantee a cure to his or her patient, no legitimate communications professional should make extravagant promises of guaranteed results.

---

2. Ask the hospital administrator or public relations/marketing director of your hospital for recommendations.

3. Check with your local medical society for names of competent firms.

4. Call the health/medical reporter or editor of your local newspaper or TV station(s) and ask whom they would recommend of the individuals or firms that contact them regularly. This is an especially good approach if you plan to engage primarily in public relations or media strategies.

5. Check with the editors of major medical publications for referrals, or check for ads by health care consulting firms in these magazines.

6. Watch locally and nationally for articles by health care marketing consultants, or articles in which consultants are quoted on marketing, public relations or promotion issues. These individuals are interviewed because they are considered knowledgeable, credible experts.

7. Look for ads by noncompeting physicians in the newspaper, local magazines, on TV or radio. Try to find those of consistently high quality that project a professional image. Call the physician(s) and ask for an introduction to their agency. Be sure to ask about their experience with the agency.

8. Check the Yellow Pages under advertising or public relations agencies. One-person shops and freelancers are also listed under "marketing," "writers" or "graphic artists."

9. Check your own contacts. Printers and typesetters can recommend a good agency or individual.

10. Still another good source is a college or university in your area. Some business and marketing professors do consulting work, and sometimes graduate students are available at reasonable rates.

11. Finally, the president of the local chapter of national advertising and public relations organizations can refer you to individuals or agencies in your community. Look for these organizations in the white pages of the directory, or check with your Chamber of Commerce. Possibilities include the American Society for Hospital Marketing and Public Relations (an organization of the American Hospital Association); the International Association of Business Communicators; the Academy for Health Care Marketing (a subsidiary of the

American Marketing Association), the Public Relations Society of America, the Direct Marketing Club, etc. They may be listed under your city or state name.

NARROWING THE CHOICES

Once you've compiled a prospect list, you're ready to narrow it down to those likely to be interested in your account, and who seem to have the interest and experience best suited to your needs. Your initial screening should start with a short letter or telephone call to each agency or individual.

Provide information up front so prospective agencies can quickly determine their interest in you as a client and their ability to serve your needs. This matchmaking is as necessary in selecting an agency as it is for you in accepting patients. You are most comfortable and competent providing care to individuals whose health or medical problems lie in your specialty field; the same is true of marketing, advertising or public relations firms, artists, and writers.

The kind of information you should be prepared to supply includes the following:

- An estimated annual budget for marketing and promotion. Maintenance budgets generally run around three percent of annual gross revenues, while aggressive start-up budgets run from five to ten percent.
- A brief statement or summary of your goals: what you hope to accomplish in revenue or patients generated, or image enhancement.
- Your practice philosophy.
- Extent of your expected involvement and that of your practice staff.

When you have gathered some names for consideration, these are some of the questions you should ask the individual/firm under consideration:

- What is their experience?
- Who are their current and former clients?
- What is their work like? You should be shown a portfolio containing samples of their work. Remember, however, that you are being shown only their best work.
- What results have they generated for clients? Look for measurable figures, not nebulous responses like "the client was very pleased," or "there was a lot of interest shown."
- Who will be your **account representative?** What is his/her experience with medical or health care clients?
- What are the rates? How are they charged—by the hour, by the project, by retainer? What is the mark-up, if any, on services they coordinate on your behalf (i.e. typesetting, printing, photography)? The industry standard is 15-20 percent. Some firms don't mark up, letting vendors bill you directly.
- How will they work with you? What is their method of meeting client needs and goals?

- Can they provide references—preferably physicians—whom you can call?
- How long has the agency or individual been in business and/or practicing health care marketing or promotion?
- If it's an agency you're considering, what are the credentials of the agency's principals? (Individual experience can offset a new company's lack of experience.)
- If a multi-person agency, how many full-time and part-time staff members do they employ, what does each do, and how long has each been with the firm? (Watch for staff turnover problems and for how much of your work may be farmed out.)
- How often will the firm meet with you to review projects and plan for future objectives and strategies?

Any qualified, reputable firm or professional should be able to respond to these questions in person or in a letter. Be sure to note how long it takes to receive the information. Although agencies are generally on their best behavior during the sales pitch stage, this will give you a good indication of how responsive they are likely to be later on.

This initial inquiry will eliminate many of the names on your list. Be sure to take the time to call a few clients of the firms or individuals you're interested in, and ask specifically about results. Your research should turn up a few prospects that you can ask for a formal presentation.

THE FORMAL MEETING

When requesting a formal meeting, don't demand speculative creative work. What you should expect is a look at samples of the prospective consultant's work, and information on how they would proceed on your account. Some agencies use a special team to pitch new accounts, so request that the person who will actually be handling your account be involved in the meeting.

Compatibility between you and your consultant is an integral part of the client/consultant relationship. It's important to find out if you are comfortable with the people you'll be working with. If a team approach is used, observe if the team seems to work well together.

Following a meeting, you should receive a written proposal or proposal letter. Check the proposal for an understanding of your goals, a concise and comprehensive plan of action, and a reasonable timetable that fits with your schedule as well as theirs. The proposal should be well-written, with benefits and budget clearly stated. Look for a clear statement of billing and charges. Without a specific financial summary, you could get some unpleasant surprises.

Finally, there should be provision for evaluation of every element of your communications plan. Not every promotional endeavor will be a resounding success, and a good agency will monitor its efforts and make changes or improvements along the way.

BEFORE YOU SELECT

Before making a final decision, consider the following points:

- Make sure your account is not too small for the firm you select.
- If there are no individuals or firms with medical or health care experience to meet your needs, understand that you will have to provide some initial education and guidance to the person/firm you select.
- Check references carefully to be sure commitments to clients, suppliers and media are honored.
- Be sure the agency will provide quotes up front for all production jobs, and that estimates are honored (as long as you haven't insisted on major changes in the job). If you have printing, typesetting, writing or design sources who have served you well in the past, ask that they be included in the bidding process if they are qualified for the project.
- Clarify ownership rights to all creative products (photos, copy, design, artwork). If possible, you want to own what you pay for so you can use it any way you wish. Otherwise, a photographer hired by you may own the rights to your photo; you'll have to get permission and/or pay every time you want to use it in a new publication.
- Don't underestimate the importance of establishing and maintaining rapport with your professional resource(s).
- Talk about fees with prospective consulting firms or individuals. Be sure you understand the method for agency compensation. Agencies generally bill in one or more of the following ways:
  1. Media commissions. A 15 percent commission for media purchases is standard.
  2. Hourly charges for agency services (or a project charge or monthly retainer to encompass a set number of hours a month).
  3. Mark-ups on purchases made for the client, generally about 20 percent for services like photography and printing.

You can usually negotiate the method by which you are billed. You don't have to accept a standard agency contract. You can negotiate an agreement that provides you with good service and the agency or individual with fair compensation.

- Begin your relationship with a written contract, recording the ground rules and avoiding misunderstanding. Be sure to include termination procedures if appropriate (generally 30, 60 or 90 days notice by either party), agency and client responsibilities, handling of and compensation for projects and services not defined in the contract, approval processes, ownership rights, billing procedures, method of compensation, and your right to review cost records for agency time and purchases made on your behalf.
- Rely on your instincts. Your money and your image are at stake. Choose someone who respects your goals, your expertise and your dollars, someone who is able to communicate and who has earned a deservedly good reputation. In turn, let them do the job you hired them to do. Respect their time and talent. Don't begrudge them a fair profit. A good professional relationship is a valuable commodity.

■ Be candid with your consultant(s). Don't keep secrets from them. Tell them everything they need to know to do a great job for you. Then let them do it. Encourage them to be candid too. You'll both benefit from it.

Note: Something new in public relations has recently emerged. It is the firm that promises to "charge you only for actual coverage generated for you." Such firms are getting extensive media coverage themselves, because it seems to be a perfect arrangement: they work tirelessly to place stories and features with the media on your behalf, and you don't pay a cent if no publicity results. What you don't learn until you contact one of these media placement firms is that they are extremely selective in the clients they take on, and will only accept as clients those individuals or businesses who have great media potential. Then, when these pre-screened clients do get coverage—on the Today Show, on Cable News Network, in *Inc.* or *Time* magazine, they charge substantial sums—anywhere from $10,000 to $100,000 per placement. There's nothing wrong with this concept; just be aware of how it differs from the standard media placement approach.

WORKING WITH YOUR CONSULTANT

The working relationship you establish could determine the success of your promotional efforts. The relationship is a delicate balance between giving the person or agency you hire the support and input they need and letting them do their job without undue interference.

To accomplish this, it's first necessary to know what to expect and how to facilitate your consultant's efforts. You already know that promotion begins with a plan, which can't be developed without the consultant's thorough knowledge of your practice. Be honest about where you stand professionally, and make sure that your consultant knows your liabilities as well as your assets. Don't put the person you're working with in the position of being surprised later by something they should have been told up front.

Don't expect specific details of your consultant's plans at the initial meeting. This is an opportunity for them to get a feel for your practice and personality. It's a time for gathering information, not providing direction. Following this session, the agency will hold its own brainstorming session, research your competition, and possibly do a more intensive assessment of your practice, patients and service area.

After completing its research, the firm or person you've hired should schedule a meeting with you at or before which you should be presented with a written plan that outlines in detail exactly what your problems and opportunities are and what can be done to combat or expand on them. They should also be able to give you a good approximation of the costs you can anticipate.

These "don'ts" will help you get the best possible work from your consultant(s):

- Don't write your own copy if you're paying them to do it. Provide input, don't be afraid to suggest, but do a fair amount of listening.
- Don't be an art critic. Commercial art and decorative art are worlds apart. Don't apply the same rules to your ad layouts that you do to the painting you have hanging over your living room sofa.
- Don't fear creativity. Promoting health services is not the same as promoting canned soup. There are more and more competing health care providers advertising the benefits of their services just as you are. It takes a creative approach to emerge from the clutter of ads and get attention without being tasteless or unprofessional.
- Don't ask your agency to imitate your competition. You can show them samples of what you like, but you want a program that reflects the unique aspects of your practice, your personality and the characteristics of the prospective patient you want to reach.
- Don't follow fads. In both public relations and other forms of promotion, certain innovations become popular for a limited period of time: exotic type faces, buzz words, offbeat slogans or phrases, a certain graphic look. But like all fads, they fade fast, and could leave your promotional effort looking very dated.
- Don't insist on starring in your own ad. Follow the objective advice of your consultant. If you're a scintillating, articulate and charismatic personality, you may be an exception to this rule. Otherwise, leave this role to a professional.
- Don't succumb to outside opinions. Trust your agency to reach your prospective audience. You're paying them to know what works.
- Don't be intimidated by your consultant. If you're given something you don't like or understand, ask for an explanation. If you're truly uncomfortable with an approach, a photo, a headline, insist on a modification or revision.

COMMUNICATION IS THE KEY

As you know, the key to an effective client/consultant relationship is communication. This requires work, but it's worth it. The "good" clients, not always the ones with the biggest budgets, often get the best creative effort. Just as physicians prefer to treat patients with high health care awareness, agencies like to work with clients with a high marketing, promotion, public relations or advertising IQ. It makes for a two-way relationship, a sharing of ideas and ultimately a productive promotion program.

Remember too, that attitude and expectations are as vital to the success of physician promotional efforts as any other element. Attitudes stem from experience and education. Open yourself to new, concentrated input; it will enhance your marketing and promotion efforts.

The Association of National Advertisers and the American Association of Advertising Agencies, in a joint study, asked their members to rate 23 factors likely to cause problems between agencies and their clients. The results apply to any form of promotion, not just advertising. And the problems described by both parties apply just as much to relationships with individual freelance artists and writers as to advertising or public relations agencies.

The clients found fault with themselves for holding too many "unproductive, unnecessary" meetings, not giving their advertising agencies enough lead time, having too many approval levels, and being unwilling to commit sufficient resources.

On the other hand, the ad agencies faulted themselves for failure to adhere to schedules, plan ahead, and ask the right questions. Clients were most frustrated by their agencies' lack of initiative, need for too much lead time, frequent personnel transfers, and failure to involve senior management often enough.

The ad agencies took their clients to task for not planning ahead, being unwilling to take chances, not adhering to schedules, and being unfamiliar with agency cost constraints.

This study was conducted in a spirit of cooperation and provides insights that should help you in your relationship with your consultant. Remember, in general, both ad agencies and their clients were satisfied with each other's performance. Figure 22-3 depicts five ways to ensure a happy client-consultant relationship.

A TEAM EFFORT

An effective, creative communications program for your practice requires hard work on the part of both consultant and the physician-client. It's a team effort. The creation of quality promotion is a four-step process requiring client cooperation and input.

FIGURE 22-3 How to Have a Happy Client-Consultant Marriage

---

1. **Talk money.** Don't avoid discussions of fees. Understand how your consultant charges, what you'll be billed for, what's included in a retainer fee.

2. **Know the terminology.** Understand what your consultant means when he/she uses terms like "comp," "market share," "CPM," or "blueline." If you don't understand, ask. Better yet, read up ahead of time—take a basic marketing course, read a marketing book.

3. **Be candid.** Say what you mean. Don't keep secrets. If you don't like something, say so. If you can't afford something, say so. If your relationship isn't comfortable, fix it or find another consultant.

4. **Loosen up.** You hire a consultant for research and creativity. Creative means innovative, exciting, relevant—not staid, safe, similar to the other guy. At the same time, if you know an approach won't work, if it's too off the wall, say so, and say why.

5. **Make a commitment.** If you're going to engage in marketing and communication, do it. Decide how much you're going to spend, for how long, and in what way. Agree on it with your consultant. Then give the consultant and the strategy a chance to work.

---

1. The first step is research, the process of gathering and organizing pertinent data in the practice and the service area. The client's responsibility is to be as candid and cooperative as possible; the agency's is to ask the right questions.
2. The second step is reviewing material and formulating strategies based on your objectives. The consultant should develop a range of strategies and objectives to be considered and refined by both parties.
3. Creating the communication/promotional strategy (brochure, ad, newsletter, etc.) is the responsibility of the consultant. It consists of developing and executing promotions based on sound strategy and positioning.
4. The review and approval phase is shared by client and agency. An internal review by the agency comes first, followed by final review by the client.

Trust your instincts in judging the work your consultant does for you. If a promotion, graphic or copy approach doesn't feel good and can't be justified by your consultant, don't use it.

PRESERVING THE RELATIONSHIP

What happens when a relationship turns sour? Twelve key public relations practitioners were asked in the June, 1985 issue of *Public Relations Journal* to name the most common reasons for losing clients. Here are the mistakes they said are most often made by PR firms.

1. Losing contact with the client. An ongoing relationship is just that; it must be nurtured. It doesn't diminish with time, or after the account is secured.
2. Lack of planning, research and direction. This is usually an indication of either a lack of interest or experience by the consultant, or not ranking high enough on an agency's client list.
3. Failure to service the account properly. Your consultants should put the same energy into keeping your account that they put into winning it.
4. Lack of staff expertise. This is usually the result of a turnover problem. Well-managed shops seldom have difficulty attracting and keeping qualified personnel.
5. Failure to establish good financial controls, inattentiveness to the details of running a business, or inaccurate bills and unexplained charges.
6. Ineffective estimation of fees. Underbidding to win an account. Or just plain inaccuracy. The "it takes more time and money than we thought" syndrome.
7. Not paying enough attention to the chemistry between the client and the account executive. If the relationship sours, it should be corrected at once.

If a Campaign Fails. Let's assume the worst: your consultant's campaign fails to produce the desired or expected results. Do you have legal recourse? According to Phoenix attorney Van O'Steen (who successfully challenged the 100-year-old ban on professional advertising before the Supreme Court), "An action against the principal for either breach of contract or negligence would be unlikely to succeed. The only possible exception would be a situation where both parties agree that the agency's right to compensation is dependent upon certain predetermined results being achieved.

"As long as the advertising agency did what it promised to do, and performed its services in a competent manner in relation to other advertisers in the community," O'Steen concludes, "the principal's only remedy is to terminate the agency contract and cease to do business with the agency in the future."

AND FINALLY . . .

You are ultimately responsible for the success or failure of your practice promotion program, just as your patients bear the ultimate responsibility for their own health and fitness. That's why the processes, procedures and relationships discussed in this chapter are so important.

If you take the time and effort to determine your needs, if you select your professional resource(s) carefully, and nurture and build a strong relationship based on honesty and communication with your consultant(s), your chances of success are good. The consultant/client relationship must not be adversarial in nature. Your objectives are identical: a successful marketing communications program that yields substantial benefits for your practice, and fair remuneration for the freelancer or firm you hire. Working with a consultant can and should be a positive, profitable experience for all concerned.

Chapter 23

And Finally . . .

A friend of ours who comes from a rather large family tells of how, when she was growing up, her mother used to call for one of her brothers or sisters. With so many children in the family, she said, her mother couldn't always pin down the name of the child she wanted, and would run through several of the siblings' names. "Mary, Lisa, Jan, Jennifer, LINDA!" she would call, her voice rising in frustration until she finally came to the name she wanted. Only then would any of the sisters or brothers pay attention, and the one being summoned would heed the call.

Marketing communication is quite similar to the process our friend's mother went through in trying to get the attention of the appropriate offspring. She called many names, but until she called the right name— thus getting the attention of that individual—it didn't matter what her message was. In the same way, the message in your marketing communication efforts must be directed at the proper audience and get their attention if it is to be accepted and acted upon.

In the preceding chapters and topics, we've tried to make the point that your *message* matters. As does your audience and the method you use to transmit your information. But most of all, the *substance* of your message matters. It matters a great deal. Marshall McLuhan is widely recalled for his observation in the early '60s that "The medium is the message." That may be true in other communication endeavors; it isn't in medical practice marketing. The content of your communication with your target audience doesn't just say something about your practice; it tells them something about medicine. Your communication gives your audience information they can use and from which they will benefit in terms of good health.

If you've read completely through to the end of this book, we trust you've gotten our message, that communication is a vital component of your medical practice in this era of competitive and environmental challenges.

Your communication efforts, if carefully planned, developed and crafted, can be very effective in attracting patients to your practice and keeping them with you. The media you choose and the words you use to convey your message are powerful. They create emotion and images. They educate and enlighten. And they persuade. Your communication efforts can even change a person's thinking.

Education and persuasion are your goals with marketing communication. This means, of course, that you have an obligation. Your obligation to the medical profession is to represent it and your peers well. To present information factually, truthfully, ethically. You have an obligation to avoid misrepresenting yourself, your skills and your services. You have an obligation to keep your knowledge and your skills current in your chosen specialty.

This responsibility to your profession extends to your patients and potential patients as well. When you communicate with your patients and the public, they will, for the most part, believe what you tell them. They will accept the evidence you present as fact. So your obligation to them is the same as it is to your profession—to tell the truth. It is also to provide high quality care in all phases of your practice, whether it's the waiting time patients encounter in your reception area, the courtesy of your staff, the diagnosis or treatment you prescribe, or the way you respond to your patients' questions during an office visit or in after-hours phone calls.

You see, as more and more physicians engage in practice marketing (and Chapter 1 laid out the statistics and trends that indicate they will), your patients and the public will become more educated. They already know more about health and wellness, more about preventing heart disease and cancer, than many doctors did just 50 years ago. They know more about the benefits of exercise and good nutrition, of avoiding overexposure to the sun and underconsumption of fiber. Yet they don't know everything they need to know about all the diseases, disorders and afflictions that visit the human population. That's why they turn to the medical profession. They acknowledge your expertise. They accept your skills and defer to your judgment.

At the same time, they have expectations, created by what they see and hear from personal experience, from neighbors and friends, the media and from the medical profession. They expect:

- Quality medical care with up-to-date equipment and techniques
- Physicians and staff members who listen to them
- Physicians and staff who treat them courteously and in a friendly manner
- Minimum waiting time.

Patients don't expect instant cures; they don't expect miracles; they don't expect their doctors to be superheroes. For the most part, the public's expectations of the medical profession are achievable—and when expectations can't be met, most people are understanding if there is a logical explanation. In other words, if you communicate with them.

What we've tried to emphasize throughout this book is that communication is a process of exchanging information. No matter what form the communication takes—newsletter, advertisement, brochure, telephone call, face to face conversation—you are listening to your audience and responding to their needs. They, in turn, listen to what you have to say, and respond in kind.

There are some, both in the medical profession and out, who dismiss marketing and its elements as all glitter and no substance. They describe it as the whipped cream without the dessert, complaining that after eating all the whipped cream, consumers will discover there's nothing there.

Having read this far, you know better. You know that marketing can occupy an honorable and rightful place in your medical practice because it ensures better care, more reasonable and compliant patients, and greater satisfaction for you, regardless of the challenges you face in your profession and in your practice.

While we were working on this book, we heard from a doctor in a small town in Louisiana. Several years ago, when the oil boom went bust, it severely flattened the economy of the oil-dependent community where he lived. A family practitioner, his practice suffered tremendously as patients began putting off getting medical care, and those who did visit him for treatment put off payment.

The physician began investigating practice opportunities elsewhere; he saw no future for his practice and his family in the economically depressed city.

Then, "I attended a practice marketing seminar at which you spoke, sponsored by the American Academy of Family Physicians," the doctor told us. "It was an eye-opener. I saw opportunities for my practice, both in my town and in surrounding communities."

He went back home and immediately contacted a television station there about doing a health program. They turned him down. Undaunted, he visited another. And another. The individual at the third TV station said "We've been thinking about getting a doctor for a regular medical program. Sure, we'll try you." Today, the family practice specialist is on TV every other week with a six minute segment on the early morning news. He runs an educational column in the local newspaper as a paid advertisement. He sends a letter of welcome to every new resident in town, outlining the services his practice offers. Recently he took a certification exam in geriatrics offered by the AAFP, because the number of elderly patients in his practice has increased substantially.

The doctor joined the Rotary Club, and now accepts numerous requests to speak to local organizations. He now has two offices offering a variety of annual screenings at affordable rates: a Healthy Heart Profile in the summer; a free flu shot program in the winter; a year-round low-cost mammogram program. Once or twice a year he opens his office doors to people who have no insurance and no money, and he diagnoses or treats them for free. He keeps his staff informed; they're enthusiastic and knowledgeable about his communication endeavors as well as his services.

How is his practice doing? It's thriving with a continued flow of new patients generated by his communication efforts, as well as referrals from current patients. In fact, his patient base has tripled since that period several years ago when he was ready to give up his practice, uproot his family, and start all over somewhere else.

There are plenty of physicians whose marketing communication has made a difference to them and to their patients. Perhaps this book will help you make a difference in your practice and with your patients.

It can. It's simply a matter of communication.

Appendix A

Physician Self-Assessment

Part A: Wants and Needs

Before an effective marketing plan can be developed and implemented, you must define exactly what you need from the practice of medicine. You can't begin a marketing plan without a direction or goal. The following outline will help you clarify your specific personal goals and give direction to your future marketing strategies.

I. PERSONAL GOALS

    A. Time Investment

       1. How many hours a week do you practice medicine? _____

       2. How many hours a week do you want to practice?

        Now? _____
        In 5 Years? _____

    B. Time Off for Self

       1. How many daytime hours a week do you take off? _____

       2. How many hours more/less a week do you need for yourself?

        Now? _____
        In 5 years? _____

    C. Time With Family

       1. How may daytime hours a week do you spend with your family? _____

       2. How many daytime hours a week would you like to spend as family time?

        Now? _____
        In 5 years? _____

    D. Financial

       1. How much money did you earn last year after taxes? $_____

       2. How much money do you want to make?

        Now? $_____
        In 5 years? $_____

       3. Assuming a 5% annual inflation rate, and a 10% yearly increase in overhead, how much will your income have to increase each year to reach your goal in 5 years? $_____

E. Retirement

1. In how many years do you want to begin to slow down? _____

2. In how many years do you want to retire? _____

II. PROFESSIONAL GOALS

A. Educational

1. Are you satisfied with your current expertise?   Yes/No

2. How many hours a month do you want to devote to continuing education? _____

3. Do you now spend that much time on continuing education?   Yes/No

4. Are there medical interests you wish to pursue that require time out of the office?   Yes/No

5. Will those interest provide new services that will benefit your patients and also increase practice income?   Yes/No

B. Teaching

1. How many hours a month do you spend teaching, either in the office or at a medical school? _____

2. Do you want to spend more time teaching?   Yes/No

3. If the answer is yes, do you take this into consideration when planning your practice and economic future?   Yes/No

C. Organizational Activities

1. How many hours a month do you spend in professional organization activities? _____

2. How many hours do you want to spend?   Now? _____
In 5 Years? _____

3. How many hours do those activities take away from your patient-care time? _____

4. Are you able to make up the time and money you lose?   Yes/No

5. Do you plan to increase your time spent in organizational activities?   Yes/No

6. If yes: By how many hours a month within 1 year? _____
By how many hours a month within 5 years? _____

D. Nonmedical Activities

1. How many hours a month do you spend on nonmedical business? _____

2. Would you like to devote more time to such activities?   Yes/No

3. If yes: Are your practice obligations, either patient-load or income loss, limiting your time for such activities?   Yes/No

III. PERSONAL PRACTICE GOALS

A. Time

1. How many hours a day do you spend in direct patient care?   _____

2. How many hours do you spend from the time you leave home until you return?   _____

3. How many minutes do you average with each patient?   _____

4. Are you satisfied with the amount of time you spend in direct patient care?   Yes/No

5. Are you satisfied with the total time per day that you devote to your practice?   Yes/No

6. Are you satisfied with the amount of time you spend with each patient?   Yes/No

B. Accessibility

1. Do you feel you are accessible by phone to your patients during the day?   Yes/No
   At night?   Yes/No
   On weekends?   Yes/No

2. Are you more or less accessible than you need to be?   More/Less

3. Within the next 5 years, do you want to change your accessibility?   Yes/No

4. If yes: Do you want to become more accessible, or less accessible?   More/Less

C. Daily Patient Load

1. How many patients do you now see in an average day?   _____

2. How many patients would you like to see?   _____

3. Will a rise in your current patient load lower your enjoyment of the practice of medicine?   Yes/No

4. Are you satisfied with your daily patient load?   Yes/No

5. Does your current patient load satisfy your economic and practice needs?   Yes/No

6. How many patients will you want/need to see per day within 5 years?   _____

D. Practice Patient Load

   1. Have you determined the actual numbers of patients and families in your practice?   Yes/No

   2. If yes: How many individual patients? How many families?   _____

   3. If no: How many patients do you think are in your practice?
      How many families?   _____ _____

   4. Do you consider those numbers adequate?   Yes/No

   5. How many new patients do you average per month?   _____

   6. Is that the number you want?   Yes/No

   7. How many patients would you like to have in your practice in 5 years?
      How many families?   _____ _____

   8. That would be a change of how many patients?
      How many families?   _____ _____

E. Patient Mixture

   1. Do you know what kinds of patients (age, socioeconomic status) make up your practice now?   Yes/No

   2. If yes complete the following:
      Average age   _____
      Average family size   _____

   3. List in order of percentages the 5 largest age groups of patients in your practice.
      a. _____
      b. _____
      c. _____
      d. _____
      e. _____

   4. List in order of frequency the 5 most prevalent disease categories you treat.
      a. _____
      b. _____
      c. _____
      d. _____
      e. _____

   5. The numbers above represent the patient and disease mixture in your practice. Do those numbers (percentages) represent the overall practice you want to have?   Yes/No

   6. If no: How would you like to see your practice mix change?
      In terms of average age: _____
      Prevalent age groups: _____
      Prevalent diseases: _____

F. New Services

1. What are the 5 major clinical services you now offer your patients?
    a. _____
    b. _____
    c. _____
    d. _____
    e. _____

2. What other services would you like to offer?
    a. _____
    b. _____
    c. _____
    d. _____
    e. _____

3. What services that you do *not* offer do you feel would be beneficial to your patients?
    a. _____
    b. _____
    c. _____
    d. _____
    e. _____

4. By priority, which of the services listed in questions 2 and 3 would benefit both your patients and your practice, either immediately or in the future?
    a. _____
    b. _____
    c. _____
    d. _____
    e. _____

G. Practice Growth

(Review your answers to Part D., Practice Patient Load.)

1. Do you have enough space to efficiently handly your current patients?   Yes/No

2. Will you need more space to handle your projected patient load in 5 years?   Yes/No

3. If you had more space now, would you be able to see more patients and still maintain your present quality of care, efficiency, and cost-effectiveness?   Yes/No

4. Are you planning to expand your physical plant within the next 5 years?   Yes/No

5. If answers to 1 through 4 are yes: Have you taken those factors into consideration in your long-range planning?   Yes/No

H. Addition of Partners

1. Do you now need a new partner?   Yes/No

2. How many new partners are you planning to
   add within 1 year? _____
   Within 5 years? _____

3. Will your current patient population support
   another partner? Yes/No

4. How many new patients will you need to add
   per month per new partner? _____

Part B: Marketing Goals

*Once analyzed, your wants and needs in Part A of this self-assessment form a
personal, professional, and practice "wish list." You may choose to leave it as just
that, as many physicians undoubtedly will. Those wants and needs, however, are
the framework for the goals in a strategic marketing plan that can help your "wish
list" come true. To see what your marketing plan goals are, use your answers in
Part A to fill in the blanks in Part B.*

I. PERSONAL GOALS

   A. Time Investment   Increase/decrease the time I invest in my practice by
                         _____ hours now, and by _____ hours in 5 years.

   B. Time for Self   Increase my time off by _____ hours now, and by
                         _____ hours within 5 years.

   C. Time with Family   Increase the time with my family each week by
                         _____ hours now, and by _____ hours within 5
                         years.

   D. Financial   Increase my income by $_____ each year for the
                         next 5 years.

   F. Retirement   Begin slowing down my practice in _____years, and
                         retire in _____ years.

II. PROFESSIONAL GOALS

   A. Educational   Increase my time spent yearly on CME by _____
                         days.

   B. Teaching   Devote _____ hours a month to teaching.

   C. Organizational   Increase/decrease my time in organizational activi-
                         ties by _____ hours a month.

                         Maximize my effectiveness in the office and time
                         with patients.

   D. Nonmedical   Devote more/less time to nonmedical business ac-
                         tivities.

III. PRACTICE GOALS

   A. Time   Increase/reduce my time in direct patient care by
                         _____ hours a day.

                         Increase/decrease the time I spend with each patient
                         by _____ minutes.

                         Increase/decrease the time I devote daily to my prac-
                         tice by _____ hours.

B. Accessibility

Increase/decrease my accessibility to my patients now.

Increase/decrease my accessibility to my patients within the next 5 years.

C. Daily Patient Load

Increase/decrease my average daily patient load by _____ patients.

See _____ patients a day within the next 5 years.

D. Practice Patient Load

Increase/decrease my practice by _____ patients/families a month to have the number I want in 5 years.

E. Patient Mix

Identify my current patient and disease mix and adjust it to my wants/needs.

F. New Services

Identify new services I want to offer and begin a plan to develop and infuse them in my practice.

G. Physical Space

Determine if my physical plant is large and flexible enough for current and future needs.

H. Addition of Partners

Measure the need for additional partners and the practice growth needed to support them.

Appendix B

Demographic Analysis

Part A: Situation Factors

Physicians often spend years deciding on a community in which to set up practice, then give little time to choosing a location within that community. When well-established doctors begin to feel the pinch of competition, they examine everything about their practice—except its location. Where your practice is located can be a critical factor in its eventual success or failure. This demographic analysis will help you set important goals to incorporate into your marketing plan. It applies equally to new physicians looking for their first location, as well as to physicians who are already well-established in their communities.

I. THE COMPETITIVE ENVIRONMENT

A. Physicians

1. How many physicians are in your current and potential practice environment?

   a. In your specialty? _____

   b. In competitive specialties? _____

   c. Others? _____

2. Are these physicians accepting new patients?

   a. In your specialty? Yes/No

   b. In competitive specialties? Yes/No

   c. Others? Yes/No

3. What is the average physician's age?

   a. In your specialty? _____

   b. In competitive specialties? _____

   c. Others? _____

4. How many new physicians have moved into the community practice area in the past 5 years?

   a. In your specialty? _____

   b. In competitive specialties? _____

   c. Others? _____

B. Nonphysicians

   1. How many nonphysician providers work independently in your community?

      a. In your specialty? _____

      b. In competitive specialties? _____

      c. Others? _____

   2. Are these providers in competition with you?   Yes/No

C. Hospitals

   1. How many hospitals are in your community? _____

   2. Do these hospitals provide competitive outpatient services? _____

      a. Emergency room?   Yes/No

      b. Primary care?   Yes/No

      c. Surgery?   Yes/No

      d. Counseling?   Yes/No

      e. Others? _____   Yes/No

      _____

   3. The following pertain to hospital policies:

      a. Is there a department for your specialty?   Yes/No

      b. Is there an "open staff" policy?   Yes/No

      c. Are privileges restricted?   Yes/No?

      d. Is there a cost-containment requirement?   Yes/No

   4. How many new physicians have been added to the staff within the past year?

      a. In your specialty? _____

      b. In competitive specialties? _____

      c. Others? _____

D. Alternative Delivery Centers

   1. Are competitive, alternative delivery centers operating in the community?   Yes/No

   2. How many:

      a. Freestanding emergency centers? _____

      b. Primary-care centers? _____

      c. Ambulatory surgical centers? _____

      d. Diagnostic testing centers? _____

      e. Industrial/workers' compensation clinics? _____

f. Others? _____

E. Alternative Delivery Systems

1. How many alternative systems function within the community? _____

   a. HMO _____

   b. IPA _____

   c. PPO _____

   d. Others _____

2. Are these systems a major competitive force within the community?

   a. HMO   Yes/No

   b. IPA   Yes/No

   c. PPO   Yes/No

   d. Others   Yes/No

3. Are these systems the trend in the community?
   If yes, are they likely to affect your practice?

   a. HMO   Yes/No

   b. IPA   Yes/No

   c. PPO   Yes/No

   d. Others   Yes/No

4. Does the medical community view these systems favorably?

   a. HMO   Yes/No

   b. IPA   Yes/No

   c. PPO   Yes/No

   d. Others   Yes/No

5. Are there plans for alternative systems in the future?   Yes/No

6. Do the major businesses/industries in the community require, or will they require, their employees to join these prepaid systems?

   a. HMO   Yes/No

   b. IPA   Yes/No

   c. PPO   Yes/No

   d. Others   Yes/No

II. COMMUNITY DEMOGRAPHICS

A. Population

1. What is the population of the community? _____

2. How did the number change in the past 5 years?

Increased by _____ Decreased by _____

3. Is the community considered transient?   Yes/No

4. What is the population of the area from which your patients do and will come?   _____

5. What is the physician-patient ratio?   _____

B. Age Distribution

   1. Pediatric

      a. Number and enrollment of nurseries and day-care centers?   _____

      b. Number of deliveries within the community per year? _____

      c. Number and enrollment of schools?   _____

   2. Demographic

      a. Number of new families that moved into the community in the past year?   _____

      b. Number of new houses/subdivisions?   _____

      c. Number of new family apartments?   _____

      d. Number of new single apartments?   _____

      e. Membership growth of area churches?   _____

      f. Number of new employment applications?   _____

   3. Geriatric

      a. Number of retirement/nursing homes?   _____

      b. Presence of older established neighborhoods?   Yes/No

      c. Number of families with older members living with them?   _____

   4. Do these age distributions correlate with the services that you provide?   Yes/No

C. Economics

   1. What is the percentage of unemployment in the area?   _____ %

   2. What are the major industries and businesses?

      a. High tech?   Yes/No

      b. Heavy industry?   Yes/No

      c. Agriculture?   Yes/No

      d. Other?   Yes/No

   3. Are new businesses opening?   Yes/No

   4. Are established businesses: Hiring? _____ or Laying Off? _____

   5. What is the average income of your practice area? $_____

III. LOCATION OF PRACTICE

A. Strategic Signs

1. Is your current/potential practice location situated near the patients (target markets) you want to affect in terms of:

    a. Age? — Yes/No

    b. Specialty? — Yes/No

    c. Income? — Yes/No

2. Is your location highly visible? — Yes/No

3. Is it near competitive alternative delivery systems? — Yes/No

4. Is it near physicians who will be competing with you? — Yes/No

5. Are competitive systems/physicians located between your office and your target populations? — Yes/No

6. Will your location allow practice expansion? — Yes/No

B. Accessibility

1. Is your setting near major transportation arteries? — Yes/No

2. Are you near public transportation? — Yes/No

3. Does traffic congestion make it difficult to get to you? — Yes/No

4. Do you have adequate parking and access for:

    a. Patients and staff? — Yes/No

    b. Handicapped patients? — Yes/No

    c. Ambulance loading? — Yes/No

C. Patient Convenience

1. Is your practice within 30 minutes of the majority of your patients? — Yes/No

2. Is it near the offices of most physicians to whom you refer patients? — Yes/No

3. Is it near the emergency room and other facilities you use? — Yes/No

4. Is it near other services, such as shopping malls, day-care centers, and businesses? — Yes/No

5. Do your patients consider your location safe and secure? — Yes/No

D. Personal Convenience

1. Is your office conveniently close to the hospitals and nursing homes you visit? — Yes/No

2. Is it convenient to your residence? — Yes/No

When you've done the research necessary to complete Part A, you're ready to prepare your analysis summary and draw up your demographic marketing goals in Part B.

Part B: Summary and Goals

I. THE COMPETITIVE ENVIRONMENT

A. Physicians

Situation Analysis: _____

Marketing Goal: _____

B. Nonphysicians

Situation Analysis: _____

Marketing Goal: _____

C. Hospitals

Situation Analysis: _____

Marketing Goal: _____

D. Alternative Delivery Centers

Situation Analysis: _____

Marketing Goal: _____

E. Alternative Delivery Systems (HMOs, PPOs, etc.)

Situation Analysis: _____

Marketing Goal: _____

II. COMMUNITY DEMOGRAPHICS

A. Population

Situation Analysis: _____

Marketing Goal: _____

B. Age Distribution

Situation Analysis: _____

Marketing Goal: _____

C. Economics

Situation Analysis: _____

Marketing Goal: _____

III. LOCATION OF PRACTICE

A. Strategic Signs

Situation Analysis: _____

Marketing Goal: _____

B. Accessibility

Situation Analysis: _____

Marketing Goal: _____

C. Patient Convenience

Situation Analysis: _____

Marketing Goal: _____

D. Personal Convenience

   Situation Analysis: _____

   Marketing Goal: _____

Appendix C

Practice Survey

Here are the major factors to include in a thorough survey of the effectiveness of a medical practice. Questions can be adapted to your own situation and needs, or you may choose to adapt the completed Patient Survey in Appendix D.

I. PATIENT ATTITUDES TOWARD:

A. Your Specialty

1. Do your patients understand what your specialty has to offer?
2. Do they understand the comprehensiveness of your care?

B. Your Physical Plant

1. Is your location convenient to the majority of your patients?
2. Is your waiting room comfortable and relaxing?
3. Are poor parking facilities a hindrance to your practice?

C. Front Office Personnel

1. Is your staff friendly and courteous?
2. Are calls handled promptly and courteously?
3. Do patients receive adequate help with their medical insurance claims?
4. Are your business policies (i.e., credit, cash, payment plans) adequately explained?

D. Nursing Personnel

1. Are your nurses friendly and courteous?
2. Are they sympathetic to patient suffering?
3. Do they give enough information to patients?

E. Doctor(s)

1. Do your patients feel you are courteous and friendly?
2. Do they feel you are interested in them as people as well as patients?
3. Do they feel you spend enough time with them?
4. Do they feel you give them enough information about their problems?
5. Do they feel other doctors in the practice (if any) give them the help and information they need?

F. Waiting Time

1. Do patients feel they spend too much time in the waiting room before seeing you?
2. Do they feel they wait too long in the examining room before you see them?

G. After-Hours and Weekend Care

1. Do patients have difficulty reaching you after hours?
2. Is your answering service prompt and courteous?
3. Are the doctors prompt in returning patients' calls?
4. If other doctors are in your practice, are your patients satisfied with their service when they're on call?
5. If doctors outside your practice are in your call rotation, are your patients satisfied with the care they provide?

H. Ancillary Services and Facilities (i.e., Lab, X-ray, Emergency Room, and Hospital)

1. Do your patients resent it when you have to use other facilities?
2. Are those other facilities convenient to your patients?
3. Are their staffs courteous and helpful to your patients?
4. Do problems arise when they bill your patients?
5. Are your patients satisfied with the hospital you use?

I. Your Fees

1. Do patients consider your fees too high?
2. Do your payment policies present problems for your patients?
3. Are your patients going to other facilities for emergency care because they see them as less expensive or more convenient?

II. PATIENT NEEDS

A. Scheduling

1. Do patients have difficulty scheduling appointments convenient to them?
2. Is your staff sympathetic to patients' scheduling needs?
3. Do patients consider your office hours convenient?

Appendix D

Patient Survey

Questionnaire Covering Letter

This is an example of the kind of covering message that should accompany your patient questionnaire. You should, of course, tailor it to your own situation.

Dear Patient:

We here at Center Street Family Practice Clinic want to provide you and your family with the highest quality health care possible in a comprehensive, compassionate, and cost-effective manner. To help us evaluate our effectiveness, we would like your opinions about us. Your answers and suggestions on the following questionnaire will help us continue to improve the health care we provide you and your family. So won't you please take a few moments to give us this important information?

Thank you,

Dr. _____ and Staff

Questionnaire

This is a patient questionnaire designed for a family practice. You can easily adapt it to your own practice.

I. ABOUT YOURSELF

Age: _____   Name (optional): _____

Sex: _____

Address: _____

Marital Status: Single _____ Married _____ Widow(er) _____

Name and Age of Spouse: _____

Names and Ages of Children: _____

Occupation: Yours _____ Spouse _____

Education: Yours _____ Spouse _____

Household Income: _____

Best Times for Appointments: _____

1. Are we the main source of health care for your family?   Yes___ No___

2. If members of your family are seeing other physicians, please tell us who and why.

Spouse _____

Children _____

Other _____

II. OUR SPECIALTY AND SERVICES

3. Do you feel you understand the specialty of our practice?   Yes___ No___

4. Do you believe you are aware of all the services we offer?   Yes___ No___

III. PHYSICAL PLANT

5. Is the location of our office convenient?   Yes___ No___

6. Do you find our waiting room comfortable?   Yes___ No___

7. Do you feel relaxed in the waiting room?   Yes___ No___

8. Are our parking facilities adequate?   Yes___ No___

9. Do you have to pay to park when you come to see us?   Yes___ No___

10. If yes, is this a hindrance to receiving your care here?   Yes___ No___

11. What changes would you make in the physical aspects of our office? _____

_____

_____

IV. FRONT OFFICE PERSONNEL

12. Do you find our front office personnel (secretary, receptionist):

Friendly?   Yes___ No___

Courteous?   Yes___ No___

13. Do you find our business personnel (office manager, bookkeeper):

Friendly?   Yes___ No___

Courteous?   Yes___ No___

14. Are your phone calls handled in a prompt, courteous manner?   Yes___ No___

15. Are you receiving adequate help with your insurance?   Yes___ No___

16. If you need help with your insurance, can we help?   Yes___ No___

17. Have you received a copy of our business policies?   Yes___ No___

18. Have our payment and billing policies been explained to your satisfaction?   Yes____ No____

19. Do our payment and billing policies create difficulties for you?   Yes____ No____

V.   NURSES

20. Do you find our nurses: Friendly/   Yes____ No____
                                         Courteous?   Yes____ No____

21. Do you feel our nurses are sympathetic to your illness?   Yes____ No____

22. Do our nurses give you enough information about their part in your care, such as telling you what your weight and blood pressure are?   Yes____ No____

VI.   DOCTORS

23. Do you find the doctor(s):   Friendly?   Yes____ No____
                                         Courteous   Yes____ No____

24. Does the doctor tell you enough about your illness?   Yes____ No____

25. Do you feel the doctor is interested in you as a person?   Yes____ No____

26. Does the doctor spend enough time with you?   Yes____ No____

27. Does the doctor give you enough health-care information, such as booklets on diet, exercise, and smoking?   Yes____ No____

28. Do you feel the doctor is interested in your health?   Yes____ No____

VII.   WAITING TIME

29. Is your wait too long in the reception area before you are called to see the doctor?   Yes____ No____

30. Do you have to wait too long in the examination room before the doctor sees you?   Yes____ No____

VII.   AFTER-HOURS AND WEEKEND CARE

31. Do you have difficulty reaching us after hours?   Yes____ No____

32. Do you know the number for our answering service?   Yes____ No____

33. Is our answering service prompt and courteous?   Yes____ No____

34. Do our doctors promptly return your calls?   Yes____ No____

35. If you see a doctor in this practice other than your regular doctor, are you as satisfied with the care you receive?   Yes____ No____

36. If doctors other than those in this practice share after-hours calls with us, are you satisfied with the care they provide?   Yes____ No____

IX. PHONE CALLS

37. Are your phone calls to the doctors during the day returned promptly?   Yes___ No___

38. Do you mind if the nurses handle some of your calls?   Yes___ No___

X. ANCILLARY SERVICES

39. Do you find it inconvenient to go someplace else for certain X-rays or lab tests?   Yes___ No___

40. Do you find the staff at these other facilities:
           Friendly?   Yes___ No___
           Courteous?   Yes___ No___
If no, at which facilities? _____

41. Is the emergency room we use convenient?   Yes___ No___
If no, which one would be more convenient? ____

42. Do you find separate billing by these other facilities inconvenient?   Yes___ No___

43. Are you satisfied with the hospital we use?   Yes___ No___

44. Is this hospital convenient for you and your family?   Yes___ No___

XI. COST OF SERVICES

45. Do you feel that our fees are:
           High?   Yes___ No___
           Average?   Yes___ No___
           Low?   Yes___ No___

46. Are you familiar with our credit and billing policies?   Yes___ No___

47. Have you used other health services (such as an emergency clinic) because you felt it would be less expensive?   Yes___ No___
If yes, which one(s)? _____

XII. SCHEDULING

48. Do you have trouble getting an appointment as soon as you would like?   Yes___ No___

49. Are our secretaries helpful in finding appointments that meet your needs?   Yes___ No___

50. Are our office hours convenient for you? If no, how could we arrange our hours to best serve you?

XIII. EDUCATIONAL INFORMATION

51. Does your doctor give you enough information about your:
           Illness?   Yes___ No___
           Medicine?   Yes___ No___
           Health?   Yes___ No___

52. Would you like more educational information from us?   Yes___ No___

53. Would you accept this information from the nurses?   Yes____ No____

54. If we had audiovisual tapes available on your problem, would you use them?   Yes____ No____

55. Would you want to get a health newsletter from us periodically?   Yes____ No____

XVI.   SERVICES OFFERED

56. Are you satisfied with the range of services provided by this practice?   Yes____ No____

57. Do you believe you know all the services we offer?   Yes____ No____

58. Are there any specific services that you would like to see us provide?   Yes____ No____

    Examples: Pediatric care?   Yes____ No____
                                  Care for elderly?   Yes____ No____
                                  Minor surgery?   Yes____ No____
                                  Diet counseling?   Yes____ No____
                                  Stress reduction?   Yes____ No____

    Others: _____

XV.   REFERRAL

59. How were you referred to this practice?
Other patients_____ Friends_____ Yellow Pages_____
Medical society_____ Another doctor_____ Our reputation_____
Other: _____

60. Are you satisfied with the care we provide to refer other people to us?   Yes____ No____

XVI.   COMMENTS

Please use the space below for any additional comments you may have.

_____

_____

_____

_____

XVII.   SIGNATURE (optional) _____

Data Analysis Method

Step 1. Record the total number of Yes and No responses by question.

    2. Record the percentages of both the Yes and No responses for each question. Calculate the percentages by dividing the number of Yes responses by the total number of responses. Do the same for the No responses.

    3. Record the Yes and No percentages for each question (see following Tabulation Sheet).

    4. Assign a marketing priority number to each question (see subsequent Data Analysis Tally) by using the following classification:

RESPONSE PERCENTAGE	PRIORITY
0 - 25	4
26 - 50	3
51 - 75	2
76 - 100	1

5. Compile lists of your marketing problems by their priorities. (See Marketing Problems and Assets Priority List, page 243.)

6. Determine and list the strengths and weaknesses of your practice. (See Top Practice Strengths and Weaknesses, page 245.)

7. You are now ready to develop a plan of action for each of your practice problems.

Tabulation Sheet
(500 Respondents)

Q	Yes	No	% Yes	% No	Q	Yes	No	% Yes	% No	Q	Yes	No	% Yes	% No
1.	400	100	80	20	21.	480	20	96	4	41.	100	400	20	80
2.	—	—	—	—	22.	420	80	84	16	42.	450	50	90	10
3.	350	150	70	30	23.	500	—	100	0	43.	500	—	100	0
4.	300	200	60	40	24.	100	400	20	80	44.	500	—	100	0
5.	400	100	80	20	25.	500	—	100	0	45.	—	—	—	—
6.	450	50	90	10	26.	150	350	30	70	46.	500	—	100	0
7.	450	50	90	10	27.	50	450	10	90	47.	450	50	90	10
8.	500	—	100	0	28.	500	—	100	0	48.	100	400	20	80
9.	480	20	96	4	29.	400	100	80	20	49.	450	50	90	10
10.	—	500	0	100	30.	100	400	20	80	50.	150	350	30	70
11.	—	—	—	—	31.	50	450	10	90	51.	—	—	—	—
12.	300	200	60	40	32.	400	100	80	20	52.	400	100	80	20
13.	300	200	60	40	33.	300	200	60	40	53.	400	100	80	20
14.	200	300	40	60	34.	350	150	70	30	54.	400	100	80	20
15.	350	150	70	30	35.	500	—	100	0	55.	500	—	100	0
16.	—	—	—	—	36.	500	—	100	0	56.	300	200	60	40
17.	100	400	20	80	37.	450	50	90	10	57.	400	100	80	20
18.	200	300	40	60	38.	300	200	60	40	58.	400	100	80	20
19.	400	100	80	20	39.	300	200	60	40	59.	—	—	—	—
20.	450	50	90	10	40.	400	100	80	20	60.	450	50	90	10

Data Analysis Tally

Area of Practice	Question	Issue Analyzed	Response Percentage	Marketing Priority
I. Demographics	1.	Treatment of entire family	No 20	4
II. Specialty	3.	Understanding of specialty	No 30	3
	4.	Awareness of range of services	No 40	3
III. Physical Plant	5.	Convenience of location	No 20	4

Area of Practice	Question	Issue Analyzed	Response Percentage		Marketing Priority
	6.	Comfort of reception area	No	10	4
	7.	Relaxing environment	No	10	4
	8.	Adequacy of parking	No	0	4
	9.	Parking charge	Yes	96	1
	10.	Parking hindrance	Yes	0	4
IV. Front Office Personnel	12.	Front office friendliness	No	40	3
		Front office courtesy	No	40	3
	13.	Business office friendliness	No	40	3
		Business office courtesy	No	40	3
	14.	Handling of phone calls	No	60	2
	15.	Help with insurance	No	30	3
	16.	Need specific help with insurance	Yes	70	2
	17.	Awareness of business policies	No	80	1
	18.	Explanation of business policies	No	60	2
	19.	Difficulty with billing policies	Yes	80	1
V. Nurses	20.	Friendliness of nursing staff	No	10	4
		Courtesy of nursing staff	No	10	4
	21.	Empathy of nursing staff	No	4	4
	22.	Health information provided by nurses	No	16	4
VI. Doctors	23.	Friendliness of doctors	No	0	4
		Courtesy of doctors	No	0	4
	24.	Information provided about illness	No	80	1
	25.	Interest in patients as people	No	0	4

Area of Practice	Question	Issue Analyzed	Response	Percentage	Marketing Priority
	26.	Enough time spent with patients	No	70	3
	27.	Health information provided	No	90	1
	28.	Interest shown in health of patients	No	0	4
VII. Waiting Time	29.	Reception area time too long	Yes	80	1
	30.	Exam room wait too long	Yes	20	4
VIII. After-Hours and Weekend Care	31.	Difficulty reaching after hours	Yes	10	4
	32.	Knowledge of how to reach after hours	No	20	4
	33.	Promptness of answering service	No	40	3
	34.	Promptness of doctors returning calls	No	30	3
	35.	Satisfaction with partners' care	No	0	4
	36.	Satisfaction with those who share calls	No	10	4
IX. Phone Calls	37.	Promptness in returning calls	No	10	4
	38.	Nurses handling calls	Yes	60	2
X. Ancillary Services	39.	Convenience of ancillary services	Yes	60	2
	40.	Friendliness of ancillary staffs	No	20	4
		Courtesy of ancillary staffs	No	20	4
	41.	Convenience of emergency room	No	80	1
	42.	Inconvenience of separate billing	Yes	90	1
	43.	Satisfaction with hospital	No	0	4
	44.	Convenience of hospital	No	0	4
XI. Cost of Services	45.	Fees too high	Yes	20	4
	46.	Understanding of credit/billing	No	0	4

Area of Practice	Question	Issue Analyzed	Response Percentage		Marketing Priority
	47.	Use of other services	Yes	90	1
XII. Scheduling	48.	Scheduling problems	Yes	20	4
	49.	Assistance with scheduling	No	10	4
	50.	Convenience of office hours	No	70	2
XIII. Educational Information	51.	Desire for information on:			
		Illness	No	70	2
		Medicines	No	60	2
		Health	No	70	2
	52.	Desire for more educational information	Yes	80	1
	53.	Nurses as providers of health information	Yes	80	1
	54.	Audiovisual aids	Yes	80	1
	55.	Newsletter	Yes	100	1
XIV. Services Offered	56.	Satisfaction with services	No	0	4
	57.	Awareness of present services	No	20	4
	58.	Desire for specific services:	Yes	80	1
		Pediatrics	Yes	70	2
		Geriatrics	Yes	60	2
		Minor surgery	Yes	40	3
		Diet counseling	Yes	50	3
		Stress reduction	Yes	10	4
XV. Referral	59.	Referral by %:			
		Friends		10	
		Patients		70	
		Yellow Pages		0	
		Medical society		5	
		Doctors		15	
		Reputation		0	
	60.	Satisfaction with practice	No	10	4

Marketing Problems and Assets Priority List
(Patient problems to address)

Have to pay for parking
Not aware of business policies
Billing policies difficult
Doctor tell more about illness
More health-care information
Too long in reception area
Emergency room inconvenient

Separate billing inconvenient
Use less expensive services
More educational information
Would use audiovisual aids
Interested in newsletter
Offer more specific services

SECOND PRIORITY

Improve telephone promptness and courtesy
Help with insurance
Explain payment and business policies
Let nurses handle calls
Ancillary services inconvenient
Give more information about illness, medicine, and health
Provide pediatric services
Provide geriatric services

THIRD PRIORITY

Don't understand specialty
Not aware of range of services
Improve front office friendliness and courtesy
Improve business office friendliness and courtesy
Want more time with doctor
Faster answers to calls
Provide diet counseling
Provide minor surgical services

FOURTH PRIORITY (Practice strengths to promote)

Treatment of entire family
Convenience of location
Comfort of reception area
Relaxing environment
Adequacy of parking
Friendliness and courtesy of nursing staff
Empathy of nursing staff
Nurses providing information
Friendliness and courtesy of physicians
Interest in patients as people
Interest in health of patients
Examining room time
Difficulty reaching after hours
Accessibility after hours
Satisfaction with partners' care
Satisfaction with those who share call
Friendliness and courtesy of ancillary staffs
Cost of care
Understand credit/billing
Scheduling appointments
Assistance with scheduling
Satisfaction with services
Awareness of services

Satisfaction with practice
Satisfaction with hospital
Convenience of hospital

Top Practice Strengths and Weaknesses

STRENGTHS TO UPHOLD	WEAKNESSES TO ADDRESS
Comprehensive Services	Paying for Parking
Convenience	Physicians not Informing Patients
Adequate Parking	Inadequate Information about Policies
Staff	Inadequate Health-Care Information
Physician Attitude	Inconvenient Emergency Room
Accessibility	Too Much Waiting Time
Pricing	Not Enough Specific Services
Scheduling	No Practice Newsletter
Overall Satisfaction	

Appendix E

FTC Policy Statement Regarding Advertising Substantiation

The Federal Trade Commission requires that advertisers must have "a reasonable basis" for advertising claims. Specifically, the FTC policy statement regarding advertising substantiation says:

"The Commission intends to continue vigorous enforcement of this existing legal requirement that advertisers substantiate express and implied claims, however conveyed, that make objective assertions about the item or service advertised. Objective claims for products or services represent explicitly or by implication that the advertiser has a reasonable basis supporting these claims. These representations of substantiation are material to consumers. That is, consumers would be less likely to rely on claims for products and services if they knew the advertiser did not have a reasonable basis for believing them to be true. Therefore, a firm's failure to possess and rely upon a reasonable basis for objective claims constitutes an unfair and deceptive act or practice in violation of Section 5 of the Federal Trade Commission Act."

STANDARDS FOR PRIOR SUBSTANTIATION

Many ads contain express or implied statements regarding the amount of support the advertiser has for the product claim. When the substantiation claim is express (e.g., "tests prove," "doctors recommend," and "studies show"), the Commission expects the firm to have at least the advertised level of substantiation. Of course, an ad may imply more substantiation than it expressly claims or may imply to consumers that the firm has a certain type of support; in such cases, the advertiser must possess the amount and type of substantiation the ad actually communicates to consumers.

Absent an express or implied reference to a certain level of support, and absent other evidence indicating what consumer expectations would be, the Commission assumes that consumers expect a "reasonable basis" for claims. The Commission's determination of what constitutes a reasonable basis depends, as it does in an unfairness analysis, on a number of factors relevant to the benefits and costs of substantiating a particular claim. These factors include: the type of claim, the product, the consequences of a false claim, the benefits of a truthful claim, the cost of developing substantiation for the claim, and the amount of substantiation experts in the field believe is reasonable. Extrinsic evidence, such as expert testimony or consumer surveys, is useful to determine what level of substantiation consumers expect to support a particular product claim and the adequacy of evidence an advertiser possesses.

One issue the Commission examined was substantiation for implied claims. Although firms are unlikely to possess substantiation for implied claims they do not believe the ad makes, they should generally be aware of reasonable interpretations and will be expected to have prior substantiation for such claims. The Commission will take care to assure that it only challenges reasonable interpretations of advertising claims.*

*Individual Commissioners have expressed differing views as to how claims should be interpreted so that advertisers are not held to outlandish or tenuous interpretations. Notwithstanding these variations in approach, the focus of all Commissioners on reasonable interpretations of claims is intended to ensure that advertisers are not required to substantiate claims that were not made.

Appendix F

How to Use a Printer

Printing sales representatives can be extremely helpful. But first it helps to have some basic information about the printing and graphics business, and to know the difference between various printers.

There are three types of print shops:

1. The quick printer. Best for simple flyers, one-color business packages (business cards/letterhead/envelopes).
2. The full-service printer. For jobs requiring complicated services such as bleeds, close registration, several ink colors, etc.
3. The two-color shop. Handles a cross-section of mid-range jobs, but not geared for the very simple or very complex printing job.

Here are some tips for getting a quality print job no matter what type of job it is or printer who does it.

1. Don't go to a two-color shop or a full-service printer for a small or very simple job. They're not geared to handle such work (although they may accept it), and their prices (higher) and turnaround time (relatively slow) will probably reflect it.
2. By the same token, don't expect a quick printer to do a high quality print job on a three-color newsletter with several screens, photos and bleeds. Again, the quick-printer may say yes to the job, but the results won't be the best.
3. Consider a *printing broker* if you want to get out of the printing game. Most larger cities have several. A broker shops around for you, getting the best price from the best place. Brokers often deal with trade shops (printers that aren't open to the public) and with printers that don't employ a sales staff. So you're not paying a marked-up price for the broker's services, and you usually will get a good deal without the hassle of price shopping.
4. But if you can't or won't use a broker, solicit at least three bids for the same job. There can be as much as 25 percent variance.

When getting bids, be sure to give all printers the same specifications. If a printer substitutes in his bid (e.g., recommends a substitute paper instead of the one specified) ask why and get a sample. Be prepared to provide bidding printers with these specifics:

- Quantity
- Size (flat and finished—folded) and number of pages if it's a multi-page piece.

- Paper stock: type, weight, and color (e.g., Strathmore text 80 pound ivory). Your layout artist or printer sales rep can help with this.
- The color of ink(s). Ink color is usually referred to by PMS number. This is a standardized color coding system used by all artists and printers. Thus when the artist specifies on your newsletter PMS 241, the printer knows exactly what ink color to mix. Also, when the job is reprinted, or the next issue is printed, the ink will match.
- Number of *stripping element*. Photos, screens, certain logos and other graphic elements must be handled separately when a printing job is being set up. The printer must know how many elements must be stripped in.
- Bleeds. A bleed is any ink that goes to the edge of the page—whether it's a block of color or a thin line. A bleed requires a larger paper, which then is cut down to the finished size.
- Type of proof required. Always request a proof of your job. A quick printer will usually give you a simple copy-machine proof; others will provide a "blue-line." Both are exact representatives of the final product; they give you the chance to check for crooked copy, photos in the wrong location, broken letters or lines, spots on the page and other errors or omissions.
- Turnaround time. Be sure to get a commitment from the printer on when he'll complete the job when you get a price quote. Ten working days turnaround is the industry standard for full-service printers, although often they can complete a non-complex job in less time. A quick-printer usually requires from 2 to 4 days for a simple job.
- Mailing or bindery requirements. If your printer will be handling mailing, he'll need to know if the job is a self-mailer or to be inserted in an envelope, if there's a Business Reply Card, where additional pieces are inserted, whether it's first class or bulk rate, etc.
- Packaging and shipping instructions (particularly if the job is not to be shipped to the billing location).

Go directly to the sales manager when requesting a printing representative. Expect an experienced, knowledgeable individual. If you don't get one, find another printer.

It's a good idea to bring the printer into the picture when you first meet with your public relations or advertising agency or designer to discuss your print job, rather than at the end when the job is completed. A good printer's rep can recommend measures that will save time, money or both, such as a special printing technique, an alternative size, a paper stock the printer has on hand and can save you money.

Don't get too many printing quotes; three are plenty. And once you've found a good, reasonably priced, dependable printer, rely on the firm for future jobs. You'll get better service when you're a steady customer, and the printer will know your needs, likes and dislikes.

Once you find a good printer, trust his or her judgment. Your printer wants to make you look good. The quality of your printed piece reflects on the printer as well.

And finally, be realistic in your task and price expectations. We recall a physician who called a printer sales rep in a panic with a big job that he needed to have printed within five days. It was an 8½" × 11" flyer to be printed in three colors on both sides. It needed typesetting, artwork and design, and was to be folded and inserted with a business reply card into an envelope. Both the BRC and envelope also had to be printed. The doctor needed a quantity of 2,000. After some quick work, the rep found a typesetter and mailhouse that could handle the job in the requested time frame. But the physician balked at the price—$700—and took the job to a printer on his own. Unfortunately, he didn't have anyone acting on his behalf to be certain the job was done properly. The postage indicia was incorrectly printed on the BRC and the post office would not accept the mailing. As a result, the whole job had to be tossed since the physician missed his deadline.

PRINTING TERMS YOU SHOULD KNOW

Letter-fold: Also called U fold. Standard business-letter fold.

Z fold: Also called accordion fold. Alternative method of folding a single-sheet printed piece.

Finished size: Size of a printed piece after it has been folded, e.g., a brochure that is $8\frac{1}{2}'' \times 11''$ opened out (flat) that is given a letter fold has a finished size of $3\frac{11}{16}'' \times 8\frac{1}{2}''$.

Embossing: Raised or relief design or type (e.g., a logo) on a page. Often it is imprinted with ink.

Blind embossing: Embossed design that is not inked.

Die cut: Design that is cut out of a page with a custom die.

Registration: Placement of two or more ink colors. Close registration refers to two or more ink colors that are very close to each other or touching, requiring exacting placement in order to avoid blurring of the final product. There is usually an added charge for close registration.

Line art: Illustration that does not need to be stripped in by the printer, as do photos (halftones) and screens. Line art can be treated like type.

Bleed: Ink that runs to the edge of the page, e.g., a rule, a photo or artwork that goes to the edge of the page is considered a *bleed*.

Coverage: Smooth, even ink application, with no light and dark in solid ink areas.

Screen: Application of ink that results in a lighter tone due to use of a screen that prevents solid coverage in the area. Using screens judiciously can give the appearance of a second color. For instance, black (100% ink coverage) can be screened back to 60% or 50% or 20% to look like grey.

Coated stock: Paper that has a polished surface. Reproduction is better, colors are crisper, photos sharper on coated stock. Coated stock is usually more costly than uncoated. Most slick magazines are printed on coated stock.

Scoring: Pre-creasing a page to prevent rippling or crinkling when folded. Heavy stock should be scored for a smooth fold.

Page: One side of a sheet.

Sheet: A piece of paper that may be folded or not. A *sheet* consists of four pages if it is folded in half. A four-page $8\frac{1}{2}'' \times 11''$ newsletter usually is printed on an $11'' \times 17''$ sheet.

Binding: How the pages of a printed piece are attached. Examples of bindings are:

Saddle stitch: Staple(s) in the fold of a printed piece. A saddle stitch binding can be used for 200 or more pages.

Velo bind: A plastic strip that is attached via heat to individual stacked pages. Can be used for thick documents, but it is best for short runs (e.g., 10 copies of a 100 page proposal).

Spiral bind: Wire binding inserted in pages that have been hole-punched.

GBC or comb binding: Similar to a spiral bind, but the binding is plastic, not wire. A GBC binding allows pages to be added or deleted if necessary.

Perfect bind: Pages are glued to a flat spine. Best for large runs. Most magazines and paperback books are perfect bound.

Color key: Indicates where ink colors are to be printed on a multi-color piece. A color key should always be requested on a four-color job, and on any 2 or more color piece where exact placement of ink colors is critical.

Typography: Headline and body copy that has been typeset. Typesetting terms you should know:

Serif: Fine-line cross strokes at the top and bottom of letters of type.

Sans Serif: Typeface without serifs.

Bullets: Series of dots, squares, etc. used to call attention to key points.

Folio: Page number. Right hand pages always have odd numbers.

Font: An assortment of type of all one style.

Justify: To adjust spacing in a line so that all lines are equally long.

Leading: Spacing between lines of type. Type that is set solid (no leading) or with very little leading is unpleasant to read.

Point: Refers to vertical type size. There are 72 points to an inch. Most body copy is set 10 or 11 point. For elderly individuals, 11 point is the minimum size you should use, and 12 point may be better (depending on application, amount of type, etc.).

Stet: A term meaning "let it stand." Used to cancel a change or correction indicated on a proof.

Runaround: Type that must fit around an illustration or headline or photo.

Appendix G

Mailing Information

There are less costly ways than first class to mail a large quantity of print material (such as newsletters, invitations and flyers). Options and requirements for these rates are listed below. Since this information is subject to change, it's best to check with the post office before determining your method of mailing.

PRE-SORT FIRST CLASS

This method is less costly than regular first class but just as speedy. It does require extra work, however.

- You must have a minimum of 500 zip-coded pieces.
- They must be pre-sorted:
    1. Ten or more pieces with the same zip code must be bundled together.
    2. Fifty or more pieces with the same three-digit zip code prefix must be grouped together.
    3. Mail that cannot be separated this way is counted toward the minimum number of pieces, but does not qualify for the lower postage rate.
- Postage may be paid for with a postage meter, a pre-printed permit, or pre-canceled stamps. Each piece must carry the words "pre-sorted first class" printed or stamped as part of or next to the meter imprint, permit imprint or pre-canceled stamp.
- There is an annual fee which is separate from the authorization fee for a permit imprint system.

THIRD CLASS BULK MAIL

This method costs substantially less than first class; however it's also substantially slower and less reliable. Mail may take up to two weeks to be delivered.

- Five-Digit Pre-sort Level:
    1. A minimum of 200 zip-coded pieces is required.
    2. Each piece must be in a bundle of 10 or more pieces to the same five-digit zip code, and must be sacked to the same five-digit zip code. Each sack must contain a minimum of 50 pieces to the same five-digit zip code. Residual pieces do not count toward the minimum number of pieces, are not eligible for the five-digit presort level, and must be charged at the "basic" level bulk rate.

- Basic Pre-sort Level:
    1. When there are 10 or more pieces with the same five-digit zip code, they must be grouped in five-digit bundles. Bundles with less than 10 pieces with the same five-digit zip code are also packaged in this manner.
    2. After making up five-digit packages, if there are pieces for a multi-zip coded office, group them together in a "city" package.
    3. When there are 10 or more pieces with the same three-digit zip code prefix after you have grouped the five-digit and "city" packages, group them together into three-digit packages. Packages containing less than 10 pieces with the same three-digit zip code prefix are also packaged in the same way, or they can be bundled together. (This is discouraged, however.)
- There is an annual *Third Class Bulk Mail* fee, separate from the authorization fee for a permit imprint system and an application fee.

Contact your local postmaster or postal service customer representative if you have fewer than 200 pieces to mail. They can suggest the best mailing system for you.

You may also wish to check with a mailing house regarding mailing your newsletter. Mailing houses can provide every service, from supplying and affixing mailing labels (yours or theirs) to metering or stamping your publication. Additionally, if you're sending something pre-sort first class, a mailing house can bundle your job in with others to assure that you have the minimum number required in each zip code zone. The following services can improve deliverability and accuracy of your mailing list:

- First Class Automatic Forwarding. All first class mail is forwarded to the new address if it has been provided to the post office. Undeliverable mail is returned to sender along with the reason for nondeliverability if a return address is shown.
- Return Requested Service. You can have printed Return Postage Guaranteed or Forwarding and Return Postage Guaranteed on the envelope to specify what is to be done with undeliverable mail. Third and fourth class mail is returned without an explanation.
- Address Correction Requested. If you print this phrase on the envelope beneath the return address, the post office will provide you with current information on the addressee's name and address. There is a charge for this service.
- Certified Mail. This provides you with proof that the mailed item has been delivered. This is a very expensive service, especially for large mailings.
- Business Reply Mail. Use this special service—available by permit—to allow the addressee to return cards, envelopes or other material without affixing postage. You pay postage (at higher than first class rates) on each item when it is delivered to you. A business reply permit requires a minimum usage each year or it will be canceled by the post office.

Appendix H

Tips for Media Interviews

Like the Boy Scouts, you must *be prepared.* Here are some tips on how to prepare for an interview.

1. Ask the reporter or interviewer to give you a general idea of the focus or theme of the article or interview when he/she calls to schedule one.

2. Try to anticipate and prepare for likely questions, particularly if the issue is sensitive or controversial. It's considered unprofessional to ask for a list of questions, but it's perfectly acceptable to ask about the types of questions or issues likely to be raised.

3. Let medical ethics be your guide during the interview. Your purpose should be to provide new information about medical techniques, treatments and therapies to the public, not to promote yourself. Avoid self-aggrandizing statements implying or stating that the quality of medical care you offer is better or the best. Instead, cite your education, your board certification and special training that can give credibility to your statements.

4. Explain your terms to the reporter when you use technical language. Avoid "medicalese" as much as possible. Chances of misunderstanding or misinterpretation are greatly reduced when you and the reporter speak a common language.

5. Say only those things that you wish to see in print or hear on the air. Going "off the record" or providing information "for background only" is risky. If you absolutely must provide unattributed information, spell out clearly at what point you are off the record and when you go back on the record.

6. When asked a tough or controversial question, or one that requires a very technical answer, take time to think about your response. It may even be appropriate to tell the reporter you'll research the question and get back to him or her if necessary.

7. If a reporter asks a question that seems to be irrelevant, you may diplomatically suggest another more pertinent question—then go ahead and answer it.

8. Avoid answering questions out of your area of expertise. Tell your interviewer it's not your specialty, and suggest others who may be able to speak on the topic.

9. If you've provided very technical or very sensitive information, you may ask the reporter to read back to you his/her notes on that area. Fill in any gaps and correct inaccuracies at that time.

10. Don't ask to review a printed piece prior to publication. Seldom will a reputable newspaper or magazine permit advance scrutiny of an article. Occasionally, however, a reporter will read back to you or show you a very technical or complex portion of an article to ensure accuracy.

11. Be sure to get the reporter's telephone number so that you can get in touch with him/her if you think of additional details after the interview.

Radio and television provide a tremendous opportunity to reach a large audience. The unique needs of the electronic media call for a somewhat different approach to interviews than print media.

1. Always provide a fact sheet prior to a radio or TV interview. It will help to ensure that the interview stays on track. It may even be acceptable to provide a list of suggested questions to be asked. To be safe, ask when you're arranging the interview if the host or producer would like a list of questions submitted prior to the interview. (Be very careful with this. Some will appreciate the effort and interpret it favorably; some may react negatively.)

2. If you haven't provided a list of questions, ask the interviewer in advance what some of the questions are, so you may phrase your responses before the interview begins.

3. Television news stories average 90 to 120 seconds, but the process of setting up for and completing the interview may take an hour or more. Making your answers as concise as possible lessens the chance of a response being edited.

4. Try to ignore cameras and microphones. Speak to your interviewer, not the camera.

5. If you're asked an unexpected or touchy question, pause to gather your thoughts. You can defuse the question with a smile or a subtly humorous answer, or try saying, "It may be more to the point to ask . . . ."

6. For a television interview, make yourself as comfortable as possible, but avoid slouching or leaning back in your chair if you're seated. If it's a swivel chair, don't swivel! Leaning slightly forward suggests interest and enthusiasm.

7. If you have enough notice for a TV interview to plan your attire, try to wear subtle or muted patterns in medium or dark tones, or a pastel blouse or shirt rather than white. Avoid black and white or strongly contrasting colors, busy or flashy patterns.

8. Radio interviews are sometimes done over the telephone and taped. Ask to be told before taping begins.

AFTER THE INTERVIEW

Improve your media relations by following a few rules of etiquette and good sense.

■ Thank the reporter or interviewer in person immediately after the interview.

■ If you've promised to check a fact, provide additional information or otherwise follow up on the interview, be sure to do so in a timely fashion.

■ Have a staff or family member or friend tape a radio or television interview so you can review it later and learn from your fumbled facts, inappropriate or overenthusiastic body language, and other visual or verbal mistakes.

■ Send a written thank-you note to the reporter or program host after the article has appeared or the program has aired. If you received positive comments from patients, colleagues or the public about an interview or article, be sure to mention it. This positive feedback is appreciated.

■ If there's an error in a print piece, inform the reporter politely, but don't expect a retraction or correction the same size or placement as the original story. Minor inaccuracies aren't worth mentioning, particularly if the general tenor of the piece is correct. Nevertheless if it's a serious or damaging error, go directly to the editor or station manager—after you've informed the reporter of the mistake.

Index

Nurses
   manpower trends for, 7
   referrals and, 106

Office
   assessing ambience of, 35, 39
   educational library in, 100–101, 103
   signage in, 70
Office manager, 79, 83, 84, 207
Open houses, 29, 84, 149
   measuring response to, 312
   publicity for, 156, 157–160
Osburn, Dan, 126
O'Steen, Van, 346
Outdoor advertising, 215, 225

Packaging, in direct mail, 301–302
Pamphlets, 97; *see also* Brochures; Educational materials; Print media
Paper stock, 68, 172
Patient education, 25
   communication and, 92–97
   need for, 93–94
   value of, 94–97
   see also Educational materials
Patients
   communicating with, 90–104
   feedback from, 23–24, 90–91
   income of, 53
   practice as perceived by, 76–77
   referrals and satisfaction of, 108–111,
      121–122
   research on composition of, 36–37
   satisfaction of, 57–58
   staff and experience of, 73–74
   time perceptions in, 91–92
Patient surveys, 24, 25, 84
   example of, 368–378
   monitoring advertising with, 317
   research with, 38
Payment sources, and computers, 197–198,
   205
Personal computers, *see* Computers
Personal relationships, 71–122
   patients and, 90–104
   referral sources and, 105–122
   staff and, 73–89
Personnel, *see* Staff
Pharmaceutical firms, 98, 100
Philosophy of practice, 168–169
Photographs
   newsletters with, 189
   print ads with, 267
Physician Marketing (publication), 14
Physician Referral Program, 119
Physicians
   competition and response of, 11
   educational materials and, 101–102

hospitals and, 10–11
   manpower trends for, 6–7, 10
   as referral sources, 107–111
   self-assessment by, 37, 352–358
Planning, 321–322
   advertising media mix and, 218–222
   goal setting and, 323–324
   process in, 321–322
Positioning, 46–59
   bundling in, 52
   definition of, 46
   developing, 49–50
   difficulty in developing, 46
   location of office and, 49–50, 53–55
   marketing mix and, 50–59
   positional advantage in, 49
   preservation in, 57–58
   price and, 52–53
   product or service used in, 51–52
   promotion and, 55–57
   repositioning in, 58
   segmentation and, 47–50
   staff and, 75
   steps in, 50
Posters, 99, 155
Postcards, 291
Practice
   assessing, *see* Research
   challenge of change in, 3–4
   computer profile of, 195–196
   marketing benefits of, 5
   modality changes in, 8
   patient perception of, 76–77
   philosophy of, 168–169
   staff and success of, 74
Practice identity, 31–70
   assessing, 33–45
   brochures and, 163
   creating, 60–70
   elements of, 60–61
   importance of, 60
   logo and, 64–67
   name and, 61–64
   positioning and, 46–59
   promotional priorities and, 327–328
   telephone techniques and, 86–88
Practice promotion
   budget for, 329–333
   challenge of, 11–17
   communication methods in, 55
   competition and, 11
   computers and, 195
   consumer attitudes on, 19
   copywriting for, 230–231
   education of physicians on, 13–14
   innovation in, 14–15
   new services and programs and, 21–23
   overview of, 18–30
   positioning strategy and, 55–57
   printed material and, 161–211